W9-DBL-242

CLINICAL
LABORATORY
ANIMAL
MEDICINE

Karen Hrapkiewicz, DVM, MS
Leticia Medina, DVM
Donald D. Holmes, DVM, MS

CLINICAL LABORATORY ANIMAL MEDICINE

AN INTRODUCTION

Second Edition

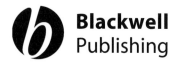
Blackwell
Publishing

Karen Hrapkiewicz, DVM, MS, is a clinical veterinarian for the Division of Laboratory Animal Resources, Wayne State University, and director of the veterinary technology program, Wayne County Community College, Detroit, Michigan. Dr. Hrapkiewicz is a Diplomate of the American College of Laboratory Animal Medicine.

Leticia Medina, DVM, is a clinical veterinarian in the Department of Comparative Medicine at Abbott Laboratories, Abbott Park, Illinois. Dr. Medina is a Diplomate of the American College of Laboratory Animal Medicine.

Donald D. Holmes, DVM, MS, retired, was author of the first edition of *Clinical Laboratory Animal Medicine* and professor of pathology and director of Laboratory Animal Resources, College of Veterinary Medicine, Oklahoma State University, Stillwater. Dr. Holmes is a Diplomate of the American College of Laboratory Animal Medicine.

© 1998 Iowa State University Press
All rights reserved

Blackwell Publishing Professional
2121 State Avenue, Ames, Iowa 50014

Orders: 1-800-862-6657
Office: 1-515-292-0140
Fax: 1-515-292-3348
Web site: www.blackwellprofessional.com

Authorization to photocopy items for internal or personal use, or the internal or personal use of specific clients, is granted by Blackwell Publishing, provided that the base fee of $.10 per copy is paid directly to the Copyright Clearance Center, 222 Rosewood Drive, Danvers, MA 01923. For those organizations that have been granted a photocopy license by CCC, a separate system of payments has been arranged. The fee code for users of the Transactional Reporting Service is 0-8138-2555-5/98 $.10.

∞ Printed on acid-free paper in the United States of America

First edition, 1984 *(through eight printings)*
Second edition, 1998

Library of Congress Cataloging-in-Publication Data

Hrapkiewicz, Karen
    Clinical laboratory animal medicine: an introduction / Karen Hrapkiewicz, Leticia Medina, Donald D. Holmes.—2nd ed.
        p.   cm.
    Rev. ed. of: Clinical laboratory animal medicine / Donald D. Holmes. 1st ed. 1984.
    Includes bibliographical references (p.   ) and index.
    ISBN 0-8138-2555-5
    1. Laboratory animals—Diseases.   2. Veterinary medicine.   I. Medina, Leticia.   II. Holmes, Donald D.   III. Title.
    SF996.5.H65   1998
    636.089—dc21   97-34537

Last digit is the print number: 9 8 7

I dedicate this book to my parents,
Theodosia and Leopold

KH

I dedicate this book to my husband, Chris, and
my daughters, Rachel and Danielle

LVM

DISCLAIMER

The dosages given in this text are derived from published literature. Many dosages, however, are empirical or based on clinical experience. Few drugs are specifically designed or licensed for use in rodents, rabbits, ferrets, and primates. Caution should be used because most uses and dosages presented herein are extra-label. The authors have made every attempt to verify all dosages and references; however, despite these efforts, errors in the original sources or in the preparation of this book may have occurred. Users of this text should evaluate all dosages prior to use to determine that they are reasonable. The authors and publisher cannot be held responsible for misuse or misapplication of the material in this book.

CONTENTS

PREFACE

THE PURPOSE of this book is to provide basic information on unique anatomic and physiologic characteristics, care and maintenance, common diseases, and recommended treatments for rodents, rabbits, ferrets, and nonhuman primates. It has been prepared as a guide for practicing veterinarians, veterinary students, veterinary technicians, research scientists, and others interested in learning about smaller mammals and nonhuman primates. Knowledge is the key to an old saying *primum non nocere*—first do no harm! To undertake medical care of a species with which one is unfamiliar can be dangerous. By gaining familiarity with the more significant, unique biologic features of laboratory animals; learning of the more commonly seen disease processes; and applying knowledge and skills acquired during professional training, veterinarians should be capable of providing health care to these animals with a reasonable degree of competence. Working with laboratory animals, whether they be kept as pets or in a research setting, can be personally satisfying and rewarding.

This second edition has been updated and substantially expanded to include new diseases, treatments, and techniques. The text has been specifically written in an easy-to-read format, with references placed at the end of each chapter. A chapter on regulations and policies governing the care and use of laboratory animals, and another on serologic testing and quality control, have been added. The formulary has been vastly expanded into a quick-reference table format that is more user friendly. The biologic and physiologic data have been reworked into a table format, and information on blood volumes has been added. Line drawings of restraint and other techniques have also been added to this edition.

This book was made possible through the support and guidance of many people. A special thanks to Dr. Donald D. Holmes, who wrote the first edition and gave us a stepping stone and place to start. The efforts of Beth Harries, L.V.T., for her creative suggestions and assistance in preparing the manuscript are gratefully acknowledged. Thanks to Robin Allen for her editing suggestions and assistance in proofreading. We extend our thanks to Ann Kennedy, L.V.T., for the line drawings. Thanks to our colleagues for their encouragement when our energy levels were low. Finally, we thank our families and friends for their patience and good nature during the writing of this text.

CLINICAL LABORATORY ANIMAL MEDICINE

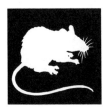

MICE

Mus musculus, the common house mouse, belongs to the order Rodentia and the family Muridae. There are over 500 outbred stocks and inbred strains of mice in the world. Adult mice usually weigh between 25 and 40 g and come in a variety of colors, including albino, black, brown, agouti, gray, and piebald. The majority of laboratory mice are albino strains, which have white coats and pink eyes.

Genetics

Three main genetic categories of mice are used in biomedical research: outbred stocks, inbred strains, and F_1 hybrids. Outbred mice are produced in a large colony where matings occur randomly among males and females from unrelated litters. Random breeding is not actually random but is carefully planned to minimize inbreeding. Outbred mice are considered to be genetically heterogeneous.

Inbred mice result from brother–sister or parent–offspring matings for 20 or more generations. Inbred mice are genetically homogeneous with greater than 97% homozygosity after 20 generations. Frequently, inbred strains are produced to select for a specific trait that will be studied, such as diabetes mellitus or anemia. Examples of important inbred strains include the athymic nude mouse, which lacks the population of T cells, and the severe combined immunodeficient (SCID) mouse, which lacks both B and T cell populations. These two strains of mice are used extensively in immunologic research because of their immunocompromised states.

F_1 hybrids are the first progeny of matings between two different inbred strains. They have the advantage of "hybrid vigor," which means they are heartier than either of the parental strains. They are also genetically identical at all loci. Inbred strains and F_1 hybrids are often chosen for research purposes because their genetic homogeneity eliminates an important variable in experimental work.

Transgenic and "knockout" mice are also used for genetic biomedical research studies. With the advent of transgenic technology in 1981, scientists are able to produce rodents that carry and express foreign genetic material. A transgenic animal is created when foreign DNA is introduced into the cells of the recipient animal during early embryonic development, thereby allowing incorporation of the genetic material into the host genome. This technology has opened the doors to allow scientists to study the complex molecular biologic effects of any gene in a living animal.

Knockout mice are produced by introducing a transgene that has been designed to include a region that is complementary to a specific gene target. Using this homologous recombination technology, scientists can, literally, knock out specific genes and then study these loss-of-function animal models or replace the gene with an alternative genetic sequence that will produce a mutant protein. Knockout mice have become powerful tools in the study of genetic diseases.

Ecologic Types

In addition to the genetic categories of mice, there are varying ecologic types that are based on microbiologic status. These are 1) germ free or axenic, which are free of all detectable microflora; 2) gnotobiotic, which have associated microflora that is known; 3) specific pathogen–free, which are free of specific pathogens; and 4) conventional, or animals with undefined microflora.

Uses

Mice make good pets if handled gently and are less prone to bite their handlers than are hamsters. Because mice are proficient breeders, pet owners should ask for same-sex pairs in order to avoid having dozens of mice in a very short time. One disadvantage of owning mice is that a musty odor is often evident in a room containing mice even when good cleaning practices are followed. Humans can develop allergies to mouse dander and urine proteins, and pet owners should be aware of this potential.

More mice are used in research than any other mammal. Mice have many attributes that make them valuable for research purposes, including a short life span, short gestation, large litter size, and great genetic diversity. The short gestation and large litter size make them valuable in studies of reproduction, teratogenicity, and genetics. A short life span permits the study of several generations over a period of a few years.

Furthermore, the anatomy, physiology, and genetics of mice have extensively been studied and are well characterized, providing a wealth of information for researchers to build upon. Mutant strains of inbred mice provide investigators with a wide variety of animal models with which to study biologic processes and diseases.

The proven safety of a product is required by the Food and Drug Administration prior to its being marketed in the United States. Companies must use the most effective ways to test the safety of a product, which currently include animal testing. Relative to other species of research animals, mice are inexpensive to purchase and easy to maintain. Thus, they are frequently used for toxicity and carcinogenicity studies of various compounds for which large numbers of animals are required to provide statistically valid data.

Behavior

Mice are social animals and do best when housed in small groups. Mice that are housed alone often gain less weight than group housed mice. When housed in social groups, mice will frequently establish a dominance hierarchy. The most dominant mouse, also called the barber mouse, will often remove the hair and whiskers from the faces and sometimes from the bodies of the other mice.

Mice are curious but not aggressive toward humans and will usually only bite their handlers when mishandled or startled. Mice also tend to be territorial. Adult males of some strains will fight if housed together, especially if overcrowded, and can inflict severe bite wounds around the genitals and along the backs of their foes. Female mice rarely fight unless defending their litters.

Although rodents are generally considered to be nocturnal animals, when housed indoors mice tend to have both active and resting periods throughout the day and night. Mice build nests in which to sleep and keep their litters.

Anatomic and Physiologic Features

General biologic and reproductive data for the mouse are listed in Table 1.1. Mice have small bodies covered in soft, dense fur; short legs; and long, thin hairless tails. Typical of rodents in general, mice have a dental formula of 2 (1/1 incisors, 0/0 canines, 0/0 premolars, 3/3 molars). The incisors are open rooted, which means that they grow continuously throughout life and are worn down by abrasion of the occlusal surface, whereas the molars have fixed roots.

Table 1.1. Biologic and reproductive data for mice	
Adult body weight	
Male	20–40 g
Female	25–40 g
Life span	1.5–3 y
Body temperature	36.5°–38°C (97.5°–100.4°F)
Heart rate	325–780 beats per minute
Respiratory rate	60–220 breaths per minute
Food consumption	12–18 g/100 g/d
Water consumption	15 mL/100 g/d
Breeding onset	
Male	50 d
Female	50–60 d
Estrous cycle length	4–5 d
Gestation period	19–21 d
Postpartum estrus	Fertile
Litter size	10–12
Weaning age	21–28 d
Breeding duration	7–9 mo
Chromosome number (diploid)	40

Source: Adapted from Harkness and Wagner (1995).

Mice have a divided stomach, consisting of a nonglandular forestomach and a glandular stomach. Their lungs consist of one large left lobe and four small right lobes. Brown fat tissue occurs in several places in the mouse, including between the scapulae. This is important in nonshivering thermogenesis during which the fat is metabolized to increase heat production in response to a cold environment.

Mice have five pairs of mammary glands: three thoracic and two abdominal. Mammary tissue is widely distributed in mice, with the glands extending well onto the sides and back. Both male and female mice have mammary glands, but the nipples are more prominent in females. Mice have open inguinal canals their entire life; therefore, to avoid herniation of abdominal organs, care should be taken to close the canals when castrating males. Males also have an os penis.

The most reliable criteria for differentiating the sexes are that the genital papilla is more prominent in the male and the distance between the anus and the genital papilla is about one and one-half to two times greater in the male. Refer to Chapter 2, Rats, Figure 2.1, for anatomy of the anogenital area. Sexing of neonatal mice requires practice but can be accomplished by comparing the anogenital distance and the size of the genital papillae.

There are several distinctive characteristics of the hematologic and urinary profiles of mice. Lymphocytes are the predominant circulating leukocyte in mice. Basophils are rarely found in the circulating blood.

Mature male mice have higher granulocyte counts than do female mice. Mouse urine is excreted a drop at a time, is highly concentrated, and contains large amounts of protein. Taurine and creatinine are also found in the urine. Urine pH is 7.3–8.5, with a mean specific gravity of 1.058. Hematologic and biochemical parameters for the mouse are listed in Appendix 1, Normal Values.

Breeding and Reproduction

A detailed description of the various breeding systems in mouse colonies is beyond the scope of this book. The following is a general overview of breeding practices. Either a monogamous (one male, one female) or a polygamous (one male, multiple females) mating system may be established, with the choice of systems dependent on a number of factors.

Mice should be bred for the first time between 7 and 8 weeks of age at a weight of 20–30 g. The normal estrous cycle of females is 4–5 days. Mice are continuously polyestrous without significant seasonal variations. For maximum productivity, breeding should begin soon after animals reach sexual maturity and be continued throughout the breeding life of the female. It may be difficult to induce females to resume breeding if the breeding cycle is interrupted.

Pheromones play an important role in the reproductive behavior of mice. Pheromones are chemical substances secreted from the body that elicit a specific behavioral reaction in the recipient by activating the olfactory system. Large groups of females housed together tend to go into anestrus and do not cycle. If these females are introduced to males or their odor, they begin to cycle and 40%–50% of the females will be in estrus within 72 hours. This synchronization of estrus is called the Whitten effect and can directly be attributed to pheromones. If a pregnant female mouse is exposed to the odor or presence of a strange male within 4 days of breeding, the existing pregnancy will often be aborted. This phenomenon is known as the Bruce effect and, like the Whitten effect, can be attributed to pheromones.

Matings can be confirmed by the presence of sperm or a vaginal plug in the female. The plug is formed by secretions from the vesicular and coagulating glands of the male. Vaginal plugs usually persist for 18–24 hours but may last up to 48 hours. Pregnant mice have an increased rate of weight gain by day 13 of gestation, marked mammary development by day 14, and a noticeably increased abdominal size. The fetuses can be palpated in mid to late gestation.

The usual gestation period in mice is 19–21 days. In lactating mice,

7

gestation is prolonged by 3–10 days owing to a delay in uterine implantation of the blastocysts. Nonfertile matings result in a pseudopregnancy, which lasts for 14 days, during which estrus and ovulation do not occur. A fertile postpartum estrus may occur 14–28 hours after parturition; otherwise, mice will resume cycling 2–5 days postweaning.

Litter size is usually 10 to 12 pups, but varies with strain and age of the mouse. To minimize cannibalism, dams and their litters should be left undisturbed for at least 2 days postpartum. Mice are altricial, in that they are blind, naked, and deaf at birth. Albino mouse pups are often called pinkies, in reference to their color. The "milk spot" in their stomach can easily be observed through their thin skin to determine whether they are nursing. By day 10, mouse pups have a full covering of fine hair and their ears are open, and by day 12, their eyes are open. The usual weaning age is 21 days but may be as long as 28 days in some smaller inbred strains. Mouse pups can begin eating solid food and drinking water by 2 weeks of age.

HUSBANDRY

Housing

Mice may be housed in shoebox-style cages constructed of a durable plastic, such as polycarbonate or polypropylene, or stainless steel. Stainless steel cages are preferable to other metals because they are easily sanitized and resist rust, but they are quite expensive. Mice may also be housed in suspended cages with grid or solid floors. Minimal space requirements for adult mice larger than 25 g are 97 cm^2 (15 in.^{2}) of floor space for each mouse and a cage height of 13 cm (5 in.). Mice tend to be proficient at escaping from their cages and do not return to them once they have escaped. To prevent escape, cages must have a cover such as a wire grid or plastic lid. Microisolator cages are commonly used to house immunosuppressed animals. These special cages have plastic lids with filters to reduce disease transmission between cages. A contact bedding material, such as wood chips, wood shavings, composite recycled paper pellets, or corncob particles should be placed in the bottom of solid shoebox cages. Softwood bedding, such as pine or cedar chips, should not be used for laboratory mice because they produce aromatic hydrocarbons that induce hepatic microsomal enzymes. An indirect bedding of absorbent material is frequently placed in waste trays located below cages with grid floors. Breeding and preweanling mice should be housed in solid-bottom cages rather than in cages with grid floors. Because of their small size, preweanling mice could fall through grid flooring and the bedding in solid-bottom cages provides young mice with the extra heat they require. Facial tissues, cotton nestlets, and soft paper towels can be provided as nesting material.

In housing mice for research purposes, rigid control of room temperature, relative humidity, ventilation, and lighting is essential. A temperature range of 18°–26°C (64°–79°F) and a relative humidity range of 30%–70% are generally recommended. It is suggested that there should be 10–15 air changes per hour to maintain adequate ventilation. A constant cycle of darkness and light should be maintained in rooms housing mice. Typically, 12–14 hours of light per day should be provided and can be controlled through automatic timers.

The required frequency of cage cleaning depends, to some extent, on the number and size of mice caged together and the amount of air movement in the room. One to three times weekly is usually adequate. Cages, water bottles, and feed hoppers should be disinfected with chemicals, hot water 61.6°–82.2°C (143°–180°F), or a combination of both. Wardrip et al. showed that when hot water is used alone, it is the combination of water temperature and time applied to the surface, known as the cumulative heat factor, that disinfects. Thus, a range of temperatures is acceptable as long as the water is applied to the surface a long enough period of time to ensure destruction of common vegetative pathogenic organisms. Higher temperatures require less contact time than lower temperatures. Detergents and chemical disinfectants enhance the effectiveness of hot water, but they must be thoroughly rinsed from all caging surfaces with fresh water.

Feeding and Watering

Mice generally consume 3–5 g of solid food per day. A nutritionally complete commercial rodent diet from a reputable company should be fed. The diet should be fresh, properly stored, and contain at least 16% protein and 4%–5% fat. The food is usually provided in the form of firm, dry pellets and fed ad libitum. The food pellets should be placed in hoppers that are either formed in the cage lid or attached to the cage wall. The practice of placing food pellets directly on the cage floor is both unsanitary and wasteful.

Adult mice drink 6–7 mL of water per day. Fresh, potable water should be available ad libitum through either water bottles with sipper tubes or automatic watering systems.

Diet supplementation is not recommended because mice may preferentially eat the supplements and not consume a well-balanced diet. An occasional fruit or seed snack to pet mice, however, is acceptable. Mice are coprophagic and will eat their own feces to recycle B vitamins and other nutrients.

TECHNIQUES

Handling and Restraint

To transfer a mouse from cage to cage, it may be picked up by the base of the tail with the fingers or with a pair of rubber-tipped forceps. Never grasp a mouse by the tip of its tail; this can result in a loss of skin and exposure of the caudal vertebrae.

To restrain a mouse, grasp the base of the tail with the thumb and forefinger of one hand and place the mouse on a surface to which it will cling, such as a wire cage lid. As the mouse attempts to move forward, quickly scruff the loose skin at the back of the neck between the thumb and forefinger of the other hand (Figure 1.1). When the skin is held properly, the mouse's head is immobilized so it cannot turn and bite. The mouse can be lifted and the tail secured between the small finger and palm of the same hand (Figure 1.2). The other hand is then free to give injections or gavage the mouse. Mechanical restrainers made of rigid plastic are commercially available and allow access to blood collection and injection sites.

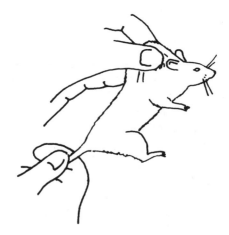

Figure 1.1. Restraint of the mouse using a two-hand grip.

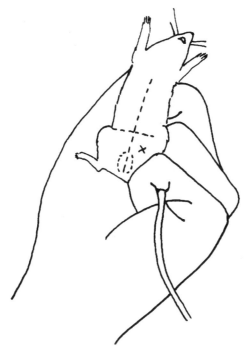

Figure 1.2. Restraint of the mouse using a one-hand grip for intraperitoneal injection. X is the injection site. Quadrants of abdomen and location of bladder are shown as *dotted lines.*

Identification

Cage cards may be used as a general means of identifying caged mice. Individual identification may be accomplished by ear punching, ear tagging, or placement of a subcutaneous microchip that allows electronic identification via a handheld scanner.

Ink tail markings and fur dyes may be used as a temporary means of identification.

Blood Collection

Collecting blood from mice can be challenging because of their small size. One of the best sites for blood collection is the retroorbital sinus. Figure 1.3 shows the anatomy of this sinus. Mice must be anesthetized for this procedure. Using the forefinger and thumb of one hand, place pressure on the top and bottom lids of one eye to keep the eye

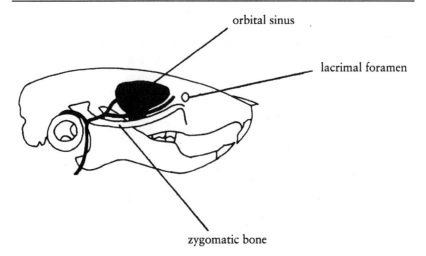

orbital sinus

lacrimal foramen

zygomatic bone

Figure 1.3. Anatomy of the retroorbital sinus in the mouse. (Adapted from Timm and Jahn 1980, Practical Methodology of the Mouse. In *Practical Methodology* [slide series], ©Regents University of California)

open and slightly proptosed. With the other hand, place the tip of a glass microcapillary tube in the medial canthus at approximately a 30°–45° angle toward the back of the eye. Figure 1.4 shows the correct angle and positioning of the tube. Using firm, steady forward pressure, quickly rotate the tube between the thumb and forefinger of the hand. This rotation will allow the tube to act as a cutting instrument through the conjunctiva at the back of the eye and enter the retroorbital sinus. Once the conjunctiva has been bypassed, the tube will come up against bone,

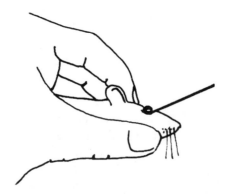

Figure 1.4. Mouse retroorbital blood collection technique.

and blood should flow into the tube by capillary action. The tube may have to be slightly withdrawn to encourage the blood to start flowing into the tube. After collecting the blood sample, withdraw the tube, close the eyelids, and place slight pressure with a gauze square to stop the flow of blood. The eyeball will not be affected when proper technique is used, as the capillary tube merely courses along the side and back of the globe.

Small amounts of blood can also be collected by capillary tube collection from the hub of a needle placed in the dorsal tail artery or lateral tail veins or from a clipped toenail. Larger blood samples can be collected from a cardiac puncture or the cranial vena cava in an anesthetized animal. Both of these procedures are invasive and can lead to death from hemorrhage into the chest cavity. To collect a terminal blood sample in euthanized mice, the axillary muscles and vessels of the arm can be cut and a Pasteur pipette can be used to collect the blood as it pools.

Approximate blood volumes for mice are listed in Table 1.2. It should be noted that white blood cell counts are highly variable. Even such factors as site of collection and time of day can influence the number of leukocytes in peripheral blood. White blood cell counts, thus, are of little value in disease diagnosis.

Urine Collection

Mice may be stimulated to urinate upon handling or upon placement on a cold surface or in a cooled plastic bag. A urine sample is best collected with a specially designed metabolic cage, which separates fecal pellets from urine.

Drug Administration

Most drug administration techniques used in small animal practice can be used with rodents when modified to fit their small size. The tendency to overdose mice and other small rodents is attributable to overestimation of their body weight. Small scales, such as a postage scale or

Table 1.2. Adult mouse blood volumes	
	Volume (mL)[a]
Total blood	1.6–3.2
Single sample	0.2–0.3
Exsanguination	1–1.5

Source: Adapted from Harkness and Wagner (1995).
[a]Values are approximate.

a triple-beam balance, are useful for obtaining accurate body weights. Dosage accuracy is increased through dilution of drugs and by use of tuberculin syringes.

Medication is frequently administered orally and is most easily accomplished by mixing the medication into the water or feed. If medications are unpalatable, 5 mL of sugar or syrup per liter can be added to the drinking water to improve the palatability. Specialized gavage needles are used to deliver a substance directly into the stomach for greater accuracy or for administering unpalatable liquids. The ball at the end of the gavage needle ensures that the needle cannot pass into the trachea. The gavage technique can be rapidly accomplished in awake mice through proper restraint and extension of the head.

Smaller-gauge needles, such as 25 or 23 gauge, should be used when giving injections. Medication can be administered through subcutaneous injections with a maximum volume of 2–3 mL. The injection is made under the loose skin over the shoulders or on the abdomen. Intramuscular injections can be given in the quadriceps muscles of the hind legs, but the volume should not exceed 0.2 mL per site. Certain drugs, such as ketamine, can cause muscle damage and nerve irritation that can lead to self-mutilation of the affected limb. Ketamine and other irritating drugs are best administered by the intraperitoneal route.

Because mice have such a small muscle mass, injectable anesthetic agents are most frequently administered into the peritoneal cavity with a maximum volume of 2–3 mL. To administer an intraperitoneal injection, the mouse should be securely restrained to minimize movement, and the injection should be administered just off of midline. Injection sites are most often placed in the lower left quadrant of the abdomen, as indicated by the "X" in Figure 1.2. Before injection, the syringe should be aspirated to ensure that the needle has not entered the bladder or intestines of the mouse.

Anesthesia, Surgery, and Postoperative Care

A variety of anesthetic and tranquilizing agents used in mice are listed in Table 1.3. Because of the small volumes of anesthetics required for mice, dilution of all injectable anesthetics is recommended. A dilution ratio of at least 1 part anesthetic to 10 parts either sterile distilled water or physiologic saline works well. The age, sex, and strain of the animal influences the dose of anesthetic needed, thus, a conservative dose is best given initially. The combination of ketamine and xylazine is frequently chosen as an injectable regimen for surgical procedures. They can be mixed and given in one injection to minimize handling stress.

Table 1.3. Anesthetic agents and tranquilizers used in mice

Drug	Dosage	Route	Reference
Inhalants			
Carbon dioxide	50%–70% mixed with O_2	Inhalation	Urbanski (1991)
Ether		Inhalation	Tarin (1972)
Halothane	1%–4% to effect	Inhalation	Tarin (1972)
Isoflurane	1%–4% to effect	Inhalation	Markovic (1993)
Methoxyflurane	0.5%–3% to effect	Inhalation	Tarin (1972)
Injectables			
Acetylpromazine	2–5 mg/kg	IP	Harkness and Wagner (1995)
Chloral hydrate	370–400 mg/kg	IP	White (1987)
Diazepam	5 mg/kg	IP	Flecknell (1987)
Ketamine	100 mg/kg	IP	White (1987)
Ketamine	100 mg/kg	IM	Flecknell (1987)
+ acetylpromazine	2.5 mg/kg	IM	
Ketamine	200 mg/kg	IM	Flecknell (1987)
+ diazepam	5 mg/kg	IP	
Ketamine	75mg/kg	IP	Flecknell (1997)
+ medetomidine	1 mg/kg	IP	
Ketamine	50 mg/kg	IP, IM	Harkness and Wagner (1995)
+ xylazine	15 mg/kg	IP, IM	
Ketamine	90–120 mg/kg	IP, IM	Harkness and Wagner (1995)
+ xylazine	10 mg/kg	IP, IM	
Ketamine	30 mg/kg	IM	O'Rourke (1994)
+ xylazine	6 mg/kg	IM	
+ acetylpromazine	1 mg/kg	IM	
Pentobarbital (diluted 1:9 in saline)	40–80 mg/kg	IP	Hughes (1981)
Propofol	26 mg/kg	IV	Harkness and Wagner (1995)
Thiopental	50 mg/kg	IP	White (1987)
Tribromoethanol (Avertin) (1.2% solution)	0.2 mL/10 g (240 mg/kg)	IP	Papaioannou and Fox (1993)

IM = intramuscular; IP = intraperitoneal; IV = intravenous.

This combination provides about 30–45 minutes of general anesthesia. Pentobarbital is sometimes used but has a narrow margin of safety, as the dosage required for surgical anesthesia is very close to the LD_{50} in most strains of rodents and rabbits. The usual duration of anesthesia following pentobarbital administration is 20–40 minutes. Tribromoethanol is another safe and effective anesthetic choice for mice. This drug must be freshly mixed, protected from light, stored in a refrigerator, and used within 48 hours for optimal effect.

Except for short procedures, inhalation anesthesia is generally impractical in a clinical setting. Isoflurane and halothane have high inherent vapor pressures and are best used in a precision vaporizer with a mask or nose-cone apparatus. Methoxyflurane has a low inherent vapor pressure and can therefore be used in a nonprecision vaporizer or a simple anesthetic chamber such as a belljar. Ether is also used but should be used with extreme caution because it is flammable, forms explosive vapor mixtures with air or oxygen, and is an irritant to the respiratory tract. A simple anesthetic chamber can be fashioned by placing a cottonball saturated with methoxyflurane or ether in the bottom of a glass beaker. A platform of hardware cloth or similar material should be placed over the cottonball to separate the patient from the anesthetic. Anesthesia is then induced by placing the mouse in the beaker and covering the beaker with a lid. When limb movement ceases and respiration is relatively slow and steady, the mouse should be removed from the chamber. If surgery is prolonged, anesthesia can be maintained by use of a nose cone made of a plastic syringe case that holds a small cottonball saturated with the anesthetic. Use of volatile anesthetics should always be performed with appropriate scavenging systems or under a fume hood to avoid exposing personnel to the anesthetic vapors.

There is rarely a need to perform surgery on a pet mouse other than a simple castration, which requires closure of the inguinal canals to prevent intestinal entrapment. There are a number of common surgical procedures performed on research mice, including hypophysectomy, adrenalectomy, thymectomy, and jugular vein or carotid artery catheterization.

Contrary to some theories, rodents are no more resistant to infection than are other mammals and surgeries should always be performed using aseptic techniques. Some research projects require multiple rodent surgical procedures to be performed in 1 day. Sterilizing several small surgical packs is not always possible when surgical instruments are limited. An alternative to multiple packs is the proper use of a cold sterilant or the use of a dry-heat glass-bead sterilizer. The glass-bead sterilizer has been shown to be the most rapid method to achieve sterilization of instruments, is easy to use, keeps the instruments dry and clean, and requires minimal bench space.

Likewise, adequate intraoperative and postoperative care is important for all animals. Rodents are particularly prone to hypothermia because of their small size. A small heating blanket or hot water bottle can be useful in maintaining the normal body temperature of a mouse during anesthesia. To help prevent drying of a rodent's eyes, an ophthalmic ointment should be used in animals that have been anesthetized with agents such as ketamine, which cause loss of the blinking reflex. Because of the high ratio of evaporative surface area to body mass, mice have a greater sensitivity to water loss than do most mammals. To help prevent dehydration, it is recommended that mice be given 1–2 mL of warm sterile saline per 100 g of body weight subcutaneously after prolonged anesthesia. Postoperative analgesics should be considered for mice that appear to be in pain or are anorexic or for procedures that are generally considered painful in larger animal species. Table 1.4 lists several analgesics that can be used in mice.

Butorphanol is recommended for mild postoperative discomfort, whereas buprenorphine works well to control acute or chronic visceral pain but causes more sedation.

Anesthetized mice should be placed on a dry paper or cloth towel for recovery. They should never be placed on small particle bedding because it can be aspirated. Use of an incubator, circulating water blanket under a cage, or heat lamp directed at one corner of the cage will help to prevent hypothermia in recovering mice. Rodents tend to cannibalize animals that appear nonresponsive. An anesthetized mouse should not be placed back into a cage with other animals until it is fully ambulatory.

Euthanasia

Methods of euthanasia should follow the 1993 American Veterinary Medical Association (AVMA) Panel on Euthanasia guidelines. These guidelines categorize each method as acceptable, conditionally acceptable, or unacceptable based on how quickly and painlessly the method causes death. The most commonly employed methods include exposure of mice to carbon dioxide in a prefilled chamber with approximately 70% carbon dioxide and administration of an overdose of an injectable

Table 1.4. Analgesic agents used in mice

Drug	Dosage	Route	Reference
Acetaminophen	1–2 mg/mL drinking water		Huerkamp (1995)
Acetylsalicylic acid	100–150 mg/kg q4h	PO	Heard (1993)
Buprenorphine	0.05–2.5 mg/kg q6–12h	SC, IP	Harkness and Wagner (1995)
Butorphanol	1–5 mg/kg q2–4h	SC	Heard (1993)
Codeine	20 mg/kg q4h	SC	Flecknell (1987)
	60–90 mg/kg	PO	Jenkins (1987)
Flunixin meglumine	2.5 mg/kg q12–24h	SC	Heard (1993)
Ibuprofen	7.5 mg/kg ~q4h	PO	Flecknell (1991)
Meperidine	20 mg/kg q2–3h	SC, IM	Heard (1993)
Syrup	0.2 mg/mL drinking water		Huerkamp (1995)
Nalbuphine	4–8 mg/kg q3h	IM	Heard (1993)
Oxymorphone	0.2–0.5 mg/kg q6–12h	SC, IM	Heard (1993)
Pentazocine	10 mg/kg q2–4h	SC	Heard (1993)

IM = intramuscular; IP = intraperitoneal; PO = per os; SC= subcutaneous.

barbiturate anesthetic. Both of these methods are categorized as acceptable by the AVMA Panel on Euthanasia guidelines. Cervical dislocation is considered to be acceptable only when performed under anesthesia.

Euthanasia of rodents should never be performed in the same room where other rodents are housed because studies have shown that this practice causes stress in the remaining animals. Noninvasive euthanasia procedures, such as carbon dioxide inhalation or pentobarbital injection, should be followed with an assurance of death procedure, such as performing a bilateral pneumothorax. This will ensure that death has occurred rather than just a deep plane of anesthesia from which the animal might later recover.

Table 1.5. Antimicrobial and antifungal agents used in mice

Drug	Dosage	Route	Reference
Amikacin	2–5 mg/kg q8–12h	SC, IM	Harkness and Wagner (1995)
Ampicillin	20–100 mg/kg q12h	PO, SC, IM	Anderson (1994)
	500 mg/L drinking water		Matsushita (1995)
Cephaloridine	10–25 mg/kg q24h	SC, IM	Anderson (1994)
Chloramphenicol	0.5 mg/mL drinking water		Burgmann and Percy (1993)
	50–200 mg/kg q8h	PO	Burgmann and Percy (1993)
	30–50 mg/kg q12h	SC	Burgmann and Percy (1993)
Ciprofloxacin	7–20 mg/kg q12h	PO	Harkness and Wagner (1995)
Doxycycline	5 mg/kg q12h	PO	Harkness and Wagner (1995)
Enrofloxacin	0.05–0.2 mg/mL drinking water for 14 d		Harkness and Wagner (1995)
	5–10 mg/kg q12h	PO, IM	Harkness and Wagner (1995)
Gentamicin	2–4 mg/kg q8–24h	SC, IM	Harkness and Wagner (1995)
Griseofulvin	25–50 mg/kg q12h for 14–60 d	PO	Harkness and Wagner (1995)
	1.5% in DMSO for 5–7 d	Topical	Harkness and Wagner (1995)
Ketoconazole	10–40 mg/kg q24h for 14 d	PO	Harkness and Wagner (1995)
Metronidazole	2.5 mg/mL drinking water for 5 d		Burgmann and Percy (1993)
	20–60 mg/kg q8–12h	PO	Harkness and Wagner (1995)
Neomycin	2.6 mg/mL drinking water		Anderson (1994)
Oxytetracycline	0.4 mg/mL drinking water		Burgmann and Percy (1993)
	10–20 mg/kg q8h	PO	Burgmann and Percy (1993)
Sulfadimethoxine	10–15 mg/kg q12h	PO	Harkness and Wagner (1995)
Sulfamerazine	1 mg/mL drinking water		Anderson (1994)
	500 mg/L drinking water		Matsushita (1995)
Sulfamethazine	1 mg/mL drinking water		Anderson (1994)
Tetracycline	2–5 mg/mL drinking water		Burgmann and Percy (1993)
	10–20 mg/kg q8–12h	PO	Burgmann and Percy (1993)
Trimethoprim/sulfa	30 mg/kg q12h	PO, IM	Harkness and Wagner (1995)
Tylosin	0.5 mg/mL drinking water		Collins (1995)
	10 mg/kg q24h	PO, SC, IM	Collins (1995)

DMSO = dimethyl sulfoxide; IM = intramuscular; PO = per os; SC = subcutaneous.

THERAPEUTIC AGENTS

Suggested mouse antimicrobial and antifungal drug dosages are listed in Table 1.5. Antiparasitic agents are listed in Table 1.6 and miscellaneous drugs are listed in Table 1.7.

Table 1.6. Antiparasitic agents used in mice

Drug	Dosage	Route	Reference
Carbamate (5%)	Twice weekly	Topical	Harkness and Wagner (1995)
Chlorpyrifos	6 g per 27 × 48 cm cage added to each bedding change, twice weekly for 3 wk	In bedding	Pence et al. (1991)
Dichlorvos	2 g per 29 × 12 cm cage added to each bedding change, once weekly for 2 wk	In bedding	Fraser (1974)
Fenbendazole	20 mg/kg q24h for 5 d	PO	Allen (1993)
	150 mg/kg of feed; provide for 7 d on, 7 d off for 3 treatments		Boivin et al. (1996)
Ivermectin	Use 1% ivermectin diluted 1:10 with tap water, delivered as a mist spray; 1–2 mL per cage once weekly for 3 wk	Topical	LeBlanc et al. (1993)
	Use 1% ivermectin at 2 mg/kg delivered as micro-dot on skin between scapulae at 10 d intervals for 2 treatments	Topical	West et al. (1992)
	8 mg/L drinking water for 4 d on, 3 d off, for 4 treatments		Klement et al. (1996)
	0.2 mg/kg q7d for 3 wk	PO, SC	Anderson (1994)
Permethrin	4 g of 0.25% dust once weekly for 4 wk	In bedding	Bean-Knudsen (1986)
	Cottonballs with 5%–7.4% (w/w) active permethrin, used as nesting material for 4 wk	In bedding	Mather and Lausen (1990)
Piperazine citrate	2–5 mg/mL drinking water for 7 d, off 7 d, repeat		Anderson (1994)
Praziquantel	6–10 mg/kg	PO	Harkness and Wagner (1995)
	140 ppm in feed for 5 d		Harkness and Wagner (1995)
Pyrethrin powder	3 times a week for 3 wk	Topical	Anderson (1994)
Thiabendazole	100–200 mg/kg	PO	Harkness and Wagner (1995)
	0.3% in feed for 7–10 d, use repeated treatments		Sebesteny (1979)

PO = per os; SC = subcutaneous.

Table 1.7. Miscellaneous agents used in mice

Drug	Dosage	Route	Reference
Atipamezole	1 mg/kg	SC, IP, IV	Flecknell (1997)
Atropine	0.05–0.1 mg/kg	SC	Harkness and Wagner (1995)
	10 mg/kg q20 min (organophosphate overdose)	SC	Harkness and Wagner (1995)
Cimetidine	5–10 mg/kg q6–12h	PO	Allen (1993)
Dexamethasone	0.5–2 mg/kg then decreasing dose q12h for 3–14 d	PO, SC	Harkness and Wagner (1995)
	0.6 mg/kg	IM	Anderson (1994)
Doxapram	5–10 mg/kg	IP, IV	Harkness (1993)
Furosemide	1–4 mg/kg q4–6h	IM	Harrenstien (1994)
Glycopyrrolate	0.01–0.02 mg/kg	SC	Huerkamp (1995)
Naloxone	0.01–0.1 mg/kg	SC, IP	Huerkamp (1995)
Prednisolone	0.5–2.2 mg/kg	SC, IM	Anderson (1994)
Vitamin K	1–10 mg/kg q24h for 4–6 d	IM	Harkness and Wagner (1995)
Yohimbine	0.5–1 mg/kg	IV	Harkness and Wagner (1995)

IM = intramuscular; IP = intraperitoneal; IV = intravenous; PO = per os; SC = subcutaneous.

BACTERIAL DISEASES

The evaluation of clinical signs in mice is difficult owing to their small size, and in many cases, histopathology and microbiology are required for a definitive diagnosis. Often, mice must be treated symptomatically, and a rather high mortality can be expected with generalized infections. A binocular loupe and an otoscope are helpful when performing physical examinations.

Pneumonia and Respiratory Diseases

Primary bacterial pneumonia is uncommon in mice unless the animals are immunologically deficient or stressed. Infection with *Mycoplasma pulmonis,* a bacterium that lacks a cell wall, may cause pneumonia in mice. Mycoplasmosis, however, is a much more serious problem in rats. Refer to Chapter 2 for a more detailed description of mycoplasmosis. Concurrent infection with Sendai virus or the cilia-associated respiratory (CAR) bacillus may result in a fatal pneumonia. Bacteria are often cultured from pneumonic lungs of mice with primary viral or mycoplasmal infections.

The CAR bacillus is a gram-negative bacillus that has been found between the cilia lining the respiratory tract of mice and other laboratory and domestic species. In mice, it appears to be opportunistic, for it has only been found in association with other respiratory pathogens. In rats, it is a more significant respiratory pathogen. Histologic changes seen in mice include a peribronchitis. Sulfamerazine or ampicillin, administered at a dose of 500 mg/L of drinking water, has been reported to eliminate colonization of the organism as well as reduce the severity of the peribronchitis. Sulfamerazine has also been reported to prevent the disease. Other bacteria occasionally associated with respiratory disease in mice include *Klebsiella pneumoniae, Corynebacterium kutscheri, Bordetella bronchiseptica,* and *Pasteurella pneumotropica.*

Clinical signs associated with pneumonia in mice include teeth chattering, labored respiration, weight loss, and conjunctivitis. Treatment with antibiotics is frequently not practical in a research colony, however, antimicrobials such as chloramphenicol, ampicillin, or oxytetracycline may be effective when circumstances justify their use.

Helicobacter spp. Infection

Several *Helicobacter* spp. have been identified that infect mice, rats, guinea pigs, rabbits, ferrets, cats, dogs, humans, and several other animal species. *Helicobacter hepaticus* is a small spiral- to rod-shaped bacterium that causes chronic active hepatitis in mice. Clinical signs are inapparent until the liver disease is nearing end stage. Gross lesions include multiple white foci in the liver that are sites of hepatic necrosis. Certain strains of mice, such as the A/JCr, are susceptible to developing hepatic tumors secondary to *H. hepaticus* infections. *H. hepaticus* has also been associated with inflammatory bowel disease in athymic and SCID mice. Other strains of *Helicobacter,* such as *Helicobacter muridarum, Helicobacter bilis,* and *Helicobacter rappini,* also inhabit the cecum and colon of mice. Antibiotic therapy for treating *Helicobacter* spp. from humans, ferrets, and cats has been shown to eradicate *H. hepaticus* successfully in mice. The therapy consists of amoxicillin or tetracycline in combination with metronidazole and bismuth given three times daily by oral gavage for 2 weeks. A recent report indicates the amoxicillin/metronidazole/bismuth therapy, administered at the dose amoxicillin 1.5–3.0 mg/d/30 g body weight (bw), metronidazole 0.69 mg/d/30 g bw, bismuth 0.185 mg/d/30 g bw, is effective when administered in the diet or by oral gavage but not when mixed in drinking water.

Tyzzer's Disease

Mice, rats, hamsters, gerbils, guinea pigs, rabbits, dogs, cats, several nonhuman primate species, and other animals are susceptible to Tyzzer's disease caused by *Clostridium piliforme*. Tyzzer's disease occurs more frequently and is usually more severe in recently weaned animals, immunosuppressed animals or those housed under unfavorable conditions. Clinical signs may include diarrhea, dehydration, and anorexia. Animals may be found dead in the absence of obvious signs of illness. Gross lesions seen at necropsy include miliary, pale foci throughout the liver and, at times, a slightly reddened lower intestinal tract. Treatment with antibiotics is frequently not effective; however, favorable results have been reported using tetracycline in the drinking water at high doses for 4–5 days.

Colonic Hyperplasia Disease

Citrobacter freundii biotype 4280 causes a disease syndrome in mice called transmissible murine colonic hyperplasia. The organism causes an enterocolitis that leads to clinical signs of diarrhea, retarded growth, ruffled fur, soft feces, and occasionally rectal prolapse. The mortality rate is variable and depends on age and strain susceptibilities with recently weaned mice having a higher mortality. The characteristic gross finding at necropsy is thickening of the distal half of the colon. Microscopically, mucosal hyperplasia, infiltration of inflammatory cells, and mucosal erosions may be evident in the affected portion of the colon. Recommended treatments include neomycin, tetracycline, and sulfamethazine.

Coryneform Hyperkeratosis in Nude Mice

Corynebacterium pseudodiptheriticum has been associated with a severe hyperkeratotic dermatitis in nude mice. The disease also causes high mortality in suckling mice. Clinical signs include dry, white flaky skin and pruritis. Definitive diagnosis requires culturing the organism on select media. There is no known treatment, and affected animals should be euthanized to prevent spread of the organism within a clean colony.

Miscellaneous Bacterial Diseases

Staphylococcus aureus infections are most frequently associated with abscesses, conjunctivitis, and superficial pyoderma, particularly around the head and face. Bite wounds are often secondarily infected with *S. aureus*. Furunculosis caused by *S. aureus* is a particularly troublesome condition in nude mice. Treatment is rarely successful.

Streptococcus spp. infections are associated with dermatitis, pharyngitis, cervical lymphadenitis, bacteremia, and a variety of other disease processes. Systemic antibiotics and improved sanitation may be beneficial in treatment.

Pseudomonas aeruginosa is frequently found in association with water and is not part of the normal microflora. Mice that are irradiated or otherwise immunologically compromised are susceptible to developing a *P. aeruginosa* septicemia. The septicemia is usually rapid, and clinical signs are limited to listlessness, anorexia, and death. Infections can be avoided by chlorinating the drinking water with sodium hypochlorite to achieve 10 ppm of free chlorine or by acidifying to a pH of 2.5–2.8 with hydrochloric acid. Acidity of the water should be tested before use.

Corynebacterium kutscheri is usually inapparent in mice, but it produces a disease in stressed or immunosuppressed mice termed pseudotuberculosis. The disease is characterized by septicemia with high mortality and produces disseminated abscesses, especially in the kidneys and liver, in surviving mice. Treatment is usually not successful.

Salmonella spp. infections were extremely common in research colonies at one time but are now rare as a result of the institution of proper management practices. Salmonellosis is rare in pet mice as well, but it is significant because of its zoonotic potential. Mice can be intermittent shedders for several months without showing clinical signs of disease.

Streptobacillus moniliformis infections are not common in mice. Epizootics are most likely to occur in mice that are housed near rats that may harbor the organism in the nasopharynx. The importance of this organism is that it has been identified as one of the causes of Rat Bite Fever, which causes an influenzalike disease in humans.

VIRAL DISEASES

☞ ### Sendai Virus

Sendai virus is a parainfluenza I virus. It is the most common cause of viral respiratory disease in mice and is the virus most likely to cause clinical disease in adult immunocompetent mice. It usually exists as an inapparent infection; however, it may produce acute disease that is sometimes fatal, particularly in suckling or weanling mice. There is a distinct strain variation in susceptibility to infection. Sendai virus infection suppresses the normal antibacterial activity of the lungs, thereby predisposing infected mice to secondary bacterial pneumonia. Clinical signs include a hunched posture, ruffled fur, dyspnea, and teeth chattering. Sendai virus has also been associated with otitis media and interna as well as exacerbations of pneumonia due to *M. pulmonis*. The severity of disease is intensified by secondary bacterial infection and immunosuppression. Antibiotics should be of benefit in preventing or eliminating secondary bacterial infection.

☞ Mouse Hepatitis Virus

Mouse hepatitis virus (MHV) is a coronavirus that is ubiquitous, highly contagious, and one of the most common viruses found in research colonies today. There are many related strains of MHV that generally fall into two disease patterns: the enteric pattern and the respiratory pattern. Enterotropic strains are much more common. Mouse hepatitis virus infections are usually enzootic and subclinical, with epizootics occurring in naive suckling mice. Clinical signs in suckling mice may include severe diarrhea, runting, an empty stomach or disappearance of the milk spot (unlike sucklings with rotavirus infection), encephalitis with tremors, and high mortality. Gross signs in adult mice include multifocal miliary white foci throughout the liver due to the necrotizing hepatitis that occurs with some strains of MHV. The most distinctive histologic finding is syncytial cells in the small intestinal mucosa and liver parenchyma. Mouse hepatitis virus does not persist in mice and can be eliminated from a colony by cessation of breeding for at least 4 weeks to allow all infected mice to clear the infection.

Epizootic Diarrhea of Infant Mice

Epizootic diarrhea of infant mice (EDIM) is a rotavirus that causes disease in suckling mice less than 2 weeks of age. It is characterized by the presence of soft, yellow feces or an accumulation of dried feces around the anus. Affected mice usually continue to nurse as evidenced by the milk spot, but their growth is often stunted. Spread of EDIM within a colony can be prevented by use of filtertop cages. No treatment exists other than supportive care.

Murine Retroviral Infection

All mice harbor both endogenous murine leukemia virus (MuLV) and endogenous murine mammary tumor virus (MuMTV) proviruses in their genome and expression of disease is mouse strain-, age-, and cell-type specific. The proviruses are transmitted genetically as inherited Mendelian characteristics.

Lymphocytic Choriomeningitis

Lymphocytic choriomeningitis virus (LCM) is an arenavirus and is the only latent virus of mice that naturally infects humans, causing an influenzalike disease. The natural reservoir of LCM is wild mice. Mice may serve as long-term asymptomatic carriers of the virus, so care should be taken when contacting tissue, feces, or urine of suspect animals.

Ectromelia (Mousepox)

Ectromelia is caused by a poxvirus and is very uncommon in the United States. It is significant when it does occur in research mice because it may be associated with high morbidity and mortality. The disease is usually introduced through imported mice, tumor transplants, or other biologic materials. This underscores the reason to serologically test all imported materials coming into a facility.

Miscellaneous Viral Infections

Mice are susceptible to a vast number of viral infections including K virus, pneumonia virus of mice, reovirus type 3, Theiler's encephalomyelitis virus, mouse adenovirus, mouse parvovirus, and lactic dehydrogenase elevating virus. These are primarily of concern as potential variables in biomedical research. Clinical signs are rarely seen in animals beyond the age of weaning. Serologic screening of research animals is routinely performed to provide the cleanest animals possible.

PARASITIC DISEASES

☞ Mites

Mites are very common in conventional mouse colonies. The degree of pathogenicity is highly variable. Light infestations are usually inapparent, whereas heavy infestations cause dermatitis, alopecia, greasy-appearing hair, and self-inflicted trauma. An allergic component may also be involved. Mite lesions must be differentiated from fight wounds, ringworm, and other skin disorders.

The more common species of pelage-inhabiting mites are *Myobia musculi, Radfordia affinis,* and *Myocoptes musculinus.* These mites may be detected by several methods including skin scrapings and applying cellophane tape to the dorsal fur and examining the tape under the microscope for nits or mites. More conclusive results are usually achieved by euthanizing the mouse and either collecting the mites as they leave the cold carcass or removing the mouse skin, placing it in a petri dish, and examining the bottom of the dish under low magnification after several hours. If mites are present, they should be transferred to a glass slide for identification.

Psorergates simplex is a follicle-inhabiting mite that produces dermal pouches that appear as small white nodules on the visceral surface of the reflected skin. These mites are rarely seen today.

Acaricides can reduce and even eliminate the mite population. Complete eradication of mites in a large mouse population, however, is difficult and requires an intensive treatment regimen. Ivermectin, given by a number of routes, and permethrin dusts have been shown to be effective in eliminating mites. Caution should be used when treating suckling mice, as they may be more sensitive to topical applications of acaricides. Other possible treatments include chlorpyrifos and fenbendazole.

☞ Pinworms

Syphacia obvelata and *Aspicularis tetraptera* inhabit the cecum and colon and are the most common nematode parasites that affect mice. *S. obvelata* is the more prevalent and troublesome. In most cases, clinical signs are absent; however, heavy infestations may lead to anal pruritis, rectal prolapse, and diarrhea. Neither species of pinworms is transmissible to humans.

The banana-shaped ova of *S. obvelata* can be detected by pressing a strip of cellophane tape to the perianal area, applying the tape to a glass slide, and examining under a microscope. The more oval eggs of *A. tetraptera* are detected by fecal examination. The most definitive diagnostic procedure involves examining the cecal contents for adult worms under a dissecting microscope.

Anthelmintics effective in treating pinworms include ivermectin, piperazine citrate, thiabendazole, and mebendazole. Complete elimination of *S. obvelata* without repopulation and strict sanitation is difficult to achieve.

Lice

Polyplax serrata, the house mouse louse, is a bloodsucking louse that causes skin irritation, anemia, and debilitation. It is uncommon in laboratory and pet mice. It can serve as the vector for *Eperythrozoon coccoides.* Ivermectin has been effectively used to eliminate lice. Dusts such as permethrin and malathion applied to the animals and the bedding are also reported to be effective against lice.

Tapeworms

Mice may harbor *Hymenolepis nana,* the dwarf tapeworm, and *Hymenolepis diminuta,* the rat tapeworm. Both species are potentially transmissible to humans. Only *H. nana,* however, is of practical public health concern because *H. diminuta* requires an intermediate host such as a grain beetle. Tapeworms are uncommon in conventional mouse colonies.

Diarrhea and retarded growth may occur with heavy infestations, but most cases are clinically silent. Infestations can be detected by the presence of ova upon fecal flotation or by observing the adults in the small intestine at necropsy. Recommended treatments include thiabendazole or praziquantel. Eradication by means other than repopulation is extremely difficult.

Flagellates

Spironucleus muris and *Giardia muris* are flagellates that occur in the small intestine and cecum. In young animals, the parasites may cause diarrhea and occasionally death, but older animals are generally asymptomatic. Treatments for giardiasis include metronidazole or oxytetracycline, which control outbreaks but do not eliminate the parasite. There are no available treatments for spironucleosis.

Rickettsia

Eperythrozoon coccoides is a rickettsial parasite of red blood cells that is rarely seen. Normally, the parasite exists in a latent state, however, splenectomy of an infected mouse will precipitate a transient parasitemia and anemia.

NEOPLASIA

The incidence and types of tumors occurring in mice are highly strain and age related. Retroviral infections play a key role in the development of most neoplasms of the lymphoreticular and hematopoietic systems, as well as of the mammary gland. Most mammary tumors are adenocarcinomas, which can produce large, firm masses on the abdomen, sides, or back of a mouse because of the wide distribution of mammary tissue.

MISCELLANEOUS CONDITIONS

☞ ### Bite Wounds

Mice, most often males, can inflict severe bite wounds to their cagemates primarily around the tail and genitals but also along the back. These wounds may become secondarily infected with *S. aureus,* which can lead to an ulcerative dermatitis with moist eczematous lesions. Bite wounds over the body must be differentiated from self-mutilation that

27

results from mange mite infestation. Treatments are usually ineffective, and euthanasia may be indicated in more severe cases. Separation of the fighters may resolve the problem.

Dehydration

Dehydration should not be overlooked as a possible cause of acute death in mice. Water may be unavailable because of an air lock in the sipper tube even when a water bottle is full. Malfunction of drinking valves in automatic watering systems can also result in a lack of water.

☞ Hair Loss

Mice frequently develop bilaterally symmetrical areas of alopecia on the muzzle caused by friction from bars on the feeder. Another cause of hair loss is barbering by cagemates, which most frequently involves hair chewing in the vibrissae or head region.

Malocclusion

Overgrowth of the incisors can occur when the jaw is maloccluded or the diet is too soft. If severe and undetected, overgrown incisors can lead to emaciation and death due to an inability to eat. Incisors can be trimmed with toenail clippers or a dental bur.

■ GENERAL REFERENCES

Sources consulted to compile the material in this chapter include *The Biology and Medicine of Rabbits and Rodents* by J.E. Harkness and J.E. Wagner, 4th edition (1995, Williams & Wilkins, 1400 North Providence Rd., Building II, Suite 5025, Media, PA 19063); *Laboratory Animal Medicine,* edited by J.G. Fox, B.J. Cohen, and F.M. Loew (1984, Academic Press, Inc., Orlando, FL 32887); *The UFAW Handbook on the Care and Management of Laboratory Animals,* 6th edition, edited by T.B. Poole (1987, Churchill Livingstone Inc., 1560 Broadway, New York, NY 10036); *Infectious Diseases of Mice and Rats* by the National Research Council (1991, National Academy Press, 2101 Constitution Ave., NW, Washington, DC 20418); and *Pathology of Laboratory Rodents and Rabbits,* by D.H. Percy and S.W. Barthold (1993, Iowa State University Press, 2121 South State Avenue, Ames, IA 50014).

■ TECHNICAL REFERENCES

Allen, D.G., J.K. Pringle, and D.A. Smith. 1993. *Handbook of Veterinary Drugs.* Philadelphia: JB Lippincott.

Anderson, N.L. 1994. Basic husbandry and medicine of pocket pets. In *Saunders Manual of Small Animal Practice,* ed. S.J. Birchard and R.G. Sherding, pp. 1363–1389. Philadelphia: WB Saunders.

AVMA (American Veterinary Medical Association) 1993. Report of the AVMA Panel on Euthanasia. *JAVMA* 202(2): 229–249.

Bean-Knudsen, D.E., J.E. Wagner, and R.D. Hall. 1986. Evaluation of the control of *Myobia musculi* infestations on laboratory mice with permethrin. *Lab Anim Sci* 36(3): 268–270.

Boivin, G.P., I. Ormsby, and J.E. Hall. 1996. Eradication of *Aspiculuris tetraptera*, using fenbendazole-medicated food. *Contemp Topics* 35(2): 69–70.

Burdette, E.C., R.A. Heckmann, and R. Ochoa. 1997. Evaluation of five treatment regimens and five diagnostic methods for murine mites (*Mycoptes musculinus* and *Myobia musculi*). *Contemp Topics* 36(2): 73–76.

Burgmann, P. and D.H. Percy. 1993. Antimicrobial drug use in rodents and rabbits. In *Antimicrobial Therapy in Veterinary Medicine*, 2nd ed., ed. J.F. Prescott and J.D. Baggot, pp. 524–541. Ames: Iowa State University Press.

Callahan, B.M., K.A. Hutchinson, A.L. Armstrong, and L.S.F. Keller. 1995. A comparison of four methods for sterilizing surgical instruments for rodent surgery. *Contemp Topics* 34(2): 57–60.

CFR (Code of Federal Regulations). 1986. Title 16 (Federal Hazardous Substances Act Regulations), Secs. 1400.40, 1400.41, and 1400.42. Washington, D.C.: Office of the Federal Register.

Collins, B.R. 1995. Antimicrobial drug use in rabbits, rodents, and other small mammals. In *Antimicrobial Therapy in Caged Birds and Exotic Pets*, pp. 3–10. Trenton, NJ: Veterinary Learning Systems.

Danneman, P.J., S. Stein, and S.O. Walshaw. 1997. Humane and practical implications of using carbon dioxide mixed with oxygen for anesthesia or euthanasia of rats. *Lab Anim Sci* 47(4): 376–385.

Flecknell, P.A. 1987. *Laboratory Animal Anesthesia*. London: Academic.

Flecknell, P.A. 1991. Post-operative analgesia in rabbits and rodents. *Lab Anim* 20(9): 34–37.

Flecknell, P.A. 1997. Medetomidine and atipamezole: Potential uses in laboratory animals. Lab Anim 26(2): 21–25.

Foltz, C.J., J.G. Fox, L. Yan, and B. Shames. 1996. Evaluation of various oral antimicrobial formulations for eradication of *Helicobacter hepaticus*. *Lab Anim Sci* 46(2): 193–197.

Foundation for Biomedical Research. 1995. Figures on Animal Research, Fiscal Year 1995.

Fraser, J., G.N. Joiner, and J.H. Jandine. 1974. The use of pelleted dichlorvos in the control of murine acariasis. *Lab Anim* 8: 271–274.

Harkness, J.E. 1993. *A Practitioner's Guide to Domestic Rodents*. Lakewood, CO: American Animal Hospital Association.

Harrenstien, L. 1994. Critical care of ferrets, rabbits, and rodents. *Semin Avian Exotic Pet Med* 3: 217–228.

Heard, D.J. 1993. Principles and techniques of anesthesia and analgesia for exotic practice. *Vet Clin North Am Small Anim Pract* 23(6): 1301–1327.

Holson, R.R. 1992. Euthanasia by decapitation: evidence that this technique produces prompt, painless unconsciousness in laboratory rodents. *Neurotoxicol Teratol* 14: 253–257.

Huerkamp, M.J. 1995. Anesthesia and postoperative management of rabbits and pocket pets. In *Kirk's Current Therapy XII—Small Animal Practice*, ed.

J.D. Bonagura, pp. 1322–1327. Philadelphia: WB Saunders.

Hughes, H.C. 1981. Anesthesia of laboratory animals. *Lab Anim* 10(5): 40–56.

Jenkins, W.L. 1987. Pharmacologic aspects of analgesic drugs in animals: an overview. *JAVMA* 191(10): 1231–1240.

Klement, P., J.M. Augustine, K.H. Delaney, G. Klement, and J.I. Weitz. 1996. An oral ivermectin regimen that eradicates pinworms (*Syphacia* spp.) in laboratory rats and mice. *Lab Anim Sci* 46(3): 286–290.

Le Blanc, S.A., R.E. Faith, and C.A. Montgomery. 1993. Use of topical ivermectin treatment for *Syphacia obvelata* in mice. *Lab Anim Sci* 43(5): 526–528.

Markovic, S.N., P.R. Night and D.M. Murasko. 1993. Inhibition of interferon stimulation of natural killer cell activity in mice anesthetized with halothane or isoflurane. *Anesthesiology* 78(4): 700–706.

Mather, T.N. and N.C.G. Lausen. 1990. A new insecticide delivery method for control of fur mite infestations in laboratory mice. *Lab Anim* 19: 25–29.

Matsushita, S. and E. Suzuki. 1995. Prevention and treatment of Cilia-associated respiratory bacillus in mice by use of antibiotics. *Lab Anim Sci* 45(5): 503–507.

NRC (National Research Council). 1996. Animal environment, housing and management. In *Guide for the Care and Use of Laboratory Animals.* Washington, DC: National Academy Press.

O'Rourke, C.M., G.K. Peter, and P.L. Junken. 1994. Evaluation of ketamine-xylazine-acepromazine as a combination anesthetic regimen in mice. *Comtemp Topics* 33: A–25.

Papaioannou, V.E. and J.G. Fox. 1993. Use and efficacy of tribromoethanol anesthesia in the mouse. *Lab Anim Sci* 43(2): 189–192.

Pence, B.C., D.S. Demick, B.C. Richard, and F. Buddingh. 1991. The efficacy and safety of chlorpyrifos (Dursban TM) for control of *Myobia musculi* infestation in mice. *Lab Anim Sci* 41(2): 139–142.

Sebesteny, A. 1979. Syrian hamsters. In *Handbook of Diseases of Laboratory Animals,* ed. J.M. Hime and P. O'Donoghue, pp. 111–136. London: Heinemann.

Skopets, B., R.P. Wilson, J.W. Griffith, and C.M. Lang. 1996. Ivermectin toxicity in young mice. *Lab Anim Sci* 46(1): 111–112.

Tarin, D. and A. Sturdee. 1972. Surgical anaesthesia of mice: evaluation of tribromoethanol, ether, halothane and methoxyflurane and development of a reliable technique. *Lab Anim* 6(1): 79–84.

Urbanski, H.F. and S.T. Kelley. 1991. Sedation by exposure to a gaseous carbon dioxide-oxygen mixture: application to studies involving small laboratory animal species. *Lab Anim Sci* 41(1): 80–82.

Wardrip, C.L., J.E. Artwohl, and B.T. Bennett. 1994. A review of the role of temperature versus time in an effective cage sanitation program. *Contemp Topics* 33(5): 66–68.

West, W.L., J.C. Schofield, and B.T. Bennett. 1992. Efficacy of the micro-dot technique for administering topical 1% ivermectin for the control of pinworms and fur mites in mice. *Contemp Topics* 31(6): 7–10.

White, W.J. and K.J. Field. 1987. Anesthesia and surgery of laboratory animals. *Vet Clin North Am Small Anim Pract* 17(5): 989–1017.

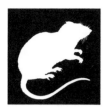

RATS

The LABORATORY RAT strains most commonly used in research are believed to be domesticated albino strains of the Norway rat, *Rattus norvegicus*. Rats, like mice, belong to the order Rodentia and the family Muridae. Adult rats generally weigh between 300 and 500 g, with males being slightly larger than females. Most laboratory rats are albino with white coats and pink eyes. There are several other color varieties including brown, black, and hooded rats, which have a dark head and shoulders with white bodies.

Genetics

Rats may be classified as outbred stocks, inbred strains or F_1 hybrids. Refer to Chapter 1, Mice, for a description of each type. Three of the most common outbred stocks of rats used in laboratories are the Sprague-Dawley, Wistar, and Long-Evans. Sprague-Dawley and Wistar rats are albinos, and the Long-Evans is a hooded rat. Two examples of inbred strains are the Fischer 344 (F344) rat and the Buffalo rat. F344 rats have a high incidence of testicular tumors, large granular lymphocytic leukemia, and retinal degeneration. They are commonly used in gerontology and long-term toxicity studies. Buffalo rats have a high incidence of autoimmune thyroiditis, also known as Hashimoto's disease.

Ecologic Types

The four ecologic types described in mice are similar for rats and include 1) germ free or axenic, 2) gnotobiotic, 3) specific pathogen–free, and 4) conventional. A description of each type is covered in Chapter 1, Mice.

Uses

Despite the fear that rats invoke in people, they actually make quiet, gentle pets that are intelligent and easily trained. They seldom bite unless provoked and do not have the distinct musty odor that is character-istic of mice. Typical of rodents, rats are extremely proficient breeders, and pet owners should purchase same-sex pairs to avoid having large numbers of rats in a very short time. Humans can develop allergies to rat dander and urine proteins.

Rats rank second only to mice in number used in biomedical re-search. Rats and mice combined account for more than 90% of all mammalian species used. Rats share most of the attributes of mice that make them valuable for research purposes, including a short life span, a short gestation length, a large litter size, great genetic diversity, low cost of purchase, and ease of maintenance. Mutant strains of inbred rats pro-vide investigators a large variety of animal models with which to study biologic processes and diseases. Hypertension, neoplasia, teratology, toxicology, embryology, and aging are several of the areas for which rats are used in research.

Behavior

Rats tend to be social animals but do well housed either singly or in small uncrowded groups. Unlike mice, rats rarely fight and males can be housed together with few problems. Females with litters may not toler-ate the company of other females. Most rat strains are docile, curious, and easily adapt to various environments. The Long-Evans and Fischer 344 strains have reputations of being more aggressive and difficult to handle. Docile behavior can be markedly improved by frequent gentle handling, especially if initiated while young. Rats will bite out of fear if they are roughly handled.

Rats are nocturnal, sleeping much of the day. They like to burrow and build nests for their young. They will escape from their cages if the lids are left off but usually return to them after a brief exploration pe-riod.

Anatomic and Physiologic Features

Biologic and reproductive data for the rat can be found in Table 2.1. Rats are much larger than mice, having conical heads and longer cylin-drical bodies, covered in thick, short fur. Their legs are short and their tails are long and sparsely haired. As with other rodents, brown fat is important in thermogenesis of rats and is found between the scapulae and in the ventral cervical region. Brown fat can be confused with sali-vary glands or lymph nodes.

The rat gastrointestinal system is anatomically similar to that of the mouse with a few notable exceptions. The dental formula 2 (1/1 in-

Table 2.1. Biologic and reproductive data for rats	
Adult body weight	
Male	300–520 g
Female	250–300 g
Life span	2.5–3.5 y
Body temperature	35.9°–37.5°C (96.6°–99.5°F)
Heart rate	250–450 beats per minute
Respiratory rate	70–115 breaths per minute
Food consumption	5–6 g/100 g/d
Water consumption	10–12 mL/100 g/d
Breeding onset	
Male	65–110 d
Female	65–110 d
Estrous cycle length	4–5 d
Gestation period	21–23 d
Postpartum estrus	Fertile
Litter size	6–12
Weaning age	21 d
Breeding duration	350–440 d
Chromosome number (diploid)	42

Sources: Adapted from Harkness and Wagner (1995); Fox, Cohen, and Loew (1984).

cisors, 0/0 canines, 0/0 premolars, 3/3 molars), continuously growing incisors, and divided stomach (aglandular forestomach, glandular stomach) are all similar. The rat, however, cannot vomit because of a fold in the limiting ridge that separates the two parts of the stomach and covers the entrance of the esophagus. Other unique features of the digestive system of rats include the absence of a gallbladder, the presence of a diffuse pancreas, and numerous salivary glands and glandlike organs in the head and neck. The cecum is highly developed and has a rumenlike function for microbial digestion of cellulose. In germ-free rats, the cecum may become greatly distended and occasionally twists on its long axis, resulting in fatal cecal torsion.

Behind the eye lies a large, pigmented, horseshoe-shaped lacrimal gland called the harderian gland. The tears secreted by this gland are high in porphyrin and can form red crusts around the eyes and nose. The lungs are similar to those in mice, consisting of one left lobe and four small right lobes.

Sexing of neonates is accomplished by comparing the anogenital distance and the size of the genital papillae. A larger genital papilla and greater anogenital distance are seen in males as compared with females, as depicted in Figure 2.1. Adult rats are readily distinguishable, as the testes are obvious in the scrotum of males. Rats, like mice, have extensive mammary tissue, ranging ventrally from the neck to the inguinal region and onto the sides and back. They have six pairs of mammary glands, three thoracic and three abdominal. The testes remain retractable throughout life because of open inguinal canals. Males have an os penis.

There are several distinctive characteristics of the hematologic and urinary profiles of rats. Lymphocytes comprise about 80% of the peripheral blood leukocyte population in rats. Basophils are rarely seen in circulation. Males generally have higher granulocyte and lymphocyte counts than do females. Rats have the ability to concentrate urine twice that of humans. Urine pH is 7.3–7.5 and the specific gravity is 1.040–1.070. Hematologic and biochemical parameters for the rat are listed in Appendix 1, Normal Values.

Breeding and Reproduction

A detailed description of the various breeding systems in rat colonies is beyond the scope of this book. The following is a general overview of breeding practices. Either a monogamous or a polygamous breeding system may be followed. With a monogamous mating system, one male and one female are permanently paired and the offspring are removed when they reach weaning age. A polygamous mating system typically entails the housing of one male and two or more females together. Pregnant females are removed prior to parturition in the polygamous mating system and returned to the breeding cage after their litters are weaned.

Rats reach puberty at 6–8 weeks, but they are normally not bred until about 3 months of age. They are continuously polyestrous, spontaneous ovulators, and have an estrous cycle length of 4–5 days. Vaginal plugs are present in the vagina for 12–24 hours after coitus and are useful to confirm matings.

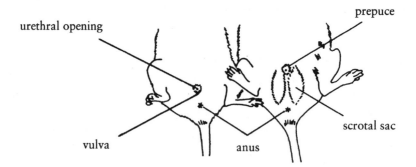

Figure 2.1. Rodent external genitalia: Female, *left*; male, *right*. (Adapted from Harkness and Wagner 1995, *The Biology and Medicine of Rabbits and Rodents*, 4th edition, Philadelphia: Williams & Wilkins)

Pheromones appear to play a less important role in the reproductive behavior of rats as compared to mice. The pheromone-mediated Bruce effect described in mice does not occur in rats. Synchronization of estrus, or the Whitten effect, does occur in rats but is not as pronounced as it is in the mouse.

The usual gestation period of a rat is 21–23 days but may be prolonged for 3–7 days in lactating rats because of delayed implantation. Rarely, nonfertile matings will result in a pseudopregnancy that lasts approximately 13 days. There is a fertile postpartum estrus; otherwise, females will resume cycling 2–4 days postweaning.

The average litter size is between six and 12 pups, but varies with strain and age of rat. It may be preferable to isolate the female for a few days before and after parturition because disturbances may cause the female to cannibalize her pups. Rat pups are born hairless, blind, and deaf. They are fully haired at 7–10 days, their ears open between 2.5 and 3.5 days, and eyes open between 7 and 14 days. Rat pups start eating solid food at about 2 weeks of age. The usual weaning age of rats is 21 days.

HUSBANDRY

Housing

Rat cages should provide each adult rat (>500 gm) with at least 452 cm^2 (70 in.^{2}) of floor space and a height of at least 18 cm (7 in.). Rats are ordinarily housed in metal cages with wire-mesh bottoms or solid-bottom shoebox-type cages constructed of plastic or stainless steel. Shoebox cages may be covered with a bonnet made from paper or a special plastic cagetop with filter called a microisolator. The cagetops reduce infectious disease transmission and minimize allergenic particulates from becoming airborne. The value of cagetops is offset to some extent by the high ammonia concentrations and increased temperature and humidity they allow to build up in the interior of the cage. A contact bedding material such as wood chips, wood shavings, composite recycled paper pellets, or corncob particles should be placed in the bottom of solid shoebox cages. Breeding animals and pups are best housed in solid-bottom cages containing wood chips or other suitable bedding material. Nesting material, such as cotton nestlets, facial tissue, or soft paper towels may be provided to pregnant dams.

The room temperature should be maintained within a range of 18°–26°C (64°–79°F) and the humidity should be between 30% and 70%. Ten to 15 air changes per hour are suggested to maintain adequate ventilation. Rats are nocturnal and must be provided with regular light:dark cycles for normal behavior and physiologic processes. In the laboratory, the light cycle is usually controlled by a timing device that provides 12–14 hours of light per day. If regular light cycles are not maintained, the circadian rhythm will be disrupted, resulting in inconsistent responses to experimental manipulation.

Rat caging should be cleaned one to three times each week depending on the number and size of rats housed in the cage. Cages, water bottles, and feed hoppers should be disinfected with chemicals, hot water 61.6°–82.2°C (143°–180°F) or a combination of both. Detergents and chemical disinfectants enhance the effectiveness of hot water, but they must be thoroughly rinsed from all caging surfaces with fresh water. Refer to Chapter 1, Mice, for a more detailed description of disinfection methods.

Feeding and Watering

Rats grow and reproduce well and can be maintained on a standard commercial rodent diet that contains at least 20%–25% protein and 4% fat. Rodent chow is usually provided in the form of firm dry blocks or pellets and offered ad libitum. Recently, however, it has been shown that restriction of caloric protein and fat, as well as feeding soy protein rather than casein, extends the life span of rats. Rats eat an average of 5–6 g/100 g of body weight per day. Food pellets can be placed either on top of the cage lid or in a hopper attached to the cage wall. Food should not be placed directly on the cage floor unless the animals are debilitated or too young to reach the hopper. Supplemental feeding is not necessary or indicated for research animals, although pet rats may enjoy an occasional fruit, vegetable, or seed treat. Rats, like most other rodents, are coprophagic.

Fresh, potable water should be made available ad libitum, either from a bottle or automatic watering system. Adult rats drink an average of 10–12 mL/100 g of body weight of water per day.

TECHNIQUES

Handling and Restraint

Rats can be transferred from cage to cage by picking them up by the base of the tail. They should not be picked up by the middle or tip of the tail, as the skin may be pulled off, creating a severe degloving injury. Rats that are used to being handled may be picked up by placing a hand under the body and then cradling the rat in the crook of the handler's elbow.

Rats can be restrained by a number of methods. One method involves holding the rat with one hand by the base of the tail and placing it on a cage lid or other surface that it can grasp. As the rat moves forward, the other hand is placed firmly over the back and rib cage, and the thumb and forefinger are placed directly behind the rat's elbows to push the legs forward so that they cross under the chin of the rat. Figure 2.2 depicts this restraint method. Care must be taken to not put too much pressure on the thorax of the rat, as that can impede respiration and cause death. Another method involves the same initial steps, but the forefinger and middle finger are placed immediately behind the mandibles to restrain the head.

Docile rats are best handled with bare or latex gloved hands. Heavy leather or chain mail gloves can be used to handle vicious rats, but are often awkward and can make rats more fearful and difficult to handle. A hand towel can be wrapped around the body of the rat to avoid the risk of the handler being bitten while giving an injection.

Clear plastic restraint bags can be bought commercially or made out of a durable freezer bag. The bags should be in the shape of a cone or cake decorating tube with an opening at the tapered end. These restraint bags are especially helpful for individuals who are working alone with large or vicious rats. The bag is held open in one hand with the tapered end pointing down. The rat is picked up by the base of the tail and is quickly lowered, head first, into the bag, so the nose is at the opening.

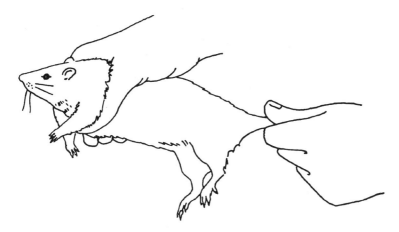

Figure 2.2. Restraint of the rat.

The rear of the bag is then gathered together, totally enclosing the rat. Injections can be given directly through the bag. Rats should only be restrained for short periods in a plastic bag, as they can quickly overheat. Rigid plastic restrainers that have openings to permit injections, blood collection, and other manipulations are also commercially available.

Identification

Cage cards are most often used as a form of general identification. There are several permanent methods to identify rats individually, including ear punching, ear tagging, tattooing the tail, or placing a subcutaneous microchip for quick electronic identification. Dyes or markers can be used as temporary identification methods.

Blood Collection

Table 2.2 lists approximate adult rat blood volumes. The retroorbital plexus is the site most commonly used for collecting small amounts of blood in rats. This procedure requires anesthesia and the use of a microhematocrit tube or Pasteur pipette to penetrate the venous plexus behind the eye. Refer to Chapter 1, Mice (Figure 1.4) for a more detailed description of the technique. The only difference in technique in the rat is that it is best to place the tube slightly dorsal to the medial canthus of the eye, rather than at the medial canthus as described in the mouse.

Other methods for obtaining small amounts of blood from a rat include capillary tube collection from the hub of a needle placed in the lateral tail veins, a snipped toenail, or from the dorsal tail artery. To facilitate blood flow to the tail, immerse it in warm water or warm it with a heat lamp for a few minutes to dilate the caudal vessels.

Larger volumes of blood may be obtained from a cardiac puncture or the cranial vena cava of an anesthetized rat. The heart can be approached from the abdomen just lateral to the xiphoid process with the needle directed at approximately a 30°–35° angle slightly to the left of midline in the rat's thorax. Alternatively, the cardiac puncture can be approached from the side, just caudal to the rat's elbow. See Figure 2.3 for location of the heart when rat is placed in lateral and dorsal recumbency.

Table 2.2. Adult rat blood volumes	
	Volume (mL)[a]
Total blood	20–40
Single sample	2–3
Exsanguination	8–12

Source: Adapted from Harkness and Wagner (1995).
[a] Values are approximate.

These procedures must be performed with a steady hand because too much movement of the needle will lacerate the heart, vessels, or lungs and result in premature death. A terminal sample can be collected from the blood that pools after laceration of the axillary vessels.

Urine Collection

Urine can be collected by placing rats in specially designed metabolism cages. These enclosures have feed and water containers outside the cage and devices for separating urine and feces below. Rats will frequently urinate and defecate when handled, enabling a sample to be collected from the table.

Drug Administration

Drug administration routes in rats are similar to those of larger mammals. Medications are routinely added to the water or feed for ease of administering to large groups of rats. If medications are unpalatable, 5 mL of sugar or syrup per liter can be added to the drinking water to

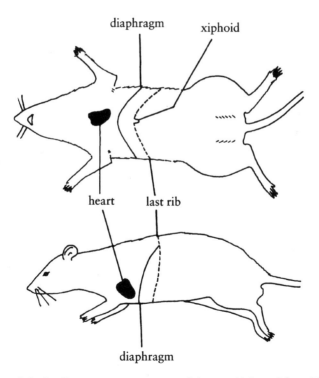

Figure 2.3. Cardiac puncture anatomy of the rat. (Adapted from Timm and Jahn 1980, Practical Methodology of the Rat. In *Practical Methodology* [slide series], ©Regents University of California)

improve the palatability. A bulbed gavage needle can be used for dosing individuals with liquid medication.

Smaller-gauge needles, such as 23 or 25 gauge, should be used for injections. Subcutaneous injections can be given in the loose skin over the back or on the abdomen with a maximum volume of 5–8 mL. Rats have such a small muscle mass that intramuscular injection volumes should be no greater than 0.3 mL. Irritation of the sciatic nerve from a misplaced injection or from certain drugs, such as ketamine, will often lead to self-mutilation of the limb. Intraperitoneal injections are preferred over intramuscular injections and should be placed in a rat's lower abdominal quadrant, just off the midline. A maximum volume of 5–10 mL should be given by the intraperitoneal route. The intraperitoneal injection technique is described in more detail in Chapter 1, Mice. Although intravenous administration of drugs is not generally practical, it is often accomplished for research purposes by surgical placement of an indwelling catheter in the jugular veins or carotid arteries. The tail vein can be used for intravenous administration in young rats; however, the tail skin of mature rats is thicker, making it more difficult to access the vein.

Anesthesia, Surgery, and Postoperative Care

Agents commonly used for anesthesia and tranquilization of rats and recommended dosages are listed in Table 2.3. Preanesthetic fasting is generally not recommended in rats unless an empty stomach is inherent to the success of the procedure. Injectable anesthetic regimens are used mainly for shorter procedures, as the depth of anesthesia is more difficult to control. The combination of ketamine and xylazine is a reasonably good choice for simple procedures. The acid pH of ketamine has been associated with muscle damage and nerve irritation and should be given preferentially through the intraperitoneal route. Pentobarbital remains a popular choice for surgical procedures despite the narrow margin between the anesthetic dose and the LD_{50}. It is safest to start with the lower end of the dose range when using this drug.

Inhalation anesthesia is generally impractical for rats in a clinical setting other than for brief periods of anesthesia. Of the inhalant anesthetic agents, isoflurane, halothane, and methoxyflurane are preferable to ether. Ether is irritating to the respiratory tract, which is particularly undesirable in rats with respiratory disease. Isoflurane and halothane require a precision vaporizer, whereas methoxyflurane and ether can be used by the open-drop method. Volatile anesthetics should always be used with appropriate waste gas scavenging systems or in a fume hood.

Table 2.3. Anesthetic agents and tranquilizers used in rats			
Drug	Dosage	Route	Reference
Inhalants			
Carbon dioxide	50%–80% CO_2 mixed with 20%–50% O_2	Inhalation	Fenwick (1989)
Ether	Ambient vaporization of ether-soaked gauze	Inhalation	Baker (1980)
Halothane	1%–3% to effect	Inhalation	Dardai (1987)
Isoflurane	1%–5% to effect	Inhalation	Dardai (1987)
Methoxyflurane	1%–3% to effect	Inhalation	Wixson (1994)
Injectables			
Alpha chloralose (5% conc.)	31–65 mg/kg	IP	White (1987)
Chloral hydrate (5% conc.)	300–450 mg/kg	IP	Silverman (1993)
Diazepam	4 mg/kg	IP	Flecknell (1987)
Fentanyl-droperidol	0.02–0.06 mL/100 g	IP	Wixson et al. (1987)
Fentanyl	0.3 mg/kg	IP	Flecknell (1997)
+ medetomidine	0.3 mg/kg	IP	
Ketamine	75–80 mg/kg	IP	Flecknell (1987)
+ acetylpromazine	2.5 mg/kg	IM	
Ketamine	40–80 mg/kg	IP	Wixson et al. (1987)
+ diazepam	5–10 mg/kg	IP	
Ketamine	75 mg/kg	IP	Flecknell (1997)
+ medetomidine	0.5 mg/kg	IP	
Ketamine	40–80 mg/kg	IP	Wixson et al. (1987)
+ xylazine	5–10 mg/kg	IP	
Pentobarbital	30–40 mg/kg	IP	Wixson et al. (1987)
Propofol	7.5–15 mg/kg	IV	Glen (1980)
Thiopental (1.25% solution)	40 mg/kg	IP	White (1987)
Tiletamine-zolazepam	20–40 mg/kg	IP	Silverman (1983)
Tiletamine-zolazepam	20–40 mg/kg	IP	Wilson (1992)
+ butorphanol	1.25–5 mg/kg	IP	
Tiletamine-zolazepam	20–40 mg/kg	IP	Wilson (1992)
+ xylazine	5–10 mg/kg	IP	
Tribromoethanol	300 mg/kg	IP	Flecknell (1987)
Urethane	1000 mg/kg	IP	Flecknell (1987)

IM = intramuscular; IP = intraperitoneal; IV = intravenous.

Refer to Chapter 1, Mice, for a more comprehensive description of different volatile anesthetic delivery systems.

Pet rats may require a simple castration or mammary tumor removal. To prevent intestinal entrapment, care should be taken to close the inguinal canals during castration. Mammary tumors are usually well encapsulated and easy to remove; however, they may reoccur. There are a number of common surgical procedures performed on research rats, including hypophysectomy, adrenalectomy, thymectomy, and jugular vein or carotid artery catheterization.

Surgeries should be performed in an aseptic manner. Care should be taken to avoid hypothermia, blood loss, and dehydration, which can lead to slow anesthetic recoveries and death. Refer to Chapter 1, Mice, for some more detailed intraoperative and postoperative management techniques.

Postanesthetic recovery of the rat includes placing it on a clean, dry cloth and not directly on small-particle bedding, which might be aspirated. Some form of heat should be provided to promote euthermia. To prevent lung congestion, the rat should be turned every 30–60 minutes until it is ambulatory. To avoid cannibalism, an anesthetized rat should not be placed back in a cage with awake cagemates until it has recovered full ambulation. Analgesics should be given for invasive surgical procedures that are known to cause pain in larger mammals. Butorphanol is recommended for mild postoperative discomfort. Buprenorphine causes more sedation but works well to control acute or chronic visceral pain. Table 2.4 lists several analgesics that can be used in rats.

Euthanasia

The use of carbon dioxide in a prefilled chamber with approximately 70% carbon dioxide or an overdose of a barbiturate solution administered intraperitoneally are acceptable methods for humane euthanasia of rats. A recent study indicates that to use CO_2 in a humane manner, one must avoid exposing conscious animals to concentrations >70%. The use of slow flow rates and non-precharged chambers are suggested to ensure a slow buildup of CO_2 in the animals' environment. Many other methods are acceptable when performed on a fully anes-

Table 2.4. Analgesic agents used in rats

Drug	Dosage	Route	Reference
Acetaminophen	1–2 mg/mL drinking water		Huerkamp (1995)
Acetylsalicylic acid	100–150 mg/kg q4h	PO	Heard (1993)
Buprenorphine	0.02–0.5 mg/kg q6–12h	SC, IP	Harkness and Wagner (1995)
	0.02 mg/mL drinking water		Cooper et al. (1997)
Butorphanol	1–5 mg/kg q2–4h	SC	Heard (1993)
Codeine	25–60 mg/kg q4h	SC	Jenkins (1987)
Flunixin meglumine	2.5 mg/kg q12–24h	SC	Heard (1993)
Ibuprofen	10–30 mg/kg ~ q4h	PO	Flecknell (1991)
Meperidine	20 mg/kg q2–3h	SC, IM	Heard (1993)
Syrup	0.2 mg/mL drinking water		Huerkamp (1995)
Nalbuphine	4–8 mg/kg q3h	IM	Heard (1993)
Oxymorphone	0.2–0.5 mg/kg q6–12h	SC, IM	Heard (1993)
Pentazocine	10 mg/kg q2–4h	SC	Heard (1993)

IM = intramusculoar; IP = intraperitoneal; PO = per os; SC = subcutaneous.

thetized animal. Occasionally, it is necessary to euthanize animals without the use of anesthetics or tranquilizers that could complicate research results. In such cases, investigators must fully justify the need for avoiding drugs and the request must be approved by an Institutional Animal Care and Use Committee. Decapitation with a guillotine is one method that is humane if properly performed. Refer to Chapter 1, Mice, for more details on euthanasia.

THERAPEUTIC AGENTS

Suggested rat antimicrobial and antifungal drug dosages are listed in Table 2.5. Antiparasitic agents are listed in Table 2.6 and miscellaneous drugs are listed in Table 2.7.

Table 2.5. Antimicrobial and antifungal agents used in rats

Drug	Dosage	Route	Reference
Ampicillin	20–100 mg/kg q12h	PO, SC, IM	Anderson (1994)
Cephaloridine	10–25 mg/kg q24h	SC, IM	Anderson (1994)
Chloramphenicol	50–200 mg/kg q8h	PO	Burgmann and Percy (1993)
	30–50 mg/kg q12h	SC, IM	Burgmann and Percy (1993)
Ciprofloxacin	7–20 mg/kg q12h	PO	Harkness and Wagner (1995)
Doxycycline	5 mg/kg q12h	PO	Harkness and Wagner (1995)
Enrofloxacin	0.05–0.2 mg/mL drinking water for 14 d		Harkness and Wagner (1995)
	5–10 mg/kg q12h	PO, IM	Harkness and Wagner (1995)
Gentamicin	2–4 mg/kg q8–24h	SC, IM	Harkness and Wagner (1995)
Griseofulvin	25–50 mg/kg q12h for 14–60 d	PO	Harkness and Wagner (1995)
	1.5% in DMSO for 5–7 d	Topical	Harkness and Wagner (1995)
Ketoconazole	10–40 mg/kg q24h for 14 d	PO	Harkness and Wagner (1995)
Metronidazole	10–40 mg/kg q24h	PO	Burgmann and Percy (1993)
Neomycin	2.6 mg/mL drinking water		Anderson (1994)
Oxytetracycline	0.4 mg/mL drinking water		Burgmann and Percy (1993)
	10–20 mg/kg q8h	PO	Burgmann and Percy (1993)
Pencillin, potassium	100,000 IU/kg q12h	IM	Russell et al. (1981)
Sulfadimethoxine	10–15 mg/kg q12h	PO	Harkness and Wagner (1995)
Sulfamerazine	1 mg/mL drinking water		Anderson (1994)
Sulfamethazine	1 mg/mL drinking water		Anderson (1994)
Sulfaquinoxaline	0.25–1 mg/mL drinking water		Burgmann and Percy (1993)
Tetracycline	2–5 mg/mL drinking water		Burgmann and Percy (1993)
	10–20 mg/kg q8–12h	PO	Burgmann and Percy (1993)
Trimethoprim-sulfa	30 mg/kg q12h	PO, IM	Harkness and Wagner (1995)
Tylosin	10 mg/kg q24h	PO, SC, IM	Collins (1995)

DMSO = dimethyl sulfoxide; IM = intramuscular; PO = per os; SC = subcutaneous.

Table 2.6. Antiparasitic agents used in rats

Drug	Dosage	Route	Reference
Carbamate (5%)	Twice weekly	Topical	Harkness and Wagner (1995)
Fenbendazole	20 mg/kg q24h for 5 d	PO	Allen (1993)
	150 mg/kg of feed; provide for 7 d on, 7 d off for 3 treatments		Boivin et al. (1996)
Ivermectin	200–400 mcg/kg every 7–10 d	PO	Harkness and Wagner (1995)
	0.2 mg/kg q7d for 3 wk	PO, SC	Anderson (1994)
	25 mg/L drinking water for 4 d on, 3 d off for 4 treatments		Klement et al. (1996)
Piperazine citrate	2–5 mg/mL drinking water for 7 d, off 7 d, repeat		Anderson (1994)
Praziquantel	6–10 mg/kg	PO	Harkness and Wagner (1995)
Pyrethrin powder	3 times a week for 3 wk	Topical	Anderson (1994)
Thiabendazole	100–200 mg/kg	PO	Harkness and Wagner (1995)

PO = per os; SC = subcutaneous.

Table 2.7. Miscellaneous agents used in rats

Drug	Dosage	Route	Reference
Atipamezole	1 mg/kg	SC, IP, IV	Flecknell (1997)
Atropine	0.05–0.1 mg/kg	SC	Harkness and Wagner (1995)
	10 mg/kg q20 min (organophosphate toxicity)	SC	Harkness and Wagner (1995)
Cimetidine	5–10 mg/kg q6–12h	PO	Allen (1993)
Dexamethasone	0.5–2 mg/kg then decreasing dose q12h for 3–14 d	PO, SC	Harkness and Wagner (1995)
Doxapram	5–10 mg/kg	IP, IV	Harkness (1993)
Furosemide	1–4 mg/kg q4–6h	IM	Harrenstien (1994)
Glycopyrrolate	0.01–0.02 mg/kg	SC	Huerkamp (1995)
Naloxone	0.01–0.1 mg/kg	SC, IP	Huerkamp (1995)
Prednisone	0.5–2.2 mg/kg	SC, IM	Anderson (1994)
Vitamin K	1–10 mg/kg q24h for 4–6 d	IM	Harkness and Wagner (1995)
Yohimbine	0.5–1 mg/kg	IV	Harkness and Wagner (1995)

IM = intramuscular; IP = intraperitoneal; IV = intravenous; PO = per os; SC = subcutaneous.

BACTERIAL DISEASES

Pneumonia and Respiratory Diseases

☞ *Mycoplasma pulmonis* is the most common and important respiratory pathogen of conventional laboratory and pet rats. It causes a chronic respiratory disease syndrome called murine respiratory mycoplasmosis (MRM). Although *M. pulmonis* is the primary etiologic agent of MRM, other viruses (e.g., Sendai, sialodacryoadenitis) and bacteria (e.g., *Streptococcus pneumoniae, Bordetella bronchiseptica,* CAR bacillus) are often recovered from the lungs of infected animals.

M. pulmonis can be transmitted by direct contact between an infected dam and her offspring, by intrauterine or sexual transfer, or by aerosol. The organism has an affinity for the epithelial cells of the respiratory tract, middle ear, and endometrium. The disease is usually subclinical and slowly progressive, with clinical signs becoming evident only when an advanced stage of disease is reached. Factors such as high ammonia levels, other respiratory pathogens, and various forms of stress have a profound effect on the clinical course and severity of the disease.

A serous or catarrhal nasal and ocular discharge may occur, but the sound of snuffling is usually more obvious than other early clinical signs. Animals with extensive pulmonary involvement may exhibit labored breathing, weight loss, lethargy, a hunched posture, and a rough haircoat. Acute deaths are usually the result of secondary bacterial infections.

Unilateral or bilateral otitis interna, characterized by the presence of a head tilt, is part of the chronic respiratory disease syndrome. The infection frequently extends up the eustachian tube into the middle ear and then to the inner ear, causing a labyrinthitis. When rats with labyrinthitis are held by the tail in a vertical position, they typically spin, rotating their bodies rapidly.

In the earliest stage, pulmonary lesions are limited to peribronchiolar lymphoid hyperplasia, visible only on microscopic examination of the lung. As the disease progresses, well-demarcated foci of firm, red–gray consolidation appear. Accumulation of inflammatory debris and mucus may result in bronchial distention, which can give the surface of the lung a "cobblestone" appearance. Diagnosis is based on history, clinical findings, gross and microscopic lesions, and isolation of *M. pulmonis* from the nasopharynx, tympanic bullae, trachea, or lungs. An enzyme-linked immunosorbent assay kit is now available for detection of *M. pulmonis* infection but can have a significant number of false-positives from cross-reactivity.

Antimicrobials added to the drinking water for periods of a week or more will suppress *M. pulmonis* infection but will not eliminate the disease. Bacterial culture and sensitivity testing are necessary to determine the most appropriate choice of antibiotics. Oxytetracycline or tetracycline in the drinking water are commonly used. For treatment of individual animals, enrofloxacin, chloramphenicol, or tylosin may be injected intramuscularly for 5 days or more. Labyrinthitis does not usually respond to treatment, but animals with pronounced head tilt will often survive for months. Elimination of this disease requires cesarean derivation of breeding stock and maintenance of animals under a barrier system.

S. pneumoniae, once a common cause of respiratory disease in young rats, today is rarely recognized in well-managed facilities. Many rats harbor the organism in the upper respiratory tract without clinical signs, and disease outbreaks can occur following stress. The disease tends to be acute to subacute and primarily affects younger animals. Affected animals exhibit depression, a serosanguinous to mucopurulent nasal discharge, a snuffling respiratory sound, dyspnea, an ocular discharge, and ruffled fur.

Gross lesions often found at necropsy include seropurulent and fibrinopurulent pleuritis, pericarditis, epicarditis, peritonitis, meningitis, otitis media and interna, metritis, and bronchopneumonia. Fibrinopurulent peritonitis and pleuritis with minimal involvement of the lung parenchyma are not uncommon.

Penicillin administered intramuscularly or oxytetracycline in the drinking water are among the more frequently used antibiotics. Many others, including ampicillin, chloramphenicol, and gentamicin, are also generally beneficial.

Naturally occurring infections of the cilia-associated respiratory (CAR) bacillus have been reported in rats, mice, rabbits, cattle, and swine. In most species, it appears to be an opportunistic invader of the respiratory tract. It may, however, cause a respiratory disease syndrome in rats with similar clinical signs and lung pathology as seen in MRM.

The CAR bacillus is found between and parallel to the cilia of the respiratory epithelium. It may be detected by using a modified Steiner silver stain of a scraping from the respiratory tract or a section of lung. The efficacy of antimicrobial therapy has not been thoroughly examined, although the organism is sensitive to procaine penicillin G, chloramphenicol, and gentamicin.

Pasteurella pneumotropica is generally latent in rats, but it is considered an opportunistic pathogen secondary to other agents such as

Sendai virus or *M. pulmonis*. Although clinical signs are usually those of pneumonia or an upper respiratory infection, abscesses of the skin, subcutaneous tissue, mammary glands, and other organs are occasionally caused by *P. pneumotropica*. Chloramphenicol may be beneficial in controlling clinical manifestations of infection. The selection of antibiotics is best based on the results of in vitro sensitivity testing. Antibiotics can control epizootics of respiratory disease but do not generally eliminate the carrier state.

Tyzzer's Disease

Clostridium piliforme is the causative agent of Tyzzer's disease. Many rat colonies have been shown to have subclinical infections with *C. piliforme*. It occasionally occurs as an acute epizootic when stressors such as poor environmental conditions or concurrent infections lead to immunosuppression. Clinical signs may include diarrhea, dehydration, and anorexia. Animals may be found dead in the absence of obvious signs of illness. Gross lesions include miliary, pale foci throughout the liver, and a slightly reddened lower intestinal tract. A definitive diagnosis may be difficult to establish and requires identification of the organism in tissues with silver, Giemsa, or periodic acid-Schiff stains. Inoculating weanling gerbils, which are highly susceptible, per os with feces from suspect animals is a useful aid in obtaining a definitive diagnosis. Oxytetracycline and tetracycline have been used to suppress an epizootic episode.

Staphylococcus sp.

Staphylococcus aureus causes a variety of lesions in rats, including ulcerative dermatitis and pododermatitis. Trimming the toenails is beneficial in eliminating the self-mutilation from scratching often associated with ulcerative dermatitis. Good sanitation procedures and, in some cases, topical or parenteral antibiotics should be used to treat staphylococcal infections. Treatment with topical antibiotics is often impractical, as rats often lick the medication off.

Miscellaneous Bacterial Infections

Corynebacterium kutscheri usually exists as a latent or subclinical infection. Stressful situations will often elicit a subacute respiratory disease with abscesses in the lungs. In chronic cases, the abscess contents in the lungs become caseous, hence the term "pseudotuberculosis." The organism is sensitive to a wide variety of antibiotics, including ampicillin, chloramphenicol, and tetracycline. If the infection exists in an acute form, the rapid course may render treatment of individual animals ineffective.

Pseudomonas aeruginosa is usually not pathogenic in immunologically competent animals. Animals may, however, become septicemic following experimental manipulations that compromise their immune system, such as radiation exposure. Chlorination (10 ppm) or acidification (2.5–2.8 pH) of the drinking water effectively protects animals against a *P. aeruginosa* septicemia.

Salmonella spp. infections are uncommon in well-managed animal facilities and pets. With the possibility of introduction by wild rodents, it should remain on the differential list for diseases of unknown etiology. Infections may exist in a subclinical form or cause acute disease with a high mortality. Salmonellosis is a concern because of its zoonotic disease potential and interspecies transmission. Rats can be asymptomatic carriers and shed the organism in the feces for many months.

Streptobacillus moniliformis is considered a commensal of low pathogenicity for rats but is capable of producing disease in mice, guinea pigs, and humans. The organism is normally found in the nasopharynx of asymptomatic rats. The disease in people is known as rat bite fever.

VIRAL DISEASES

Sialodacryoadenitis Virus

Sialodacryoadenitis virus is a highly contagious coronavirus that causes inflammation of the salivary and lacrimal glands. It is antigenically related to the mouse hepatitis viruses and rat coronavirus. The virus is widespread in the rat population and may even be found in the colonies of reputable breeders. Clinical disease usually occurs either as an endemic infection of breeding colonies or as an explosive outbreak among nonimmune young rats. It is known to exacerbate respiratory disease attributable to *M. pulmonis*. The usual signs of infection are eye squinting, swelling of the ventral cervical region and jaw, and protrusion of the eye. Keratoconjunctivitis is the only clinical sign of infection in some outbreaks. Affected rats usually remain active and continue to eat. Although sialodacryoadenitis virus may spread rapidly in a susceptible colony, mortality is usually very low. Treatment is not indicated unless protrusion of the eyeball leads to keratitis for which a topical ophthalmic preparation is indicated. Generally, the swelling subsides in 10–14 days and the rat returns to normal. There is no carrier state, but rats that are reinfected may show no clinical signs yet shed the virus for several weeks.

Hantaviruses

Several hantaviruses have been recognized in wild rats including the Hantaan virus and the Four Corners virus. Wild rodents serve as the primary reservoir hosts for hantaviruses but show no clinical disease. Most major wild rat populations in the United States are infected with hantaviruses.

The virus is shed in the saliva, urine, and feces of infected rodents for an unknown duration and may, in fact, be persistently shed. Transmission may occur through bites, aerosols, direct contact with contaminated fomites, or ingestion of contaminated food and water. The disease in people is called hemorrhagic fever with renal syndrome (HFRS). Clinical signs include high fever, malaise, myalgia, headaches, diarrhea, vomiting, proteinuria, oliguria, hemorrhaging, and death. Wild rodents should be prevented from colonizing areas where people live and work.

Infectious Diarrhea of Infant Rats

Infectious diarrhea of infant rats (IDIR) is a rotavirus that causes disease in suckling rats. It usually occurs at less than 2 weeks of age and is characterized by the presence of soft yellow feces or an accumulation of dried feces around the anus. Affected rats usually continue to nurse as evidenced by the "milk spot," but their growth is often stunted. No treatment exists other than supportive care.

Miscellaneous Viral Infections

A number of viruses, including rat parvovirus, cytomegalovirus, rat coronavirus, adenovirus, and Sendai virus, produce naturally occurring infections in rats, but infections are usually subclinical. Latent or indigenous viruses that may be activated by stress or alter the response of animals to experimental procedures are nevertheless of concern in the research laboratory. The majority of rodents purchased for research are actually rigorously screened for all known viruses and are determined to be pathogen–free, or viral antibody–free, thus presenting the cleanest animals possible.

PARASITIC DISEASES

Mites

Several mites can cause disease in rats. *Radfordia ensifera,* the fur mite of rats, can cause pruritus, hair loss, and debilitation with heavy infestations. *Notoedres muris,* a rare mange mite that burrows into the deeper layers of the epidermis, can produce red papules or reddened and thickened skin. Mite infestations are effectively treated by ivermectin, permethrin dusts, and other miticidal preparations. Caution should be used when treating suckling rats, for they have been shown to be more sensitive to the neurotoxic effects of ivermectin.

☞ ## Pinworms

Syphacia muris, S. obvelata, and *Aspicularis tetraptera* are the pinworms of rats, with *S. muris* being the most common. None ordinarily cause clinical symptoms. The eggs of *S. muris* and *S. obvelata* may be detected in infected rats by microscopic examination of cellophane tape pressed against the perianal region. A negative perianal tape test should be followed by examination of the cecum and colon contents under a dissecting microscope for adult worms. *A. tetraptera* infections are diagnosed by the presence of eggs in the feces or adult worms in the intestine. Sound management practices are required to prevent the introduction of pinworms into a colony. Ivermectin, fenbendazole, and piperazine are used in treatment, but pinworms are very difficult to eradicate.

Lice

Polyplax spinulosa, the spined rat louse, is a bloodsucking louse commonly seen in wild rats. *P. spinulosa* causes skin irritation, anemia, and debilitation. It can transmit the blood parasite *Haemobartonella muris.* Ivermectin has been effectively used to eliminate lice. Permethrin dust applied to the animals and the bedding is also reported to be effective.

Tapeworms

The rat is a definitive host for *Hymenolepis nana,* the dwarf tapeworm, and *H. diminuta,* the rat tapeworm. These worms are pathogenic only with heavy infestations. *H. nana* is of concern because of its direct life cycle, interspecies transmission, and zoonotic potential. Prevention of hymenolepid infections requires strict sanitation practices and elimination of vectors. Praziquantel and thiabendazole are reported to be effective in treating rat tapeworms. Total eradication in large rat populations is difficult to achieve without repopulation.

Flagellates

Spironucleus muris and *Giardia muris* are pathogenic flagellates that are occasionally found in the small intestine. Clinical disease is most likely to occur in young or immunosuppressed animals. Control depends on good sanitation practices. Treatment with metronidazole or oxytetracycline is reported to be effective for *G. muris*.

Urinary Bladder Worm

Trichosomoides crassicauda may be found in the urinary bladder or renal pelvis of rats. It is usually of no clinical significance. Treatment with ivermectin is effective.

Rickettsia

Haemobartonella muris was once common in laboratory rats, but is now only found in wild rats. Infections are almost always inapparent, and organisms are not seen in the peripheral blood unless an animal is splenectomized.

☞ NEOPLASIA

Spontaneous neoplasms involving essentially every organ have been reported. The incidence depends to a large extent on the particular stock or strain and age of animals examined.

Mammary Tumors

Mammary tumors are very common in most stocks of laboratory rats. Because of the distribution of mammary tissue, the tumors may occur over a wide area of the body and may reach enormous sizes. These tumors are usually classified as fibroadenomas, are well encapsulated, and do not metastasize. Surgical removal is feasible, and prospects of recovery are favorable. Tumors can, however, reoccur.

Keratoacanthoma

Keratoacanthomas are benign tumors of the skin that can become quite large. They appear as proliferations of keratin or horny growths anywhere on the skin. No treatment is required, as these tumors will eventually fall off and the skin will heal uneventfully.

Large Granular Lymphocytic Leukemia

Large granular lymphocytic leukemia is a major cause of death in aging F344 rats. A leucocytosis of up to 180,000/µL may occur. Clinical signs include weight loss, anemia, jaundice, and depression. Gross findings include marked splenomegaly with moderate hepatomegaly and lymphadenopathy. Histologically, a diffuse infiltration of large malig-

51

nant lymphocytes throughout many organs including the spleen, liver, lymph nodes, and lungs is seen.

Pituitary Adenomas

Pituitary adenomas occur frequently in old rats, particularly in Sprague-Dawley and Wistar rats. These tumors can grow very large and compress adjacent central nervous system tissue. Clinical signs include severe depression, incoordination, torticollis, and death.

Zymbal's Gland Tumors

Tumors of the Zymbal's gland, which is located at the base of the ear, occur with some frequency in rats. The tumor tends to be locally invasive but not metastatic.

MISCELLANEOUS CONDITIONS

Adynamic Ileus

The intraperitoneal administration of high concentrations of chloral hydrate may result in adynamic ileus. Affected animals exhibit abdominal distention and lethargy prior to death. Lesser concentrations of chloral hydrate, such as 5%, may minimize or eliminate this adverse effect.

☞ ## Chromodacryorrhea

The harderian gland in the rat orbit secretes porphyrins. When secretion becomes excessive, tears containing porphyrin run down the nasolacrimal duct and form a red crust around the eyes and nose. This reddish material resembles blood. The amount of secretion increases with age and under forms of stress such as shipping. Old rats or rats with pneumonia may have obvious signs of chromodacryorrhea. Treatment specifically for chromodacryorrhea is not indicated. The presence of excess secretions, however, may suggest the possibility of some other underlying disease.

☞ ## Chronic Progressive Glomerulonephropathy

Chronic progressive glomerulonephropathy (CPN) is a common old age disease of some rat stocks, such as the Sprague-Dawley. Several factors may play a role in the development of CPN, including age, sex, strain, and diet. Clinical signs may include weight loss, unkempt haircoats, and acute death from renal failure. There is marked proteinuria. Grossly, the renal cortices are pitted and irregular.

Dehydration

Dehydration should not be overlooked as a possible cause of acute death in rats. Water may be unavailable because of an air lock in the sipper tube even when a water bottle is full. Malfunction of drinking valves in automatic watering systems can also result in a lack of water.

Dermatophytosis (Ringworm)

Ringworm in rats is usually caused by *Trichophyton mentagrophytes*. Infection may cause widespread skin lesions in a colony or may produce asymptomatic carriers. Systemic mycoses are extremely rare in rats.

☞ ## Malocclusion

Overgrowth of the incisors can occur when the jaw is maloccluded or the diet is too soft. If severe and undetected, overgrown incisors can lead to emaciation and death due to an inability to eat. Rodent incisors can be trimmed with toenail clippers or a dental bur.

Polyarteritis Nodosa

Polyarteritis nodosa is a chronic degenerative disease of aging rats, especially in Sprague-Dawley and spontaneously hypertensive rats (SHR). At necropsy, gross findings include segmental thickening and marked tortuosity of the medium-sized arteries of the mesentery, pancreas, pancreaticoduodenal artery, and testes. The cause of these lesions has not been determined but may be an immunologically mediated response.

Ringtail

Ringtail is caused by housing suckling or preweaned rats at low (≤20%) ambient relative humidity. It is usually seen in the winter months when heating systems are in use. Ringtail appears as one or more annular constrictions of the tail. Distal to the constriction, the tail may become edematous or necrotic. If the tail is sloughed, the stump will usually heal without complication. Ringtail can be prevented by providing solid-bottomed cages with adequate bedding and maintaining the relative humidity at approximately 50%.

Spontaneous Radiculoneuropathy

Radiculoneuropathy is a spontaneous aging disease of rats that involves degeneration of the spinal roots and concurrent atrophy of the skeletal muscles of the lumbar region and hindlimbs. Affected animals exhibit posterior weakness or paresis.

■ GENERAL REFERENCES

Sources consulted to compile the material in this chapter include *The Biology and Medicine of Rabbits and Rodents* by J.E. Harkness and J.E. Wagner, 4th edition (1995, Williams & Wilkins, 1400 North Providence Rd., Building II, Suite 5025, Media, PA 19063); *Laboratory Animal Medicine*, edited by J.G. Fox, B.J. Cohen, and F.M. Loew (1984, Academic Press, Inc., Orlando, FL 32887); *The Laboratory Rat Volume I, Biology and Diseases*, edited by H.J. Baker, J.R. Lindsey, and S.H. Weisbroth (1979, Academic Press, Inc., Orlando, FL 32887); *The Laboratory Rat Volume II, Research Applications*, edited by H.J. Baker, J.R. Lindsey, and S.H. Weisbroth (1980, Academic Press, Inc., Orlando, FL 32887); *The UFAW Handbook on the Care and Management of Laboratory Animals*, 6th edition, edited by T.B. Poole (1987, Churchill Livingstone Inc., 1560 Broadway, New York, NY 10036); *Infectious Diseases of Mice and Rats* by the National Research Council (1991, National Academy Press, 2101 Constitution Ave., NW, Washington, DC 20418); and *Pathology of Laboratory Rodents and Rabbits*, by D.H. Percy and S.W. Barthold (1993, Iowa State University Press, 2121 South State Avenue, Ames, IA 50014).

■ TECHNICAL REFERENCES

Allen, D.G., J.K. Pringle, and D.A. Smith. 1993. *Handbook of Veterinary Drugs.* Philadelphia: JB Lippincott.

Anderson, N.L. 1994. Basic husbandry and medicine of pocket pets. In *Saunders Manual of Small Animal Practice,* ed. S.J. Birchard and R.G. Sherding, pp. 1363–1389. Philadelphia: WB Saunders.

Boivin, G.P., I. Ormsby, and J.E. Hall. 1996. Eradication of *Aspicularis tetraptera,* using fenbendazole-medicated food. *Contemp Topics* 35(2): 69–70.

Burgmann, P. and D.H. Percy. 1993. Antimicrobial drug use in rodents and rabbits. In *Antimicrobial Therapy in Veterinary Medicine,* 2nd ed., ed. J.F. Prescott and J.D. Baggot, pp. 524–541. Ames: Iowa State University Press.

Collins, B.R. 1995. Antimicrobial drug use in rabbits, rodents, and other small mammals. In *Antimicrobial Therapy in Caged Birds and Exotic Pets,* pp. 3–10. Trenton, NJ: Veterinary Learning Systems.

Cooper, D.M., D. DeLong, and C.S. Gillette. 1997. Analgesic efficacy of acetaminophen and buprenorphine administered in the drinking water of rats. *Contemp Topics* 36(3): 58–62.

Danneman, P.J., and T.D. Mandrell. 1997. Evaluation of five agents/methods for anesthesia of neonatal rats. *Lab Anim Sci* 47(4): 386–395.

Dardai, E. and J.E. Heavner. 1987. Respiratory and cardiovascular effects of halothane, isoflurane and enflurane delivered via a Jackson-Rees breathing system in temperature controlled and uncontrolled rats. *Methods Find Exp Clin Pharmacol* 9(11): 717–720.

Fenwick, D.C. and J.K. Blackshaw. 1989. Carbon dioxide as a short-term restraint anaesthetic in rats with subclinical respiratory disease. *Lab Anim* 23(3): 220–228.

Flecknell, P.A. 1987. *Laboratory Animal Anesthesia.* London: Academic.

Flecknell, P.A. 1991. Postoperative analgesia in rabbits and rodents. *Lab Anim* 20(9): 34–37.

Flecknell, P.A. 1997. Medetomidine and atipamezole: Potential uses in laboratory animals. *Lab Anim* 26(2): 21–25.

Foundation for Biomedical Research. 1995. Figures on Animal Research, Fiscal Year 1995.

Glen, J.B. 1980. Animal studies of the anaesthetic activity of ICI 35 868. *Br J Anaesth* 52(8): 731–742.

Harkness, J.E. 1993. *A Practitioner's Guide to Domestic Rodents.* Lakewood, CO: American Animal Hospital Association.

Harrenstien, L. 1994. Critical care of ferrets, rabbits, and rodents. *Semin Avian Exotic Pet Med* 3: 217–228.

Heard, D.J. 1993. Principles and techniques of anesthesia and analgesia for exotic practice. *Vet Clin North Am Small Anim Pract* 23(6): 1301–1327.

Huerkamp, M.J. 1995. Anesthesia and postoperative management of rabbits and pocket pets. In *Kirk's Current Veterinary Therapy XII: Small Animal Practice,* ed. J.D. Bonagura, pp. 1322–1327. Philadelphia: WB Saunders.

Jenkins, W.L. 1987. Pharmacologic aspects of analgesic drugs in animals: an overview. *JAVMA* 191(10): 1231–1240.

Klement, P., J.M. Augustine, K.H. Delaney, G. Klement, and J.I. Weitz. 1996. An oral ivermectin regimen that eradicates pinworms (*Syphacia* spp.) in laboratory rats and mice. *Lab Anim Sci* 46(3): 286–290.

NRC (National Research Council). 1996. Animal environment, housing and management. In *Guide for Care and Use of Laboratory Animals.* Washington, DC: National Academy Press.

Poul, J.-M. 1988. Effects of perinatal ivermectin exposure on behavioral development of rats. *Neurotoxicol Teratol* 10(3): 267–272.

Russell, R.J., D.K. Johnson, and J.A. Stunkard. 1981. *A Guide to Diagnosis, Treatment, and Husbandry of Pet Rabbits and Rodents.* Edwardsville, KS: Veterinary Medicine.

Silverman, J. and W.W. Muir. 1993. A review of laboratory animal anesthesia with chloral hydrate and chloralose. *Lab Anim Sci* 43(3): 210–216.

Silverman, J., M. Huhndorf, M. Balk, and G. Slater. 1983. Evaluation of a combination of tiletamine and zolazepam as an anesthetic for laboratory rodents. *Lab Anim Sci* 33(5): 457–460.

White, W.J. and K.J. Field. 1987. Anesthesia and surgery of laboratory animals. *Vet Clin North Am Small Anim Pract* 17(5): 989–1017.

Wilson, R.P., I.S. Zagon, D.R. Larach, and C.M. Lang. 1992. Antinociceptive properties of tiletamine-zolazepam improved by addition of xylazine or butorphanol. *Pharmacol Biochem Behav* 43(4): 1129–1133.

Wixson, S.K. 1994. Rabbits and rodents: anesthesia and analgesia. In *Research*

Animal Anesthesia, Analgesia and Surgery, ed. A.C. Smith and M.M. Swindle, pp. 59–92. Greenbelt, MD: Scientists Center for Animal Welfare.

Wixson, S.K., W.J. White, H.C. Hughes, Jr., C.M. Lang, and W. K. Marshall. 1987. A comparison of pentobarbital, fentanyl-droperidol, ketamine-xylazine and ketamine-diazepam anesthesia in adult male rats. *Lab Anim Sci* 37(6): 726–730.

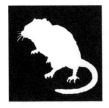

GERBILS

THE MONGOLIAN GERBIL is a rodent of the family Cricetidae and a relative of the hamster. Its scientific name is *Meriones unguiculatus,* which translates into "mammal having claws." The Mongolian gerbil is also known as the jird, the sand rat, or desert rat. It is native to desert regions of China and Mongolia. Gerbils are intermediate in size between mice and hamsters. Adults typically weigh 55–100 g, with males being slightly larger than females. The most common coat color is the agouti, which has a light buff to white ventrum with mixed white, yellow, and black hairs dorsally, giving it an overall brown color. Gerbils may also be black, gray, white, cinnamon, dove, or piebald.

Uses

Gerbils have several favorable attributes that make them a popular rodent pet. They are clean, friendly, easy to handle and tame, rarely bite, and are nearly odor free. They make an interesting pocket pet as they are very curious and tend to be quite active.

Gerbils are useful in a number of research areas including parasitology, radiobiology, toxicology, auditory, lipid metabolism, and infectious disease research. They are an important animal model for stroke research because they have an incomplete circle of Willis, which is the major arterial vascular supply to the base of the brain. This unique anatomic feature makes it possible to create ipsilateral cerebral ischemia by unilateral carotid ligation. Gerbils are also an important model for the study of epilepsy, as they have a high incidence of spontaneous epileptiform seizures.

Behavior

Gerbils are social animals and, under normal circumstances, live peacefully in same-sex or mixed-sex groups. They may fight if crowded or if grouped as adults. Gerbils are active burrowers and, in their natural desert environment, will construct elaborate tunnels with multiple entrances, nesting rooms, and food chambers. They tend to be most active in the evening, with short periods of activity during the day. Gerbils frequently sit upright on their hind limbs in an inquisitive stance. When caged, a common activity is to scratch repeatedly a bottom corner of their cage with their front paws and back push bedding material with their hind limbs. Gerbils attract attention or express aggressiveness by thumping their hind limbs to create a drumming sound. They generally mate for life, forming stable breeding pairs. Both sexes nest build and take an active role in parenting.

Anatomic and Physiologic Features

Gerbil biologic and reproductive data can be found in Table 3.1. The body conformation of the gerbil is longer and more slender than the hamster. Gerbils are characterized by a long tail that is fully furred with a tuft of longer hairs on the end. They have prominent ears; large, slightly protruding eyes; strong claws for burrowing; and elongated hind limbs used for jumping or maintaining a semierect posture. Both sexes have an elliptical, ventral midline sebaceous gland with overlying coarse orange hair. This marking gland is, however, more prominent in the male. Their dental formula is typical of rodents: 2 (1/1 incisors, no canines or premolars, and 3/3 molars). Only the incisors continuously grow. The stomach consists of a nonglandular forestomach and a glandular stomach. The adrenal glands are very large relative to the total body weight and are approximately four times larger than those of the rat. Gerbils have a great capacity for temperature regulation and water and electrolyte conservation.

Sexing gerbils is fairly easy because the male has a prominent, darkly pigmented scrotum and a substantially greater anogenital distance than the female. The female has three body openings in the anogenital region: the urinary papilla, vagina, and anus. Newborn gerbils can be sexed by anogenital distance and by noting the male's larger genital papilla. Females have four pairs of teats.

There are several distinctive characteristics of the hematologic and urinary profiles of gerbils. Gerbils frequently exhibit lipemia and hypercholesterolemia even when fed standard rodent diets. The lipemia can be accentuated by feeding high-fat chows or sunflower seeds. The life span of their red blood cells is relatively short, approximately 9–10 days. It is common to see large numbers of reticulocytes and erythrocytes with basophilic stippling in the peripheral blood, especially in young animals. Lymphocytes are the predominant leukocyte. Gerbils produce small

Table 3.1. Biologic and reproductive data for gerbils	
Adult body weight	
Male	65–100 g
Female	55–85 g
Life span	3–4 y
Body temperature	37°–38.5°C (98.6°–101.3°F)
Heart rate	360 beats per minute
Respiratory rate	70–120 breaths per minute
Food consumption	5–8 g/100 g/d
Water consumption	4–7 mL/100 g/d
Breeding onset	
Male	70–85 d
Female	65–85 d
Estrous cycle length	4–6 d
Gestation period	24–26 d
Postpartum estrus	Fertile
Litter size	3–7
Weaning age	20–30 d
Breeding duration	12–17 mo
Chromosome number (diploid)	44

Source: Adapted from Harkness and Wagner (1995) and Anderson (1994).

quantities of highly concentrated urine. Selected hematologic and biochemical values are listed in Appendix 1, Normal Values.

Breeding and Reproduction

Gerbils breed readily throughout the year, but they are not as prolific as mice. They are inclined to periods of nonbreeding, especially during the winter. Controlling light cycles to supply 12–14 hours of light per day, providing tin cans for hideaways, changing the bedding type, or housing in an opaque cage may encourage nonbreeding gerbils to resume breeding. Pairs should be formed at 8 weeks of age or earlier and should not be separated unless they are incompatible. Breeding pairs are usually monogamous and, if they lose their mate, they will generally not accept another. In comparison to other rodents, puberty occurs later in gerbils. They should be bred when they are 10–12 weeks of age. Gerbils are polyestrous, spontaneous ovulators, with an estrous cycle length of 4–6 days. They have a fertile postpartum estrus. A female in estrus acts restless and may have a congested vulva. The behavior of the two sexes is a better guide to the presence of estrus than are vaginal smears, as the changes in the vaginal epithelium are not obvious as in the mouse or rat. Breeding usually occurs in the late evening. The female is actively pursued by the excited male until she stands to allow mounting. Copulation is characterized by multiple intromissions. A vaginal plug is formed during mating, but it is not readily detectable for it is small and lies deep in the vagina. Gestation lasts 24–26 days in a nonlactating gerbil. If the female is bred while suckling a large litter, implantation may be delayed and gestation may be as long as 42 days. The average litter size is five. Newborns are rarely abandoned or cannibalized, except if the litter is small. Development of young is somewhat slower in gerbils than in mice or rats. Young gerbils start eating solid foods around 2 weeks of age. It may be helpful to soak the dry food pellets when feeding young. Care should be taken to ensure that they can reach the food hopper and water supply. Gerbils are weaned at 20–30 days of age.

HUSBANDRY

Housing

Gerbils are best housed in rigid plastic or metal rodent cages with a solid floor and deep bedding. Glass aquariums are popular and work well for pet gerbils. The enclosure should be at least 15 cm (6 in.) in height to provide the animals adequate space to sit upright. Each adult gerbil should be provided with 230 cm^2 (36 in.^{2}) floor area. The cage needs to have a secure lid and be designed to prevent escape. Gerbils are active gnawers and burrowers, and although they do not climb well, they are capable of jumping. An escaped gerbil generally returns to its cage or moves to the middle of a room rather than hide. Hardwood chips, wood shavings, composite recycled paper pellets, and sand are satisfactory for bedding. Cedar is not recommended because it is irritating to the skin and mucous membranes. Bedding depth should be at least 2 cm (1 in.) to facilitate nest building and burrowing activity. The recommended temperature range for gerbils in a research facility is 18°–26° C (64°–79° F) with a relative humidity between 30% and 50%. Humidity in excess of 50% causes the gerbil's haircoat to become matted and wet. Ventilation should provide 10–15 air changes per hour. The light cycle is usually controlled by a timing device to provide 12 hours of light per day. Exercise wheels, tubes and boxes for hiding, and shreddable materials for nesting can be used to provide environmental enrichment. Commercial synthetic small-rodent nesting fiber should not be used, for it can wind around the feet or teeth or cause impactions if ingested. Gerbil caging requires less cleaning than do the cages of other rodents as they produce only a few drops of urine daily and their fecal pellets are small, dry, and hard. Cages, bottles, and feed hoppers can be disinfected with chemicals, hot water 61.6°–82.2° C (143°–180°F), or a combination of both. Detergents and chemical disinfectants enhance the effectiveness of hot water, but they must be thoroughly rinsed from the surfaces of the item. Refer to Chapter 1, Mice, for a more detailed description of disinfection methods.

Feeding and Watering

Gerbils should be fed a pelleted rodent chow that contains 16%–22% protein. Gerbils eat an average of 5–8 g/100 g of body weight per day. Diet should be provided in a food hopper ad libitum. Although gerbils prefer sunflower seeds to pelleted chows, these are not satisfactory as a total diet. Sunflower seeds are low in calcium and high in fat and do not meet the nutritional needs of the species. A seed mixture with chopped foods such as lettuce, spinach, apple, and carrot may be given once weekly in a supplementary manner. Gerbils, especially females, typically will hoard food. Gerbils should be provided with fresh, potable water ad libitum. Water can be provided by bottle or automatic watering system. Adult gerbils drink an average of 4–7 mL/100 g of body weight per day.

TECHNIQUES

Handling and Restraint

Although not inclined to bite, gerbils are quick and capable of leaping great distances in an effort to escape. A gerbil may be lifted from its cage by grasping the base of the tail. Care must be taken not to grasp the tip of the tail, as the skin may slip off (referred to as degloving) to expose the vertebrae. A gerbil can also be scooped up in the palm of the hand; however, it should be held firmly. To restrain for examination or manipulation, first hold the base of the tail with one hand, then grasp the scruff of the neck with the other hand as shown in Figure 3.1. Alternatively, the gerbil may be grasped by placing a hand over the gerbil's back to enclose the body firmly, as shown in Figure 3.2. Gerbils resist being placed on their back and tend to struggle. Injections or manipulations are more readily accomplished when animals are held in an upright position.

Identification

Cage cards are most often used as a form of general identification. There are several permanent methods to identify gerbils individually, including ear punching, ear tagging, or placement of a subcutaneous microchip for quick electronic identification. Dyes or markers can be used as temporary identification methods.

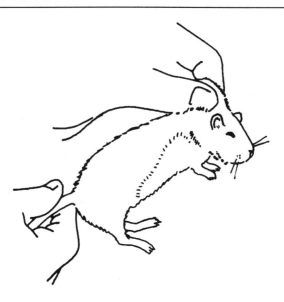

Figure 3.1. Two-hand method of gerbil restraint. (Adapted from Harkness and Wagner 1995, *The Biology and Medicine of Rabbits and Rodents,* 4th edition, Philadelphia: Williams & Wilkins)

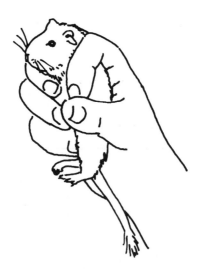

Figure 3.2. One-hand method of gerbil restraint.

Blood Collection

Small amounts of blood are best obtained by retroorbital bleeding under anesthesia, from the lateral metatarsal vein, or by capillary tube collection from a clipped toenail. Larger blood samples can be obtained via cardiac puncture in an anesthetized animal. This procedure is risky and normally reserved for an animal that is not expected to survive. The approximate blood volumes of the adult gerbil are listed in Table 3.2.

Urine Collection

Collecting urine from a gerbil can be a challenge because of the small quantities that are produced daily. Handling stress commonly causes gerbils to urinate.

Drug Administration

Small scales are useful for obtaining accurate body weights to calculate a medication dose. Dosage accuracy is increased through dilution of drugs and by use of a tuberculin syringe. Most drug administration techniques used in small animal practice can be used with gerbils when modified to fit their small size. Medication can be administered orally by mixing the medication in the water or feed. If medications are unpalatable, 5 mL of sugar or syrup per liter can be added to the drinking water to improve the palatability. If more accurate dosing is necessary, an eyedropper or a gavage needle may be used. Smaller-gauge needles, such as 23 or 25 gauge, should be used for injections. Medication can be administered by subcutaneous injection using the skin over the shoulders provided that the administered agent is not excessively irritating. A maximum volume of 3–4 mL is suggested. Because gerbils have such small muscle mass, intramuscular injection volumes should be no greater than 0.1 mL. Because of the risk of accidental sciatic nerve injury, small muscle mass, and stress of restraint, the intraperitoneal route of drug administration is recommended over the intramuscular route. Intraperitoneal injections, with a maximum volume of 2–3 mL, should be given

Table 3.2. Adult gerbil blood volumes	
	Volume (mL)[a]
Total blood	4.4–8.0
Single sample	0.5–1.0
Exsanguination	2–4

Source: Adapted from Harkness and Wagner (1995).
[a]Values are approximate.

in the lower quadrant of the abdomen, lateral to the midline. Although technically challenging, the lateral metatarsal vein can be used for intravenous injections.

Anesthesia, Surgery, and Postoperative Care

A variety of agents that can be used to tranquilize and anesthetize gerbils are listed in Table 3.3. Preanesthetic fasting is not recommended, as the gerbil has a high metabolic rate and there is potential for inducing hypoglycemia and hypothermia. The use of acetylpromazine in this species is not recommended as it lowers the seizure threshold. Single-injection anesthesia techniques are generally used to minimize handling stress. Ketamine plus xylazine or ketamine plus diazepam administered by the intraperitoneal route produce fairly consistent anesthesia. Inhalation anesthesia is generally impractical in a clinical setting other than for brief anesthesia. Gerbils can be placed in an induction chamber or masked down with an inhalation agent delivered from a precision va-

Table 3.3. Anesthetic agents and tranquilizers used in gerbils

Drug	Dosage	Route	Reference
Inhalants			
Halothane	1%–4% to effect	Inhalation	Wixson (1994)
Isoflurane	1%–4% to effect	Inhalation	Wixson (1994)
Methoxyflurane	1%–3% to effect	Inhalation	Norris (1981)
Injectables			
Alphaxalone-alphadolone (Saffan)	80–120 mg/kg	IP	Flecknell (1983)
Fentanyl-fluanisone (Hypnorm)	0.1–1 mg/kg	IP	Flecknell (1987)
Fentanyl	0.05 mg/kg	SC	Flecknell (1983)
+ metomidate	50 mg/kg	SC	
Ketamine	50 mg/kg	IP	Harkness and Wagner
+ diazepam	5–10 mg/kg	IP	(1995)
Ketamine	75 mg/kg	IP	Flecknell (1997)
+ medetomidine	0.5 mg/kg	IP	
Ketamine	50 mg/kg	IP	Harkness and Wagner
+ xylazine	2 mg/kg	IP	(1995)
Pentobarbital	60 mg/kg up to 6 mg maximum	IP	Norris (1987)
Tiletamine-zolazepam	20 mg/kg	IP	Huerkamp (1995)
+ xylazine	10 mg/kg	IP	
Tribromoethanol	250–300 mg/kg	IP	Flecknell (1987)

IP = intraperitoneal; SC = subcutaneous.

porizer. When using inhalation agents, care must be used to scavenge anesthetic gases to ensure the safety of personnel working with the animal or in the general area. Methoxyflurane can be used safely by the open-drop method in a small chamber or nose cone made from a syringe casing. When using an open-drop method, care must be taken to prevent physical contact of the animal with the anesthetic liquid. Halothane and isoflurane should only be used in precision vaporizers and not by the open-drop method, as lethal concentrations of gases can be rapidly reached at room temperature.

Gerbils may show an idiosyncratic writhing before entering a surgical plane of anesthesia. This should not be confused with light anesthesia. The depth of anesthesia can be determined by using a combination of reflexes such as the righting reflex, pedal withdrawal reflex, and the abdominal pinch reflex. Muscle tone and purposeful movement in response to surgical stimuli may also be used as indicators of anesthetic depth. Ocular position and the palpebral reflex are inconsistent and unreliable indicators of anesthetic depth.

While anesthetized, gerbils should have bland ophthalmic ointment placed in their eyes to prevent exposure keratitis. Use of a circulating-water heating pad promotes euthermia and is recommended.

Pet gerbils may require a simple castration, tail amputation, or growth removal. Care should be taken to close the inguinal canals during castration to prevent intestinal entrapment. In research, one of the most common surgical procedures is to produce cerebral infarction. Suture lines are carefully placed around a carotid artery and the gerbil is allowed to recover. Several days postoperatively when the animal is stabilized, a stroke can be produced by pulling on the suture to create unilateral ligation of the common carotid artery. Surgeries should be performed in an aseptic manner. Prevention of blood loss is an important consideration.

The anesthetized gerbil should be placed on a clean, dry paper or cloth towel and recovered in an escape proof incubator. Alternatively, a circulating-water heating pad or heat lamp placed outside the cage can be used to prevent hypothermia. Small-particle bedding materials are contraindicated in recovery cages because they can stick to the eyes, nose, and mouth of the recovering animal. A nonambulatory animal should be turned every 30–60 minutes to prevent hypostatic lung congestion. Table 3.4 lists analgesics than can be used. Butorphanol is recommended for mild postoperative discomfort. Buprenorphine works well to control acute or chronic visceral pain but causes more sedation.

Table 3.4. Analgesic agents used in gerbils			
Drug	Dosage	Route	Reference
Acetaminophen	1–2 mg/mL drinking water		Huerkamp (1995)
Acetylsalicylic acid	100–150 mg/kg q4h	PO	Heard (1993)
Buprenorphine	0.1–0.2 mg/kg q8h	SC	Harkness and Wagner (1995)
Butorphanol	1–5 mg/kg q2–4h	SC	Heard (1993)
Meperidine	20 mg/kg q2–3h	SC, IM	Heard (1993)
Syrup	0.2 mg/mL drinking water		Huerkamp (1995)
Nalbuphine	4–8 mg/kg q3h	IM	Heard (1993)
Oxymorphone	0.2–0.5 mg/kg q6–12h	SC, IM	Heard (1993)
Pentazocine	10 mg/kg q2–4h	SC	Heard (1993)

IM = intramuscular; PO = per os; SC = subcutaneous.

Euthanasia

Suitable methods of euthanasia include the use of carbon dioxide (approximately 70%) in a prefilled chamber, overdose of an inhalant anesthetic, and sodium pentobarbital administered intraperitoneally at three to four times the anesthetic dose. Refer to Chapter 1, Mice, for more details on euthanasia.

THERAPEUTIC AGENTS

Suggested gerbil antimicrobial and antifungal drug doses are listed in Table 3.5. Antiparasitic agents are listed in Table 3.6 and miscellaneous drugs are listed in Table 3.7.

Table 3.5. Antimicrobial and antifungal agents used in gerbils

Drug	Dosage	Route	Reference
Amikacin	2–5 mg/kg q8–12h	SC, IM	Harkness and Wagner (1995)
Ampicillin	6–30 mg/kg q8h	PO	Anderson (1994)
Cephaloridine	30 mg/kg q12h	IM	Flecknell (1987)
Chloramphenicol	50–200 mg/kg q8h	PO	Burgmann and Percy (1993)
	30–50 mg/kg q12h	SC, IM	Burgmann and Percy (1993)
Ciprofloxacin	7–20 mg/kg q12h	PO	Harkness and Wagner (1995)
Doxycycline	2.5 mg/kg q12h	PO	Allen (1993)
Enrofloxacin	0.05–0.2 mg/mL drinking water for 14 d		Harkness and Wagner (1995)
	5–10 mg/kg q12h	PO, IM	Harkness and Wagner (1995)
Gentamicin	2–4 mg/kg q8–24h	SC, IM	Harkness and Wagner (1995)
Griseofulvin	25–50 mg/kg q12h for 14–60 d	PO	Harkness and Wagner (1995)
	1.5% in DMSO for 5–7 d	Topical	Harkness and Wagner (1995)
Metronidazole	7.5 mg/70–90g animal q8h	PO	Collins (1995)
Neomycin	2.6 mg/mL drinking water		Anderson (1994)
	100 mg/kg q24h	PO	Burgmann and Percy (1993)
Oxytetracycline	0.8 mg/mL drinking water		Burgmann and Percy (1993)
	10 mg/kg q8h	PO	Burgmann and Percy (1993)
Sulfadimethoxine	10–15 mg/kg q12h	PO	Harkness and Wagner (1995)
Sulfamerazine	0.8 mg/mL drinking water		Anderson (1994)
Sulfamethazine	0.8 mg/mL drinking water		Anderson (1994)
Sulfaquinoxaline	1 mg/mL drinking water		Collins (1995)
Tetracycline	2–5 mg/mL drinking water		Burgmann and Percy (1993)
	10–20 mg/kg q8–12h	PO	Burgmann and Percy (1993)
Trimethoprim/sulfa	30 mg/kg q12h	PO, IM	Harkness and Wagner (1995)
Tylosin	0.5 mg/mL drinking water		Collins (1995)
	10 mg/kg q24h	PO, SC, IM	Collins (1995)

DMSO = dimethyl sulfoxide; IM = intramuscular; PO = per os; SC = subcutaneous.

Table 3.6. Antiparasitic agents used in gerbils

Drug	Dosage	Route	Reference
Amitraz	1.4 mL/L water using cottonball application q14d for 3 to 6 treatments	Topical	Harkness and Wagner (1995)
Fenbendazole	20 mg/kg q24h for 5 d	PO	Allen (1993)
Ivermectin	0.2 mg/kg q7d for 3 wk	PO, SC	Anderson (1994)
Piperazine citrate	2–5 mg/mL drinking water for 7 d, off 7 d, repeat		Anderson (1994)
Praziquantel	30 mg/kg q14d for 3 treatments	PO	Burke (1995)
Pyrethrin powder	3 times per week for 3 wk	Topical	Anderson (1994)
Thiabendazole	100 mg/kg q24h for 5 d	PO	Allen (1993)

PO = per os; SC = subcutaneous.

Table 3.7. Miscellaneous agents used in gerbils

Drug	Dosage	Route	Reference
Atipamezole	1 mg/kg	SC, IP, IV	Flecknell (1997)
Atropine	0.05–0.1 mg/kg	SC	Harkness and Wagner (1995)
Cimetidine	5–10 mg/kg q6–12h	PO	Allen (1993)
Doxapram	5–10 mg/kg	IV, IP	Harkness (1993)
Flunixin meglumine	2.5 mg/kg q12–24h	SC	Heard (1993)
Glycopyrrolate	0.01–0.02 mg/kg	SC	Huerkamp (1995)
Naloxone	0.01–0.1 mg/kg	SC, IP	Huerkamp (1995)
Vitamin K	1–10 mg/kg q24h for 4–6 d	IM	Harkness and Wagner (1995)
Yohimbine	0.5–1.0 mg/kg	IV	Harkness and Wagner (1995)

IM = intramuscular; IP = intraperitoneal; IV = intravenous; PO = per os; SC = subcutaneous.

BACTERIAL DISEASES

Salmonella spp. and *Bordetella bronchiseptica* are potential problems in gerbils primarily from interspecies transmission. Contact with species known to carry these organisms should be avoided. Adult gerbils are fairly resistant to *Salmonella;* however, disease has been observed in young gerbils. Although *B. bronchiseptica* has not been reported to cause naturally occurring disease, young gerbils inoculated experimentally with the bacterium develop severe disease with high mortality.

Tyzzer's Disease

Tyzzer's disease, caused by *Clostridium piliforme,* is a common disease of gerbils. The disease is most frequently seen at weaning age, but adults can be affected. Mortality is high in young animals 3–7 weeks of age. Poor sanitation and stress are important contributing factors of disease. Affected animals typically have a rough haircoat, are lethargic and anorexic, and die within 1–3 days. Diarrhea may be absent or mild in gerbils, in contrast to other species, which show a profuse watery diarrhea. Transmission is thought to be fecal–oral. Characteristically, infected animals have enlarged livers with numerous gray, white, or yellow foci, 1–2 mm in diameter. Edema and hemorrhage of the intestines, particularly in the ileocecal area, may also be present. Oxytetracycline or tetracycline can be used to suppress infection. Supplemental fluid therapy can be provided if indicated. In an outbreak, it is best to isolate ill animals and cull them. Infectious spores can remain in the environment for prolonged periods of time. All cages, feeding, and watering equipment should be sterilized.

Staphylococcal and Streptococcal Infections

ß-Hemolytic *Staphylococcus aureus* has been associated with a diffuse dermatitis in young gerbils. The face, feet, legs, and ventral body surface are affected. Bite wounds from aggression, nose abrasions from burrowing, and the ventral sebaceous gland can become infected with *Staphylococcus* spp., *Streptococcus* spp., and other bacteria. Topical treatment with nitrofurazone ointment or other antibacterial preparation applied daily is often beneficial. Chloramphenicol, tetracycline, or sulfonamides can be used for parenteral treatment.

VIRAL DISEASES

Clinically significant viral infections are not currently recognized to be a problem.

PARASITIC DISEASES

Demodex

Alopecia and dermatitis associated with *Demodex* spp. have been reported in gerbils. Demodex infestations are not regarded to be a problem in clinically healthy animals. Old age and debilitation are considered to be important predisposing factors. Gerbils can be treated in a similar fashion as hamsters with a dilute solution of amitraz applied topically with a cotton ball.

Pinworms

Gerbils can become infected with several species of oxyurids including *Syphacia* spp. from mice and rats. None cause clinical problems. Ivermectin, piperazine, or thiabendazole are effective treatments.

Tapeworms

Cestodiasis in gerbils is normally subclinical; however, severe infections with the dwarf tapeworm, *Hymenolepis nana,* have been reported. Infections have been associated with debilitation and diarrhea. *H. nana* is a concern because of its direct life cycle, transmission to other rodents, and zoonotic potential. Praziquantel or thiabendazole are effective treatments.

NEOPLASIA

The incidence of spontaneous tumors is relatively low in the gerbil. Neoplasms occur primarily in aged gerbils over 2 years old. The most commonly recognized neoplasms in gerbils are ovarian, adrenocortical, and cutaneous tumors.

MISCELLANEOUS CONDITIONS

Nasal Dermatitis (Sore Nose)

☞ Nasal dermatitis, or sore nose, is most commonly encountered in recently weaned and adult gerbils. Affected animals have alopecia around the external nares and upper labial region with a varying degree of red–brown, moist dermatitis. Chemical irritation of the skin by porphyrin-containing harderian gland secretions is thought to be the primary cause. Mechanical trauma due to excessive burrowing may be an important contributing factor. Secondary infections with *Staphylococcus* spp. are common. Using sand or clay bedding material rather than wood shavings or chips, cleaning the face, application of a topical ointment, and removing stress factors may be helpful in treating the condition.

Degloving

☞ The tail is especially sensitive to degloving wounds, particularly if it is handled roughly or by the tip. If the tail is degloved, it should be amputated at the level of the break and the skin sutured closed.

Tail Barbering

Gerbils will barber each other if bored or if housed in overcrowded conditions. The hair of a subordinate animal is chewed off around the base of the tail or along the tail in a closely shaved pattern.

Epileptiform Seizures

☞ Gerbils exhibit spontaneous epileptiform seizures that vary from hypnotic and cataleptic to grand mal. The seizures may be initiated by handling, stress, or novel environment. Typically, the episodes are brief, lasting up to a few minutes. Animals resume normal activity soon afterward and show no ill effects. Treatment is not recommended.

Chromodacryorrhea

The harderian gland in the orbit produces porphyrin. The porphyrins are normally removed by grooming; however, when there is excessive secretion, a red crust appears in the medial canthus of the eye or on the end of the nose. Animals that are stressed or ill commonly exhibit these "red tears."

Streptomycin Toxicity

Gerbils do not develop the fatal gram-negative bacterial enterotoxemia associated with penicillin and other antibiotics having similar action, as is seen in hamsters and guinea pigs. Streptomycin, however, has been reported to have a direct toxic effect. The margin of safety for streptomycin is low in this species and thus not recommended.

Malocclusion

Malocclusion is rarely a problem in the gerbil but may occur as a result of upper incisor loss with overgrowth of the lower teeth. Trimming the teeth with toenail clippers or a dental bur may be necessary to prevent overgrowth.

Cystic Ovaries

Cystic ovaries are very common in females over 2 years of age and can be associated with reduced litter size or infertility.

Chronic Interstitial Nephritis

Aged gerbils are susceptible to chronic interstitial nephritis. Clinical signs include polyuria, polydipsia, and weight loss.

Aural Cholesteatoma

Spontaneous aural cholesteatomas frequently occur in gerbils over 2 years of age. Clinical signs include head tilt and keratin mass accumulation in the external ear canal.

Ocular Proptosis

Aged gerbils can develop ocular proptosis including protrusion of the nictitating membrane.

■ GENERAL REFERENCES

Sources consulted to compile the material in this chapter include *The Biology and Medicine of Rabbits and Rodents* by J.E. Harkness and J.E. Wagner, 4th edition (1995, Williams & Wilkins, 1400 North Providence Rd., Building II, Suite 5025, Media, PA 19063); *Laboratory Animal Medicine,* edited by J.G. Fox, B.J. Cohen, and F.M. Loew (1984, Academic Press, Inc., Orlando, FL 32887); and *Pathology of Laboratory Rodents and Rabbits,* by D.H. Percy and

S.W. Barthold (1993, Iowa State University Press, 2121 South State Avenue, Ames, IA 50014).

■ TECHNICAL REFERENCES

Allen, D.G., J.K. Pringle, and D.A. Smith. 1993. *Handbook of Veterinary Drugs.* Philadelphia: JB Lippincott.

Anderson, N.L. 1994. Basic husbandry and medicine of pocket pets. In *Saunders Manual of Small Animal Practice,* ed. S.J. Birchard and R.G. Sherding, pp. 1363–1389. Philadelphia: WB Saunders.

Burgmann, P. and D.H. Percy. 1993. Antimicrobial drug use in rodents and rabbits. In *Antimicrobial Therapy in Veterinary Medicine,* 2nd ed., ed. J.F. Prescott and J.D. Baggot, pp. 524–541. Ames: Iowa State University Press.

Burke, T.J. 1995. "Wet tail" in hamsters and other diarrheas of small rodents. In *Kirk's Current Veterinary Therapy XII—Small Animal Practice,* ed. J.D. Bonagura, pp. 1336–1339. Philadelphia: WB Saunders.

Collins, B.R. 1995. Antimicrobial drug use in rabbits, rodents, and other small mammals. In *Antimicrobial Therapy in Caged Birds and Exotic Pets,* pp. 3–10. Trenton, NJ: Veterinary Learning Systems.

Flecknell, P.A. 1987. *Laboratory Animal Anesthesia.* London: Academic.

Flecknell, P.A. 1997. Medetomidine and atipamezole: Potential uses in laboratory animals. *Lab Anim* 26(2): 21–25.

Flecknell, P.A., M. John, M. Mitchell, and C. Shurey. 1983. Injectable anaesthetic techniques in 2 species of gerbil (*Meriones libycus* and *Meriones unguiculatus*). *Lab Anim* 17: 118–122.

Harkness, J.E. 1993. *A Practitioner's Guide to Domestic Rodents.* Lakewood, CO: American Animal Hospital Association.

Heard, D.J. 1993. Principles and techniques of anesthesia and analgesia for exotic practice. *Vet Clin North Am Small Anim Pract* 23: 1301–1327.

Huerkamp, M.J. 1995. Anesthesia and postoperative management of rabbits and pocket pets. In *Kirk's Current Veterinary Therapy XII—Small Animal Practice,* ed. J.D. Bonagura, pp. 1322–1327. Philadelphia: WB Saunders.

Norris, M.L. 1981. Portable anaesthetic apparatus designed to induce and maintain surgical anaesthesia methoxyflurane inhalation in the Mongolian gerbil *(Meriones unguiculatus).* *Lab Anim* 15(2): 153–155.

Norris, M.L. 1987. Gerbils. In *UFAW Handbook on the Care and Management of Laboratory Animals,* 6th ed. New York: Churchill Livingstone.

Wixson, S.K. 1994. Rabbits and rodents: anesthesia and analgesia. In *Research Animal Anesthesia, Analgesia and Surgery,* ed. A.C. Smith and M.M. Swindle, pp. 59–92. Greenbelt, MD: Scientists Center for Animal Welfare.

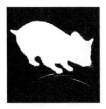

HAMSTERS

4

Hamsters are rodents of the family Cricetidae. There are over 50 species, subspecies, and varieties of hamsters. Only two are found in any significant number in captivity as pets or in laboratories. These are the Golden or Syrian hamster (*Mesocricetus auratus*) and the Chinese, or striped hamster (*Cricetulus griseus*). The Syrian is by far the most popular hamster, and the specific information provided in this chapter refers primarily to it. It weighs approximately 120 g and comes in a variety of colors including reddish–golden brown with gray ventrum, cinnamon, cream, white, piebald, albino, and a long-haired variety called teddy bear. The Chinese hamster is much smaller than the Syrian and weighs approximately 30 g and is gray–brown with a dark stripe down the back.

Uses

Hamsters are popular as pets and are important research animals. Their small size, ease of taming, low care requirements, and relative freedom from spontaneous diseases are positive attributes. Syrian hamsters have proven valuable in a number of areas of biomedical research particularly in studies of infectious disease, cancer, immunology, hypothermia, dental caries, reproductive physiology, cardiomyopathy, and thrombosis. Chinese hamsters are utilized as a model of type 1 juvenile-onset diabetes and in cytogenetic studies, which take advantage of their low diploid chromosome number of 22. Both Syrian and Chinese hamsters have been used in radiobiology research, as they are radioresistant.

Behavior

Hamsters tend to be solitary, rather than social animals. Studies have shown that group housing is stressful and can lead to aggression and obesity. Hamsters are generally aggressive and territorial toward unfamiliar hamsters of either sex. Females, in particular, are prone to fight or kill other hamsters especially when pregnant or lactating. Hamsters are less apt to fight if housed together at the time of weaning or before they are sexually mature. Pet hamsters that are aggressive toward one another should be provided with hiding places in their cage or they may be anesthetized and awakened together in a neutral area. Hamsters frequently exhibit agonistic postures, but are not naturally aggressive to their handlers. If suddenly disturbed or if handled roughly they will bite. They are easily tamed if handled gently and repeatedly.

In their natural desert environment, hamsters live in deep tunnels that provide them with a cooler temperature and higher humidity. Like most rodents, they are nocturnal and are quite inactive during the day. They are sound sleepers and, upon casual observation, may appear dead. Normal hamsters are active and spend time storing and transporting food in their distensible cheek pouches. When exercise wheels are provided, they readily run on them. They are reported to run up to 8 km (5 mi) per day. They make very little noise except to chatter or screech when hurt, frightened, or fighting.

The hamster is considered a permissive hibernator, as it has the option of hibernating or not depending upon conditions. Low light intensity, short day lengths, quietness, and cooler temperatures of approximately 8°C (46°F) induce hibernation. During this period of tupor, the hamster has a decreased body temperature with extremely slow respirations and heart rate, yet remains sensitive to touch. Hibernation is not continuous, but consists of 2–3 days of tupor alternating with short periods of arousal to normal alertness.

Anatomic and Physiologic Features

General biologic and reproductive data for the hamster are listed in Table 4.1. The hamster has a chunky body with short legs, bright beady black eyes, prominent dark ears, and a stubby tail. It has a large amount of very loose skin that is covered with dense, soft, short fur. Hamsters have well-developed buccal or cheek pouches that run along the lateral side of the neck and head and extend back to the shoulder region. The cheek pouches are devoid of glands and appear to be immunologically privileged sites.

Typical of rodents, hamsters have a dental formula of 2 (1/1 open-rooted incisors, no canines or premolars, and 3/3 molars with fixed roots). The teeth turn yellow–orange with age. The stomach is distinctly compartmentalized into a forestomach and a glandular stomach. The nonglandular forestomach acts like a rumen and has a higher pH than

Table 4.1. Biologic and reproductive data for hamsters

Adult body weight	
Male	85–130 g
Female	95–150 g
Life span	18–24 mo
Body temperature	37°–38°C (98.6°–100.4°F)
Heart rate	250–500 beats per minute
Respiratory rate	35–135 breaths per minute
Food consumption	8–12 g/100g/d
Water consumption	8–10 mL/100g/d
Breeding onset	
Male	10–14 wk
Female	6–10 wk
Estrous cycle length	4 d
Gestation period	15–16 d
Postpartum estrus	Infertile
Litter size	5–9
Weaning age	21 d
Breeding duration	10–12 mo
Chromosome number (diploid)	44

Source: Adapted from Harkness and Wagner (1995) and Van Hoosier and McPherson (1987).

the glandular stomach. The digestive tract suggests an adaptation for water conservation having a long duodenum and jejunum, short ileum, large cecum, and long colon. The lungs consist of a large single left lobe and five smaller lobes on the right side. The hamster kidney has an extremely long papilla that extends out into the ureter, which makes it possible to collect in vivo urine samples from single collecting tubules.

Hamsters have prominent deposits of brown adipose tissue, the majority of which is located ventral to and between the scapulae. This tissue plays a thermogenic role, particularly in hibernating or newborn hamsters. Two flank, or costovertebral, glands are present in both sexes but are much more developed in the male. These sebaceous glands are darkly pigmented spots with roughened skin and coarse hairs located in the flank region. The glands are used to mark territory and are involved in mating behavior.

Differentiation between adult males and females is rather simple and can be determined without handling the animal. When viewed from above, the rear margin of the male hamster is rounded because of the scrotal sac, whereas the female posterior is pointed toward the tail. Adult males have prominent testicles. Adult females are larger than males. Males have a greater anogenital distance than do females. Applying gentle pressure to the rear of the male's abdomen will cause the testicles to protrude. Newborns can be sexed by comparing the anogenital distance. The distance is greater in the male, and the genital papilla of the male is more prominent than that of the female. Female hamsters usually have six to seven pairs of mammary glands. Male hamsters have large seminal vesicles located laterally to the bladder that resemble a ram's horns.

There are several distinctive characteristics of the hematologic and urinary profiles of hamsters. Leukocyte counts are 5000–10,000/µL, with the lymphocyte being the most dominant leukocyte. Polychromasia is relatively common in hamster erythrocytes. Hamster urine has a basic pH and appears turbid and milky because of the large number of small crystals it contains. Selected hematologic and biochemical values are listed in Appendix 1, Normal Values.

Breeding and Reproduction

Hamsters are usually bred for the first time between 6 and 8 weeks of age at a weight of 80–100 g. The female hamster is continuously polyestrous, cycling every 4 days. There is a normal seasonal breeding quiescence, however, in the winter months. Ovulation is spontaneous and follows lordosis onset by approximately 8 hours. A white stringy, opaque postovulatory discharge is present on the 2nd day of the cycle. This discharge indicates the hamster has reached peak estrus the day before and can be used to predict the best time to breed. The female can be successfully mated in the evening of the 3rd day after the observance of the postovulatory discharge.

Except for the period of estrus, the female will usually attack a newly introduced male. Because of this belligerent attitude, it is best to watch the pair closely for compatibility and to leave them together for only 30 minutes. When a receptive female is placed with a male, after a short getting-acquainted period, she assumes a lordosis posture, arching her back downward. Mating is characterized by repeated intromissions and ejaculations. Signs of pregnancy include a distended abdomen and rapid weight gain at 10 days. Pregnancy can be confirmed by the absence of postovulatory discharge on days 5 and 9 after mating. If the discharge is present, the female is having normal estrous cycles. The postpartum estrus is usually anovulatory.

The gestation period, the shortest of any of the common laboratory animals, is on the average 16 days. Litter size is usually five to nine. The babies are born with sharp incisor teeth and are hairless. Their ears open at 4–5 days of age and eyes open at 14–16 days. Young start eating food and drinking water when they are 7–10 days of age. Care should be taken to ensure the young can reach the water supply and are provided with food on the floor of the cage. Young are weaned at 3 weeks of age. A fertile estrus follows weaning by 2–18 days.

Cannibalism of the young and litter abandonment are common during the first pregnancy and the first week postpartum. To reduce this risk, the female should be placed in a clean cage with clean bedding, food, and nesting material at 14 days after mating. The addition of bits of apple or lettuce to the diet prior to parturition is advocated by some as a means of preventing cannibalism. Opaque caging and a quiet area are also helpful. For the next 7–10 days, which is the critical postdelivery period, the mother and young should be disturbed as little as possible.

HUSBANDRY

Housing

A variety of caging used for other laboratory rodents are satisfactory; however, hamsters prefer solid-bottom cages with contact bedding. An adult hamster, over 100 g, requires a floor area of at least 123 cm² (19 in.²) and a cage height of at least 15 cm (6 in.). Caging materials should be carefully selected to preclude destruction and escape, as hamsters are noted escape artists. They frequently will dislodge cage lids and/or gnaw on caging materials, escape, and live for months hiding in a house. They do not return to their cages as may rats and gerbils. Rigid plastic and stainless or galvanized steel are acceptable caging materials. Hardwood chips, wood shavings, ground corn cobs, or recycled composite pellets can be used as bedding materials. Exercise wheels and a variety of tubelike toys can be used to enrich the environment. Facial tissue paper can be used as nesting material. Commercial, synthetic small-rodent nesting fiber should not be used, for it can wind around the feet or teeth, or cause an impaction if ingested.

Suggested environmental parameters for housing hamsters include a temperature between 18° and 26°C (64° and 79°F), a relative humidity between 30% and 70%, and 10–15 air changes per hour. Typically, 14 hours of light per day should be provided and can be controlled by automatic timers.

Hamsters are fastidious in that they will utilize different locations of the cage in which to store food, urinate, and defecate. Weekly cleaning of the cage usually suffices as hamsters produce little waste or odor.

Cages, bottles, and feed hoppers should be disinfected with chemicals, hot water 61.6°–82.2°C (143°–180°F) or a combination of both. Detergents and chemical disinfectants enhance the effectiveness of hot water, but they must be thoroughly rinsed from all caging surfaces with fresh water. Soaking or rinsing the cages with an acid solution may be helpful to remove urine scale buildup. Refer to Chapter 1, Mice, for a more detailed description of disinfection methods.

Feeding and Watering

Fresh, properly stored commercial pelleted rodent diets that contain at least 16% protein and 4%–5% fat are adequate for hamsters. Hamsters eat an average of 8–12 g/100 g of body weight per day. Diet can be provided in a slotted, sheet metal hopper or a wire mesh feeder. Slot widths of less than 11 mm in food hoppers should be avoided, as hamsters have difficulty reaching food because of their broad noses. Hamsters hoard food and will frequently remove pellets from the feeder and store them on the floor or in a corner of the cage. According to the Animal Welfare Act, it is permissible to place pelleted feed on the floor of a primary enclosure for this species. Although hamsters enjoy fruits and vegetables, it is neither necessary nor suggested to supplement their diets. Treats sold in pet shops are frequently low in protein and may not be adequate diets for growth and reproduction. Fresh potable water should be available ad libitum. Water can be provided by bottle or automatic watering system. Hamsters drink an average of 8–10 mL/100 g of body weight of water per day. They are coprophagic and may be observed bending their body when defecating to eat feces. Coprophagy serves to recycle B vitamins and other nutrients.

TECHNIQUES

Handling and Restraint

To avoid getting bitten by a hamster, it is important to make sure it is awake and expects to be picked up. A hamster can be moved from one cage to another by cupping the hands under the animal and gently scooping it up or by putting a small tin can in the cage that the hamster will enter. A hamster may be restrained by picking it up by the loose skin at the scruff of the neck as shown in Figure 4.1 or using the whole hand grip as shown in Figure 4.2. The loose skin must be securely gathered to immobilize the hamster fully. The use of protective gloves and forceps are not recommended to handle hamsters because they may cause the animals to develop aggressive behavior.

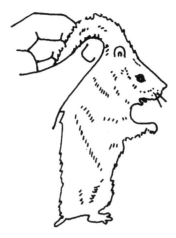

Figure 4.1. Restraint of the hamster using scruff-of-the-neck grip. (Adapted from Harkness and Wagner 1995, *The Biology and Medicine of Rabbits and Rodents,* 4th edition, Philadelphia: Williams & Wilkins)

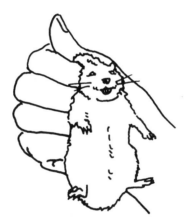

Figure 4.2. Restraint of the hamster using whole-hand grip.

Identification

Cage cards are most often used as a form of general identification. Ear punching, ear tagging, or microchip implantation may be used to identify individual animals permanently. Dyes or markers can be used as temporary identification methods.

Blood Collection

Small amounts of blood can be obtained by retroorbital bleeding under anesthesia, by capillary tube collection from limb veins or a clipped toenail, and from the jugular or femoral vein. The retroorbital bleeding technique is similar to the technique described in Chapter 1, Mice; however, the lateral or the medial canthus of the eye may be used. When using the lateral canthus technique, the capillary tube should be directed medially, but not anteriorly, as the sinus is located in the posterior part of the orbit. Larger blood samples can be obtained via cardiac puncture in an anesthetized animal. Cardiac sampling is associated with significant mortality and should be used only in animals not expected to survive the procedure. Approximate blood volumes of adult hamsters are listed in Table 4.2.

Urine Collection

Urine may be collected using a metabolic cage that separates the urine and fecal pellets. Other methods include holding the hamster, placing it on a cold metal surface or in a plastic cooled bag, and waiting for it to urinate.

Drug Administration

Small scales are useful for obtaining accurate body weights to calculate the medication dose. Dosage accuracy is increased through dilution of drugs and by use of a tuberculin syringe. Most drug administration techniques used in small animal practice can be used with hamsters when modified to fit their smaller size. Medications can be administered orally by mixing them in the water or feed. If medications are unpalatable, 5 mL of sugar or syrup per liter can be added to the drinking water to improve the palatability. If more accurate dosing is necessary, an eyedropper or a gavage needle may be used. Smaller-gauge needles, such as 23 or 25 gauge, should be used for injections. Medications can also be administered by subcutaneous injection, with a maximum volume of 3–4 mL, using the loose skin over the shoulders. Intramuscular injec-

Table 4.2. Adult hamster blood volumes	
	Volume (mL)[a]
Total blood	6.8–12
Single sample	0.5–1.2
Exsanguination	3–5

Source: Adapted from Harkness and Wagner (1995).
[a]Values are approximate.

tions are not frequently used because hamsters have such small muscle mass. Another drawback to using the intramuscular route is that certain drugs such as ketamine can cause muscle necrosis and nerve irritation that can lead to self-mutilation of the affected limb. A maximum volume of 0.1 mL is recommended for the intramuscular route. Medications and injectable anesthetics are more commonly administered by the intraperitoneal route. A maximum volume of 3–4 mL is suggested. When making an intraperitoneal injection, the animal's head should be tilted downward. The injection is made immediately to the right or left of the midline in the lower half of the abdomen. Intravenous injections are most frequently made into the cephalic vein, the jugular vein, or into the lateral metatarsal vein.

Anesthesia, Surgery, and Postoperative Care

A variety of agents that can be used to tranquilize and anesthetize hamsters are listed in Table 4.3. Preanesthetic fasting is not recommended because the hamster has a high metabolic rate and there is potential for inducing hypoglycemia and hypothermia. Single-injection anesthesia techniques are generally used to minimize handling stress. Ketamine combined with xylazine and administered by the intraperitoneal route provides fairly consistent anesthesia. Ketamine can also be combined with an inhalant anesthetic such as methoxyflurane. Fentanyl–droperidol combination is not recommended in this species because of unwanted central nervous system stimulation.

Inhalation anesthesia is generally impractical for hamsters in a clinical setting other than for brief periods of anesthesia. Due to the difficulty in intubating hamsters, inhalation agents are generally delivered by a nose cone or face mask. When using inhalation agents, care must be used to scavenge anesthetic gases to ensure the safety of personnel working with the animal or in the general area. Methoxyflurane can be used safely by the open-drop method in a small chamber or nose cone made from a syringe casing. Halothane and isoflurane should only be used in precision vaporizers and not by the open-drop method because lethal concentrations of gases can be rapidly reached at room temperature.

The depth of anesthesia can be determined by using the righting reflex, muscle tone, pedal withdrawal reflex, or abdominal pinch reflex. It is helpful to have a small face mask that can be used to deliver oxygen in an emergency. A drop of doxapram can be placed under the tongue to stimulate respirations.

While anesthetized, hamsters should have bland ophthalmic ointment placed in their eyes to prevent exposure keratitis. Use of a circulating-water heating pad promotes euthermia and is recommended. Surgery should be done in an aseptic manner. Prevention of blood loss is an important consideration.

Surgery is done more often for experimental than for therapeutic purposes. Nephrectomy, adrenalectomy, thymectomy, and ovariectomy are a few of the surgeries performed in research. Female hamsters are ovariectomized to utilize their ova for an in vitro test. The hamster egg is the only rodent ovum that will accept sperm from any other species. Thus, it can be used to test the ability of human sperm to penetrate an egg. There is rarely a need to perform surgery on a pet hamster, other than a simple castration.

The anesthetized hamster should be placed on a clean, dry paper or cloth towel and recovered in an escape-proof incubator. Alternatively, a circulating-water heating pad or heat lamp placed outside the cage can be used to prevent hypothermia. Small-particle bedding materials are contraindicated in recovery cages because they can stick to the eyes, nose, and mouth of the recovering animal. A nonambulatory animal should be turned every 30 to 60 minutes to prevent hypostatic lung congestion. Table 4.4 lists analgesics that can be used if indicated. Butorphanol is recommended for mild postoperative discomfort. Buprenorphine works well to control acute or chronic visceral pain but causes more sedation.

Euthanasia

Suitable methods of euthanasia include the use of carbon dioxide (approximately 70%) in a prefilled chamber, overdose of an inhalant anesthetic, and sodium pentobarbital administered intraperitoneally at three to four times the anesthetic dose. Refer to Chapter 1, Mice, for further details on euthanasia.

Table 4.3. Anesthetic agents and tranquilizers used in hamsters

Drug	Dosage	Route	Reference
Inhalants			
Halothane	1%–4% to effect	Inhalation	Wixson (1994)
Isoflurane	1%–4% to effect	Inhalation	Wixson (1994)
Methoxyflurane	1%–3% to effect	Inhalation	Wixson (1994)
Injectables			
Alphadolone-alphaxalone (Saffan)	150 mg/kg	IP	Flecknell (1987)
Chloral hydrate	270–360 mg/kg	IP	Hughes (1981)
Fentanyl-droperidol	Not recommended because of induction of CNS abnormalities		Thayer (1972)
Fentanyl-fluanisone (Hypnorm)	1 mL/kg (of a 1/10 dilution of Hypnorm)	IP	Flecknell (1987)
Ketamine	200 mg/kg	IP	White (1987)
Ketamine	150 mg/kg	IM	Flecknell (1987)
+ acetylpromazine	5 mg/kg	IM	
Ketamine	40–100 mg/kg	IP	Harkness and
+ diazepam	5 mg/kg	IP	Wagner (1995)
Ketamine	100 mg/kg	IP	Flecknell (1997)
+ medetomidine	0.25 mg/kg	IP	
Ketamine	80–100 mg/kg	IP	Curl (1983)
+ xylazine	7–10 mg/kg	IP	
Methohexital	2–4 mL/kg	IP	White (1987)
+ diazepam (combined in a mixture containing 7.5 mg/mL methohexital + 1.25 mg/mL diazepam)			
Pentobarbital	70–90 mg/kg	IP	White (1987)
Tiletamine-zolazepam	Not recommended		Silverman (1983)
Tiletamine-zolazepam	20–30 mg/kg	IP	Forsythe (1992)
+ xylazine	10 mg/kg	IP	
Urethane (50% w/v)	150 mg/100 g	IP	Reid (1989)

IM = intramuscular; IP = intraperitoneal.

Table 4.4. Analgesic agents used in hamsters

Drug	Dosage	Route	Reference
Acetaminophen	1–2 mg/mL drinking water		Huerkamp (1995)
Acetylsalicylic acid	100–150 mg/kg q4h	PO	Heard (1993)
Buprenorphine	0.5 mg/kg q8h	SC	Harkness and Wagner (1995)
Butorphanol	1–5 mg/kg q2–4h	SC	Heard (1993)
Flunixin meglumine	2.5 mg/kg q12–24h	SC	Heard (1993)
Meperidine	20 mg/kg q2–3h	SC, IM	Heard (1993)
Syrup	0.2 mg/mL drinking water		Huerkamp (1995)
Nalbuphine	4–8 mg/kg q3h	IM	Heard (1993)
Oxymorphone	0.2–0.5 mg/kg q6–12h	SC, IM	Heard (1993)
Pentazocine	10 mg/kg q2–4h	SC	Heard (1993)

IM = intramuscular; PO = per os; SC = subcutaneous.

83

THERAPEUTIC AGENTS

Suggested hamster antimicrobial and antifungal drug dosages are listed in Table 4.5. Antiparasitic agents are listed in Table 4.6 and miscellaneous drugs are listed in Table 4.7.

Table 4.5.   Antimicrobial and antifungal agents used in hamsters

Drug	Dosage	Route	Reference
Amikacin	2–5 mg/kg q8–12h	SC, IM	Harkness and Wagner (1995)
Ampicillin	Do not use		
Cephaloridine	10–25 mg/kg q24h	SC, IM	Anderson (1994)
Chloramphenicol	50–200 mg/kg q8h	PO	Burgmann and Percy (1993)
	30–50 mg/kg q12h	IM, SC	Burgmann and Percy (1993)
Ciprofloxacin	7–20 mg/kg q12h	PO	Harkness and Wagner (1995)
Doxycyline	2.5 mg/kg q12h	PO	Allen (1993)
Enrofloxacin	5–10 mg/kg q12h	PO, IM	Harkness and Wagner (1995)
	0.05–0.2 mg/mL drinking water for 14 d		Harkness and Wagner (1995)
Erythromycin	0.13 mg/mL drinking water continuously		Burke (1995)
Gentamicin	5 mg/kg q24h	IM, SC	Anderson (1994)
Griseofulvin	25–50 mg/kg q12h for 14–60 d	PO	Harkness and Wagner (1995)
	1.5% in DMSO for 5–7 d	Topical	Harkness and Wagner (1995)
Metronidazole	7.5 mg/70–90 g animal q8h	PO	Collins (1995)
Neomycin	100 mg/kg q24h	PO	Burgmann and Percy (1993)
	0.5 mg/mL drinking water		Anderson (1994)
Oxytetracycline	0.25–1 mg/mL drinking water		Burgmann and Percy (1993)
Sulfadimethoxine	10–15 mg/kg q12h	PO	Harkness and Wagner (1995)
Sulfamerazine	1 mg/mL drinking water		Anderson (1994)
Sulfamethazine	1 mg/mL drinking water		Anderson (1994)
Sulfaquinoxaline	1 mg/mL drinking water		Burgmann and Percy (1993)
Tetracycline	10–20 mg/kg q8–12h	PO	Burgmann and Percy (1993)
	0.4 mg/mL drinking water		Burgmann and Percy (1993)
Trimethoprim-sulfadiazine	30 mg/kg q12h	PO, IM	Harkness and Wagner (1995)
Trimethoprim-sulfamethoxazole	15 mg/kg q12h	PO	Anderson (1994)
Tylosin	2–8 mg/kg q12h	IM, SC, PO	Burgmann and Percy (1993)
	500 mg/L drinking water		Burgmann and Percy (1993)
Vancomycin	20 mg/kg for 3+ mo	PO	Boss et al. (1994)

DMSO = Dimethyl sulfoxide; IM = intramuscular; PO = per os; SC = subcutaneous.

Table 4.6. Antiparasitic agents used in hamsters

Drug	Dosage	Route	Reference
Amitraz	1.4 mL/L water using cottonball application q14d for 3–6 treatments	Topical	Harkness and Wagner (1995)
Carbamate (5%)	Twice weekly	Topical	Harkness and Wagner (1995)
Fenbendazole	20 mg/kg q24h for 5 d	PO	Allen (1993)
Ivermectin	0.2–0.4 mg/kg q7–10d	PO	Harkness and Wagner (1995)
	0.2–0.5 mg/kg q14d for 3 treatments	SC, PO	Anderson (1994)
Piperazine citrate	2–5 mg/mL drinking water for 7 d, off 7 d, then repeat		Anderson (1994)
Praziquantel	6–10 mg/kg	PO	Harkness and Wagner (1995)
Pyrethrin powder	Three times a week for 3 wk	Topical	Anderson (1994)
Thiabendazole	100–200 mg/kg	PO	Harkness and Wagner (1995)

PO = per os; SC = subcutaneous.

Table 4.7. Miscellaneous agents used in hamsters

Drug	Dosage	Route	Reference
Atipamezole	1 mg/kg	SC, IP, IV	Flecknell (1997)
Atropine	0.05–0.1 mg/kg	SC	Harkness and Wagner (1995)
	10 mg/kg q20 min for organophosphate overdose	SC	Harkness and Wagner (1995)
Cimetidine	5–10 mg/kg q6–12h	PO	Allen et al. (1993)
Dexamethasone	0.5–2.0 mg/kg then decreasing dose 2h for 3–14 d	PO, SC	Harkness and Wagner (1995)
	0.6 mg/kg	IM	Anderson (1994)
Doxapram	5–10 mg/kg	IP, IV	Harkness (1993)
Furosemide	1–4 mg/kg q4–6h	IM	Harrenstien (1994)
Glycopyrrolate	0.01–0.02 mg/kg	SC	Huerkamp (1995)
Lactobacilli	Administer during antibiotic treatment period, then 5–7 d beyond cessation	PO	Collins (1995)
Loperamide hydrochloride (Imodium A–D)	0.1 mg/kg q8h for 3 d then q24h for 2 d, give in 1 mL of water	PO	Harkness and Wagner (1995)
Naloxone	0.01–0.10 mg/kg	SC, IP	Huerkamp (1995)
Prednisone	0.5–2.2 mg/kg	SC, IM	Anderson (1994)
Vitamin D	200–400 IU/kg	SC, IM	Anderson (1994)
Vitamin E-selenium (Bo-Se)	0.1 mL/100–250 g	SC	Anderson (1994)
Vitamin K	1–10 mg/kg q24h for 4–6d	IM	Harkness and Wagner (1995)
Yohimbine	0.5–1 mg/kg	IV	Harkness and Wagner (1995)

IM = intramuscular; IP = intraperitoneal; IV = intravenous; PO = per os; SC = subcutaneous.

BACTERIAL DISEASES

Antibiotic-Associated Enterocolitis

☞   The potential value of treating a hamster with a microbial agent must be carefully weighed against the risk of inducing antibiotic-associated enterocolitis. Care must be used in selecting the antibiotic and length of therapy. Discrepancies exist among reports of antimicrobial use in hamsters. Many antimicrobial agents are highly toxic for hamsters, even when the agent is given in a single, minute dose. Lincomycin, clindamycin, ampicillin, vancomycin, erythromycin, cephalosporins, gentamicin, and penicillin all have been associated with enterocolitis.

The specific cause of antimicrobial toxicity is primarily thought to be toxins from *Clostridium difficile*. Hamster intestinal flora is predominantly of the bacterial genera *Lactobacillus* and *Bacteroides* with few coliforms. This normal flora is thought to have a protective role against toxins. After certain antimicrobial agents are given, the intestinal flora changes to predominantly coliforms. Alteration of the normal microbial flora is thought to play a major role in the cause of antibiotic-associated enterocolitis. Clinical signs are similar regardless of the antimicrobial agent involved and include anorexia, ruffled fur, dehydration, and profuse diarrhea. Most hamsters die within 4–10 days. The characteristic gross lesion on necropsy is a hemorrhagic ileocolitis in hamsters. Anderson suggests treating by discontinuing antibiotics, providing a *Lactobacillus* supplement, and giving supportive care. Gram-negative antibiotics should be continued if a specific gram-negative pathogen is cultured. It has been reported that hamsters could be protected against fatal *C. difficile* enteritis by long-term, daily oral administration of 20 mg/kg vancomycin.

Proliferative Ileitis (Transmissible Ileal Hyperplasia or Wet Tail)

☞   Proliferative ileitis is the most common spontaneous disease of hamsters. The causative agent is a *Desulfovibrio* sp., a *Campylobacter*-like organism. Disease is usually confined to young animals, 3–8 weeks of age. The agents are transmitted by the fecal–oral route. Mortality is often high. Stress plays an important role in susceptibility to clinical disease, with weaning, improper diet, transportation, crowding, and poor sanitation serving as significant predisposing factors. Clinical signs include unkempt haircoat; anorexia; moistened perineal area; foul-smelling, watery diarrhea; and dehydration. On abdominal palpation, the animal frequently seems uncomfortable and the bowel loops are often found to be distended. Intussusceptions and rectal prolapses can occur. Typical gross necropsy lesions include gas and yellow diarrhea in the distal intestinal tract, as well as an ileum that is segmentally thickened and edematous.

Prognosis is grave. To be effective, antibiotics must be administered early in the course of disease. Tetracycline and neomycin have been used with moderate success. Metronidazole and chloramphenicol have also been recommended. Erythromycin provided in the drinking water and supplied continuously, and tetracycline added to the drinking water for 10 days, have been reported to reduce mortality during an outbreak. Administration of warmed fluids intraperitoneally or subcutaneously and increasing the room temperature may be helpful. Supportive therapy with whole milk or buttermilk has been reported to be beneficial. Quarantine of affected hamsters and good sanitation practices are useful in controlling proliferative ileitis. The importance of correcting any management problems and eliminating stress factors should not be overlooked.

Campylobacteriosis

There is a relatively high incidence of hamsters that carry *Campylobacter jejuni*. Most hamsters are asymptomatic. Hamsters should be considered as a potential source for human infections. Erythromycin administered orally is the drug of choice for treatment of humans with *C. jejuni* diarrhea.

Abscesses and Skin Ulceration

Abscesses and skin ulceration are frequently caused by *Staphylococcus aureus*. Other less common organisms include *Streptococcus* spp. and *Pasteurella pneumotropica*. Systemic chloramphenicol and tetracycline can be used with local treatment of the area.

Pneumonia

Streptococcus spp. and *P. pneumotropica* infections may cause pneumonia. The illness is usually acute, with affected animals exhibiting sneezing, dyspnea, ocular discharge, and depression. Chloramphenicol and tetracycline are useful antibiotics to treat pneumonia.

VIRAL DISEASES

Hamsters are susceptible to infection by a number of murine viruses such as Sendai virus and pneumonia virus of mice; however, clinical disease is rarely recognized.

Lymphocytic Choriomeningitis

The natural host of this virus is the wild mouse. Infection can be transmitted readily to other species such as the hamster. Lymphocytic choriomeningitis (LCM) is an important public health consideration, as the virus may be transmitted from infected animals to humans through saliva by biting, on contact with feces and urine, or through infected murine tissues and cell lines. In the 1970s, hamsters were the source of several hundred human cases in the United States. In the hamster, LCM is almost always subclinical. In humans, signs vary from subclinical to influenzalike symptoms and, rarely, to meningitis.

PARASITIC DISEASES

Demodex

Two species of mites, *Demodex criceti* and *D. aurati,* occur in hamsters. The mites are normally of low pathogenicity. Disease is normally seen in older animals, particularly males, and is usually secondary to another systemic disease. Affected hamsters may have a rough haircoat, scaly and scabby dermatitis, and areas of alopecia over the back, neck, and rump. Demodex mites can be difficult to detect. A deep skin scraping is suggested. It is best to bathe the hamster in a mild soap and towel dry, prior to treating with a dilute solution of amitraz. Apply the solution using a cotton ball and allow it to dry on the animal. Dipping is not suggested.

Pinworms

Hamsters can be infected by *Syphacia* species. Pinworms apparently are of low pathogenicity; however, they may affect certain research projects and may be a problem with interspecies transmission. Ivermectin, piperazine, and thiabendazole are reported to be effective treatments.

Tapeworms

Several species of *Hymenolepis* readily infect hamsters. In small numbers, tapeworms are relatively nonpathogenic. Heavy infestations can cause diarrhea. Colonies of hamsters have been frequently found to be infected with *H. nana.* Infections with *H. nana* are a concern because of its direct life cycle, transmission to other rodents, and zoonotic potential. Recommended treatments include praziquantel or thiabendazole.

Protozoa

Numerous protozoa including *Spironucleus* spp., *Trichomonas* spp., and *Giardia* spp., are found in the intestines but are of no clinical significance.

NEOPLASIA

The incidence of spontaneous tumors in hamsters is relatively low. The majority of tumors are benign and frequently arise from the endocrine system or alimentary tract.

MISCELLANEOUS CONDITIONS

Rupture of Eye

Hamsters are prone to rupture of the eye secondary to trauma or infection. Enucleation is suggested, but care should be taken to control hemorrhage. Surgical absorbable gelatin sponge placed in the socket enhances clot formation.

Malocclusion

Malocclusion and overgrowth of incisors occasionally occur in hamsters because of traumatic or genetic reasons. Overgrowth of teeth can result in weight loss and starvation if the condition persists. Sharp toenail trimmers or a dental bur may be used to shorten overgrown incisors.

Alopecia

Diets low in protein may cause alopecia. Diets should contain at least 16% protein.

Bedding-Associated Dermatitis

A dermatitis that primarily affects the foot pads and digits has been reported in hamsters housed on wood shavings. Lesions may spread to the legs and shoulders.

Cage Paralysis Syndrome

Paralysis is most frequently the result of injuries sustained when animals are dropped onto a hard surface. A nutritional myopathy caused by a vitamin deficiency can occur in hamsters fed all seed diets or table scraps and deprived of exercise. In mild cases, the hamster is able to move the hind legs but cannot support their weight. In more advanced cases, the hamster may have posterior paresis. Nutritional improvement, supplementation with vitamin E, and opportunity to exercise are usually curative.

Bone Fractures and Trauma

External splinting is often not satisfactory for fracture repair. Stainless steel hypodermic needles used as intramedullary pins may be preferable for repair of fractured long bones. Fine stainless steel wire is preferable to other material for suturing lacerations, as it is not gnawed out as quickly.

Nephrosis

Degenerative renal disease is a common problem in aged hamsters and is an important cause of mortality. Females are more commonly affected. Amyloid deposition frequently occurs concurrently.

Amyloidosis

☞ Hamsters have a high incidence of amyloidosis. Renal amyloidosis is a common problem in aged hamsters, particularly females. Signs frequently seen are edema and ascites.

Atrial Thrombosis

☞ Geriatric hamsters frequently suffer from atrial thrombosis. Most thromboses occur in the left atrium and are secondary to degenerative cardiomyopathy and amyloidosis. Hamsters often present with severe dyspnea. Anderson has reported temporary improvement in some hamsters treated with digitalis using a cat dose and furosemide.

Polycystic Disease

Aged hamsters frequently develop cysts in the liver. Less frequently, cysts are found in the pancreas, epididymis, and seminal vesicles. No clinical signs are associated with the cysts.

■ GENERAL REFERENCES

Sources consulted to compile the material in this chapter include *The Hamster in Biomedical Research,* edited by G.L. Van Hoosier, Jr., and C.W. McPherson (1987, Academic Press, Inc., Orlando, FL 32887); *The Biology and Medicine of Rabbits and Rodents* by J.E. Harkness and J.E. Wagner, 4th edition (1995, Williams & Wilkins, 1400 North Providence Rd., Building II, Suite 5025,

Media, PA 19063); *Laboratory Animal Medicine,* edited by J.F. Fox, B.J. Cohen, and F.M. Loew (1984, Academic Press, Inc., Orlando, FL 32887); *The UFAW Handbook on the Care and Management of Laboratory Animals,* 6th edition, edited by T.B. Poole (1987, Churchill Livingstone Inc., 1560 Broadway, New York, NY 10036); and *Pathology of Laboratory Rodents and Rabbits* by D.H. Percy and S.W. Barthold (1993, Iowa State University Press, 2121 South State Avenue, Ames, IA 50014).

■ TECHNICAL REFERENCES

Allen, D.G., J.K. Pringle, and D.A. Smith. 1993. *Handbook of Veterinary Drugs.* Philadelphia: JB Lippincott.

Anderson, N.L. 1994. Basic husbandry and medicine of pocket pets. In *Saunders Manual of Small Animal Practice,* ed. J.S. Birchard and R.G. Sherding, pp. 1363–1389. Philadelphia: WB Saunders.

Boss, S.M., C.L. Gries, B.K. Kirchner, G.D. Smith, and P.C. Francis. 1994. Use of vancomycin hydrochloride for treatment of *Clostridium difficile* enteritis in Syrian hamsters. *Lab Anim Sci* 44(1): 31–37.

Burgmann, P. and D.H. Percy. 1993. Antimicrobial drug use in rodents and rabbits. In *Antimicrobial Therapy in Veterinary Medicine,* 2d ed., ed. J.F. Prescott and J.D. Baggot, pp. 524–541. Ames: Iowa State University Press.

Burke, T.J. 1995. "Wet tail" in hamsters and other diarrheas of small rodents. In *Kirk's Current Veterinary Therapy XII: Small Animal Practice,* ed. J.D. Bonagura, pp. 1336–1339. Philadelphia: WB Saunders.

Collins, B.R. 1995. Antimicrobial drug use in rabbits, rodents, and other small mammals. In *Antimicrobial Therapy in Caged Birds and Exotic Pets,* pp. 3–10. Trenton, NJ: Veterinary Learning Systems.

Curl, J.L. and L.J. Peters. 1983. Ketamine hydrochloride and xylazine hydrochloride anaesthesia in the golden hamster *(Mesocricetus auratus). Lab Anim* 17: 290–293.

Flecknell, P.A. 1987. *Laboratory Animal Anesthesia.* London: Academic.

Flecknell, P.A. 1997. Medetomidine and atipamezole: Potential uses in laboratory animals. *Lab Anim* 26(2): 21–25.

Forsythe, D.B., A.J. Payton, D. Dixson, et al. 1992. Evaluation of Telazol-xylazine as an anesthetic combination for use in Syrian hamsters. *Lab Anim Sci* 42(5): 497–502.

Harkness, J.E. 1993. *A Practitioner's Guide to Domestic Rodents.* Lakewood, CO: American Animal Hospital Association.

Harrenstien, L. 1994. Critical care of ferrets, rabbits, and rodents. *Semin Avian Exotic Pet Med* 3: 217–228.

Heard, D.J. 1993. Principles and techniques of anesthesia and analgesia for exotic practice. *Vet Clin North Am Small Anim Pract* 23: 1301–1327.

Huerkamp, M.J. 1995. Anesthesia and postoperative management of rabbits and pocket pets. In *Kirk's Current Veterinary Therapy XII: Small Animal Practice,* ed. J.D. Bonagura, pp. 1322–1327. Philadelphia: WB Saunders.

Hughes, H.C. 1981. Anesthesia of laboratory animals. *Lab Anim* 10(5): 40–56.

Meshorer, A. 1976. Leg lesions in hamsters caused by wood shavings. *Lab Anim Sci* 26: 827–29.

Peace, T.A., K.V. Brock, and H.F. Stills, Jr. 1994. Comparative analysis of the 16S rRNA gene sequence of the putative agent of proliferative ileitis of hamsters. *Int J Syst Bacteriol* 44(4): 832–835.

Reid, W.D., C. Davies, P.D. Pare, and R.L. Pardy. 1989. An effective combination of anaesthetics for 6-hour experimentation in the golden Syrian hamster. *Lab Anim* 23: 156–162.

Silverman, J., M. Huhndorf, M. Balk, and G. Slater. 1983. Evaluation of a combination of tiletamine and zolazepam as an anesthetic for laboratory rodents. *Lab Anim Sci* 33(5): 457–460.

Thayer, C.B., S. Lowe, and W.C. Rubright. 1972. Clinical evaluation of a combination of droperidol and fentanyl as an anesthetic for the rat and hamster. *JAVMA* 161: 665–668.

White, W.J. and K.J. Field. 1987. Anesthesia and surgery of laboratory animals. *Vet Clin North Am Small Anim Pract* 17(5): 989–1017.

Wixson, S.K. 1994. Rabbits and rodents: Anesthesia and analgesia. In *Research Animal Anesthesia, Analgesia and Surgery,* ed. A.C. Smith and M.M. Swindle, pp. 59–92. Greenbelt, MD: Scientists Center for Animal Welfare.

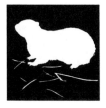

GUINEA PIGS

GUINEA PIGS are hystricomorph (hedgehoglike) rodents origi-
nating from South America. Although they belong to the order Rodentia, guinea pigs are more closely related to porcupines and chinchillas
than to mice and rats. Recent data, based on the construction of a molecular phylogentic tree, suggest the guinea pig may belong to an order
distinct from Rodentia. The guinea pig is also known as a cavy, which is
derived from its scientific name, *Cavia porcellus*. There are three main
varieties of guinea pigs: English, Abyssinian, and Peruvian. They can be
distinguished by the length, texture, and direction of hair growth. English guinea pigs have uniformly short, straight hair. They are the most
common type seen as a pet or in a research setting. There are a number
of outbred stocks (Dunkan-Hartley, Hartley) and inbred strains (Strain
2, Strain 13) of English guinea pigs. Abyssinian guinea pigs have short,
coarse hair arranged in whorls or rosettes, which gives them an untidy
appearance. Peruvian guinea pigs, or rag mops, have long, fine, silky
hair. Guinea pigs may be monocolored, bicolored, or tricolored. Many
color and coat patterns are possible because the varieties can interbreed.

Uses

The docile nature of guinea pigs accounts for their popularity as
pets. Guinea pigs seldom bite or scratch and will respond to attention
with frequent and gentle handling. On the other hand, they tend to be
messy, living up to their name of "pig" by scattering food and bedding.
The development of human allergies to guinea pigs is not uncommon.

Although not as popular as other rodents, guinea pigs nevertheless
have left their mark as research animals. In the English language, the
term "guinea pig" is synonymous with the term "research subject."
They have several attributes, including size, availability, and tractable
disposition, that make them desirable research animals. They share several features with humans such as the need for vitamin C and suscepti-

bility to tuberculosis. Guinea pigs are used primarily in studies involving immunology, infectious disease, audiology, nutrition, and toxicology. They are a well-established model of anaphylaxis. Sensitized animals have a high incidence of anaphylaxis when injected with a small amount of antigen and subsequently develop lethal brochiolar constriction in response to histamine release.

Behavior

Guinea pigs are communal animals that live together amicably. When housed in groups, guinea pigs establish male-dominated social hierarchies. Once the hierarchy is formed, the group is usually stable. Introduction of a new male into a group, however, can provoke fighting. Dominant animals will frequently chew and barber the hair of subordinate cagemates. Barbering is also associated with boredom and overcrowding. Adults, especially boars, will chew the ears of the young.

Guinea pigs are active during daylight hours and eat frequently. They are generally calm but are sensitive and easily excited by sudden noise or changes in their environment. They tend to freeze at unfamiliar sounds and scatter when exposed to sudden movements. The immobility reaction can last from several seconds to 20 minutes. The scatter reaction can involve stampeding, jumping, or rapid circling of their cage. Guinea pigs exhibit a Preyer or pinna reflex and will cock their ears in response to sound. Vocalization appears to play an important part in their behavior. At least 11 different vocalizations have been recorded, some of which are inaudible to humans. They will whistle in anticipation of feeding, chut and purr during social interactions, and squeal or scream when injured or fearful. Guinea pigs develop rigid habits and dislike change. Any change in food or water may cause a guinea pig to stop eating.

Anatomic and Physiologic Features

Guinea pig biologic and reproductive data are listed in Table 5.1. Guinea pigs have a compact body with short legs and no tail. Unlike other common laboratory rodents, guinea pigs have four digits on the forelimbs and three digits on their hind limbs. Their dental formula, 2 (1/1 incisors, 0/0 canines, 1/1 premolars, and 3/3 molars), is unique for rodents, as most do not have premolars. All of their teeth are open rooted and erupt continuously. Guinea pigs have large tympanic bullae, which makes it easier to access internal structures of the ear. The thymus of the guinea pig surrounds the trachea, rather than being located in the thoracic cavity overlying the heart, as it is in other rodents. The pharynx

Table 5.1. Biologic and reproductive data for guinea pigs	
Adult body weight	
Male	900–1200 g
Female	700–900 g
Life span	4–5 y
Body temperature	37.2°–39.5°C (99°–103.1°F)
Heart rate	230–380 beats per minute
Respiratory rate	42–104 breaths per minute
Food consumption	6 g/100 g/d
Water consumption	10 mL/100 g/d
Breeding onset	
Male	3–4 mo (600–700g)
Female	2–3 mo (350–450g)
Estrous cycle length	15–17 d
Gestation period	59–72 d
Postpartum estrus	Fertile
Litter size	2–5
Weaning age	14–21 d
Breeding duration	18–48 mo
Chromosome number (diploid)	64

Source: Adapted from Harkness and Wagner (1995).

has a unique anatomy. The soft palate is continuous with the base of the tongue and has a hole in it, called the palatal ostium. This is the only opening from the oropharynx to the remainder of the pharynx. The right lung has four lobes and the left lung has three lobes. The adrenal glands are bilobed and large. The guinea pig has an undivided stomach and a capacious cecum and colon. The large intestine occupies most of the abdominal cavity. Guinea pigs are strongly coprophagic and will eat feces directly from the anus or from the cage floor. They have marking glands located circumanally and on their rump and are often seen walking or sitting with the glands pressed against a surface.

☞ The guinea pig is the only common laboratory animal, other than nonhuman primates, which resembles the human in its dietary requirement of vitamin C. Guinea pigs lack L-gulonolactone oxidase, an enzyme required for the synthesis of vitamin C, and thus require vitamin C in their diet.

Sexing is done by manipulation and visualization. Male guinea pigs are larger than females. They have large testes and a penis that is easily extruded from the preputial sheath. The inguinal canals remain open in the male. Both sexes possess one pair of mammary glands in the inguinal region; however, the male's nipples are smaller. Females have a Y-shaped genital–anal opening in contrast to the male's slit-shaped opening. The female guinea pig has a vaginal closure membrane that is only open during estrus and parturition.

Compared with other rodents, the packed cell volume, erythrocytes, and hemoglobin levels of the guinea pig are relatively low. Typical of rodents, the lymphocyte is the dominant leukocyte. Guinea pigs have heterophils (neutrophils) with distinct eosinophilic cytoplasmic granules like those of the rabbit. Sex chromatin drumsticks can be seen on granulocytes in the sow's blood. The guinea pig has a unique leukocyte, the Kurloff cell. The Kurloff cell is a mononuclear lymphocyte with a large intracytoplasmic inclusion that proliferates with estrogenic stimulation. Kurloff cells are found in highest numbers in the placenta and are thought to function as killer cells. Guinea pigs, especially mature sows, are an excellent source of complement that has high activity. Complement is involved naturally in immunologic reactions and is a necessary reagent used in serologic testing. Guinea pigs have opaque, creamy yellow urine. The urine has an alkaline pH of 8–9 and contains crystals. Selected hematologic and biochemical values are listed in Appendix 1, Normal Values.

Breeding and Reproduction

The sow, female guinea pig, is usually bred at 2–3 months, which corresponds to a weight of 350–450 g. It is important that the sow be bred prior to 7 months of age to prevent permanent fusion of the pelvic symphysis, which often results in dystocia. The boar, male guinea pig, is bred at 3–4 months of age or 600–700 g body weight. The sow is a nonseasonal, continuously polyestrous breeder. The estrous cycle lasts 15–17 days. Detection of estrus is not necessary unless timed matings are desired, as guinea pigs are normally pair housed for mating. When the sow is in estrus, she will exhibit lordosis, characterized by extension of all four legs, straightening and arching of the back, and elevation of the pubic area. Pregnancy can be confirmed by palpating the fetal mass at 14–21 days of gestation. The body weight may nearly double in a pregnant sow. During the last week of gestation, the pelvic symphysis relaxes and separates. The gestation period ranges from 59 to 72 days, with an average of 68 days. The gestation length varies inversely with the size of the litter, being longer for small litters and shorter for large litters. Guinea pigs do not build nests. Farrowing normally takes approximately 30 minutes. Young are precocious, as they are born fully haired, with teeth, and their eyes and ears open. They begin eating solid food during the 1st week of life and are nearly self-sufficient by 4–5 days of age. Guinea pigs can be weaned at 14–21 days or when they weigh approximately 180 g.

HUSBANDRY

Housing

Guinea pigs may be housed individually or grouped in a colony arrangement. Cages may be solid plastic or metal with solid, metal-slat, or wire-grid flooring. To reduce limb injuries, solid-bottom cages with bedding are preferred. If guinea pigs are raised on wire, they learn to walk with ease. Inexperienced guinea pigs placed onto wire often fall through the mesh, lacerating or fracturing their limbs. Because guinea pigs are not inclined to climb or jump, they can be kept in open-top boxes provided the sides are at least 25 cm (10 in.) high. Rectangular cages are preferred over square, as they tend to discourage the stampede response. Adult animals should be provided with at least 652 cm^2 (101 in.^{2}) of floor space per animal. The bedding material should be as dust free as possible. Wood shavings, corn cobs, shredded paper, or other material of plant origin can be used. Guinea pigs are housed at temperatures between 18° and 26°C (64° and 79°F), with 21°C (70°F) recommended. Having a compact body, they can tolerate low temperatures better than high temperatures, especially if the humidity is high. Avoiding temperature fluctuations and drafts is most important. The environmental humidity should be maintained between 30% and 70%, with 10–15 air changes per hour. Typically, 12 hours of light per day are provided, which can be controlled through automatic timers. Guinea pigs should not be housed with animal species such as rabbits, cats, and dogs that may carry *Bordetella bronchiseptica* subclinically, as guinea pigs are susceptible to infection. Cages should be cleaned at least once weekly, as guinea pigs tend to be messy. Cages, water bottles, and feed hoppers should be disinfected with chemicals, hot water 61.6°–82.2°C (143°–180°F), or a combination of both. A weak acidic solution may be helpful to remove urine scale. Detergents and chemical disinfectants enhance the effectiveness of hot water, but they must be thoroughly rinsed from all caging surfaces with fresh water. Refer to Chapter 1, Mice, for a more detailed description of disinfection methods.

Feeding and Watering

Commercial pelleted diets manufactured specifically for guinea pigs should be fed ad libitum. It is important that the food be freshly milled, properly stored, and used within 90 days of milling to ensure adequate vitamin C content. Guinea pigs eat an average of 6 g/100 g of body ☞ weight per day. Feed is best provided in self-feeders mounted on the cage wall, as guinea pigs tend to sit, sleep, and defecate in bowls placed on the cage floor. Good-quality hay can be provided as a supplement to reduce boredom and decrease barbering. If the amount of vitamin C in the formulated feed is questionable or inadequate, ascorbic acid may be added to the drinking water or provided as a food supplement. Water fortified with ascorbic acid should be provided in glass or plastic bottles rather than metal containers or open bowls to prolong the activity of the added vitamin. Kale, parsley, beet greens, kiwi fruit, broccoli, orange, or cabbage are good sources of vitamin C and can be fed in small amounts not to exceed 10% to 15% by weight of the pelleted diet. Fresh fruits and vegetables should be cleaned by rinsing thoroughly with water before they are fed. If supplements are fed, unused portions should be removed daily. Hay and supplements can be a source of pathogenic organisms. Fresh potable water should be available ad libitum by bottle or automatic watering system. Adult guinea pigs drink an average of 10 mL/100 g of body weight per day. Water bowls or crocks placed on the cage floor should not be used, as they readily become contaminated with feces and bedding. Guinea pigs are untidy water drinkers. Rather than lick, they chew on and play with sipper tubes and valves and will waste a significant amount of water. Guinea pigs will also blow food up the sipper tube and foul the water supply. The use of automatic water systems with valves located outside the cage is thus more advantageous.

TECHNIQUES

Handling and Restraint

Guinea pigs should be handled gently but firmly. They should be lifted by grasping under the trunk with one hand while supporting the rear quarters with the other hand. Restraint of the guinea pig is shown in Figure 5.1. Support is particularly important with adults and pregnant animals. Grabbing a guinea pig too firmly around the thorax or abdomen can impede breathing and cause injury to the lungs or liver.

Identification

Cage cards or color pattern records can be used to identify guinea pigs. Permanent individual animal identification can be accomplished by ear notching, ear tagging, tattooing, or microchip placement. Dyes and markers can be used for temporary identification.

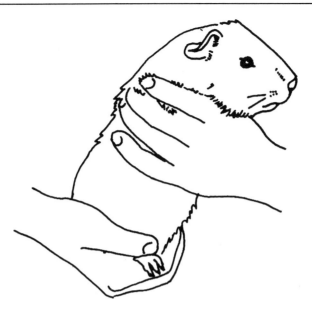

Figure 5.1. Restraint of the guinea pig. (Adapted from Harkness and Wagner 1995, *The Biology and Medicine of Rabbits and Rodents,* 4th edition, Philadelphia: Williams & Wilkins)

Blood Collection

Guinea pigs lack readily accessible peripheral veins. Small amounts of blood can be obtained from a toenail bed, the marginal ear vein, saphenous vein, or cephalic vein. Larger quantities of blood can be obtained from the cranial vena cava, femoral artery or vein, or directly from the heart. The guinea pig must be sedated to obtain blood from the cranial vena cava or femoral vessels and must be anesthetized when using the heart. Cardiac punctures involve a significant element of risk. A catheter can also be implanted into the jugular vein to collect blood samples. Approximate blood volumes for guinea pigs are listed in Table 5.2.

Table 5.2. Adult guinea pig blood volumes	
	Volume (mL)[a]
Total blood	40–80
Single sample	4–8
Exsanguination	15–30

Source: Adapted from Harkness and Wagner (1995).
[a]Values are approximate.

99

Urine Collection

Urine may be collected by using a metabolic cage, gentle digital pressure on the bladder, cystocentesis, or placing the animal on a cold, clean surface.

Drug Administration

Palatable drugs can be incorporated into the food or water, but guinea pigs will often refuse food or water with an unfamiliar taste. If medications are unpalatable, 5 mL of sugar or syrup per liter can be added to the drinking water to improve the palatability. Liquids can be administered orally using a small syringe or dosing needle. Subcutaneous injections require some force, as guinea pig skin is tough, especially over the neck and back. A maximum volume of 5–10 mL is recommended per site. Intramuscular injections with a maximum volume of 0.5 mL may be given in the quadriceps muscle to avoid the sciatic nerve. Intraperitoneal injections are made lateral to the midline in the lower left quadrant of the abdomen after tilting the guinea pig's head toward the floor. This position shifts the abdominal organs forward and helps to prevent inadvertent injection into the intestine. A maximum volume of 5–8 mL can be given by the intraperitoneal route. Intravenous injections can be made using the saphenous vein, the cephalic vein, or the marginal ear vein. The penile vein and lingual vein can also be used but are technically challenging.

Anesthesia, Surgery, and Postoperative Care

☞ Guinea pigs should be fasted for 3–6 hours before anesthetizing to decrease the amount of ingesta in the cecum and stomach. A variety of agents that can be used to tranquilize and anesthetize guinea pigs are listed in Table 5.3. Anesthesia in the guinea pig is difficult for a number of reasons. Guinea pigs have a variable response to drugs, thus, there is a wide range of dosages for various agents reported in the literature. When utilizing injectable agents, care must be used in calculating the dose. The body weight can be misleading on account of the large cecum and contents of the intestinal tract or fetal mass. Guinea pigs can be difficult to monitor when anesthetized. Under some anesthetics such as pentobarbital and volatile agents, guinea pigs exhibit a peculiar squirming muscle movement that does not signify return to consciousness. Several agents, such as fentanyl-droperidol and ketamine-xylazine, injected by the intramuscular route have been noted to cause muscle necrosis and/or self-mutilation of the injected limb. When using these agents, use

Table 5.3. Anesthetic agents and tranquilizers used in guinea pigs			
Drug	Dosage	Route	Reference
Inhalants			
Halothane	0.5%–4% to effect	Inhalation	Harkness and Wagner (1995)
Isoflurane	2%–5% to effect	Inhalation	Harkness and Wagner (1995)
Methoxyflurane	0.5%–3% to effect	Inhalation	Harkness and Wagner (1995)
Injectables			
Acetylpromazine	0.5–1 mg/kg	IM	Harkness and Wagner (1995)
Chloral hydrate	400 mg/kg	IP	White (1987)
Diazepam	0.5–3 mg/kg	IM	Anderson (1994)
Fentanyl-droperidol	0.22–0.88 mL/kg	IM	Anderson (1994)
Ketamine	25–55 mg/kg	IM	Harkness and Wagner (1995)
+ acetylpromazine	0.75–3 mg/kg	IM	
Ketamine	20–30 mg/kg	IM	Quesenberry (1994)
+ diazepam	1–2 mg/kg	IM	
Ketamine	60–100 mg/kg	IM	Gilroy (1980)
+ diazepam	5–8 mg/kg	IM	
Ketamine	40 mg/kg	IP	Flecknell (1997)
+ medetomidine	0.5 mg/kg	IP	
Ketamine	40 mg/kg	IP	Brown et al. (1989)
+ xylazine	2 mg/kg	IM	
Ketamine	22–64 mg/kg,	IM	Anderson (1994)
+ xylazine	2–5 mg/kg	IM	
+ acetylpromazine	0.75 mg/kg	IM	
Pentobarbital	25–35 mg/kg	IP	Harkness and Wagner (1995)
Tiletamine-zolazepam	20–40 mg/kg	IM	Mason (1997)
Urethane	1500 mg/kg	IV, IP	Flecknell (1987)

IM = intramuscular; IP = intraperitoneal; IV = intravenous.

the lowest dose possible and dilute and/or reduce the amount injected per site. Utilization of the intraperitoneal route of drug administration is suggested. Lidocaine hydrochloride 1% with 1:200,000 epinephrine used as a local anesthetic has been found to be helpful in overcoming the analgesic shortcomings of injectable anesthetic agents.

Face masks are often used to administer inhalation agents because it is difficult to intubate guinea pigs owing to the anatomy of the pharynx, small size of their trachea, and difficulty in visualizing the area. Isoflurane and halothane require a precision vaporizer, whereas methoxyflurane can be used by the open-drop method. Methoxyflurane is a good anesthetic agent; however, it stimulates salivation, and premedication with atropine is suggested. Halothane has been associated with hepatitis and/or hepatic necrosis in hypoxic guinea pigs. Inhalant anesthetics should always be used with appropriate waste gas scavenging systems.

The ear pinch, respiratory rate, and heart rate can be used to monitor the depth of anesthesia. Palpebral reflexes, eyeball position, and toe-

101

pinch reflexes are not reliable indicators of depth of anesthesia in this species.

While anesthetized, guinea pigs should have bland ophthalmic ointment placed in their eyes to prevent exposure keratitis. Use of a circulating-water heating pad promotes euthermia and is recommended.

Pet guinea pigs may require a simple castration or cesarean section. Castration can be done using the same technique as in rabbits. The most common surgery performed on a research guinea pig involves the inner ear.

Surgery should be performed in an aseptic manner. Postoperative care should include hydration of the anesthetized animal with warmed saline-dextrose solutions, a method to prevent hypothermia, turning the animal every 30 minutes to prevent hypostatic pulmonary congestion, and stimulation to return to normal feeding. Analgesics should be administered when pain is observed or expected to occur. Table 5.4 lists analgesics that can be used in this species. Butorphanol is recommended for mild postoperative discomfort. Buprenorphine works well to control acute or chronic visceral pain.

Euthanasia

Suitable methods for euthanasia include an overdose of inhalation anesthetic agent, pentobarbital (150–200 mg/kg) or other euthanasia solution given by the intravenous or intraperitoneal route, and carbon dioxide (approximately 70%) in a prefilled chamber. Refer to Chapter 1, Mice, for more information on appropriate euthanasia methods.

Table 5.4. Analgesic agents used in guinea pigs

Drug	Dosage	Route	Reference
Acetaminophen	1–2 mg/mL drinking water		Huerkamp (1995)
Acetylsalicylic acid	50–100 mg/kg q4h	PO	Heard (1993)
Buprenorphine	0.05–0.5 mg/kg q6–12h	SC	Wixson (1994)
Butorphanol	2 mg/kg q2–4h	SC	Heard (1993)
Flunixin meglumine	2.5–5 mg/kg q12–24h	SC	Heard (1993)
Ibuprofen	10 mg/kg q4h	PO	Harkness and Wagner (1995)
Meperidine	20 mg/kg q2–3h	SC, IM	Heard (1993)
Syrup	0.2 mg/mL drinking water		Huerkamp (1995)
Nalbuphine	1–2 mg/kg q3h	IM	Heard (1993)
Oxymorphone	0.2–0.5 mg/kg q6–12h	SC, IM	Heard (1993)
Pentazocine	10 mg/kg q2–4h	SC	Heard (1993)

IM = intramuscular; PO = per os; SC = subcutaneous.

THERAPEUTIC AGENTS

Suggested guinea pig antimicrobial and antifungal drug dosages are listed in Table 5.5. Antiparasitic agents are listed in Table 5.6, and miscellaneous agents are listed in Table 5.7.

Table 5.5. Antimicrobial and antifungal agents used in guinea pigs

Drug	Dosage	Route	Reference
Amikacin	2–5 mg/kg q8–12h	SC, IM	Harkness and Wagner (1995)
Ceftiofur sodium	1 mg/kg q24h	IM	Harkness (1993)
Cephalexin	50 mg/kg q24h	IM	Richardson (1992)
Cephaloridine	10–25 mg/kg q8–24h	IM	Anderson (1994)
Chloramphenicol	50 mg/kg q12h	PO	Burgmann and Percy (1993)
	30–50 mg/kg q12h	SC, IM	Burgmann and Percy (1993)
Ciprofloxacin	7–20 mg/kg q12h	PO	Harkness and Wagner (1995)
Doxycycline	2.5mg/kg q12h	PO	Allen (1993)
Enrofloxacin	0.05–0.2 mg/mL drinking water for 14 d		Harkness and Wagner (1995)
	5–10 mg/kg q12h	PO, IM	Harkness and Wagner (1995)
Gentamicin	2–4 mg/kg q8–24h	SC, IM	Harkness and Wagner (1995)
Griseofulvin	25–50 mg/kg q12h for 14–60 d	PO	Harkness and Wagner (1995)
	1.5% in DMSO for 5–7 d	Topical	Harkness and Wagner (1995)
Neomycin	12–16 mg/kg q12h	PO	Anderson (1994)
Sulfadimethoxine	10–15 mg/kg q12h	PO	Harkness and Wagner (1995)
Sulfamerazine	1 mg/mL drinking water		Anderson (1994)
Sulfamethazine	1 mg/mL drinking water		Anderson (1994)
Sulfaquinoxaline	1 mg/mL drinking water		Collins (1995)
Tetracycline	10–20 mg/kg q8–12h	PO	Burgmann and Percy (1993)
Trimethoprim-sulfa	30 mg/kg q12h	PO, IM	Harkness and Wagner (1995)

DMSO = dimethyl sulfoxide; IM = intramuscular, PO = per os; SC = subcutaneous.

Table 5.6. Antiparasitic agents used in guinea pigs

Drug	Dosage	Route	Reference
Carbaryl powder (5%)	Dust q7d for 3 wk	Topical	Anderson (1994)
Fenbendazole	20 mg/kg q24h for 5 d	PO	Allen (1993)
Ivermectin	0.2 mg/kg q7d for 3 wk	PO, SC	Anderson (1994)
	500 µg/kg, repeat in 7 d	SC	McKellar et al. (1992)
Lime sulfur dip	Dilute 1:40 with water, dip q7d for 6 wk	Topical	Anderson (1994)
Metronidazole	10–40 mg/kg q24h	PO	Collins (1995)
Piperazine citrate	2–5 mg/mL drinking water for 7 d, off 7 d, repeat		Anderson (1994)
Praziquantel	6–10 mg/kg	PO	Harkness and Wagner (1995)
Pyrethrin powder	Dust q7d for 3 wk	Topical	Anderson (1994)
Thiabendazole	100 mg/kg q24h for 5 d	PO	Allen (1993)

PO = per os; SC = subcutaneous.

Table 5.7.	Miscellaneous agents used in guinea pigs		
Drug	Dosage	Route	Reference
Atipamezole	1 mg/kg	SC, IP, IV	Flecknell (1997)
Atropine	0.05–0.1 mg/kg	SC	Harkness and Wagner (1995)
	10 mg/kg q20 min (for organo-phosphate toxicity)	SC	Harkness and Wagner (1995)
Betamethasone	0.1–0.2 mL	IM, SC	Richardson (1992)
Chlorpheniramine	5 mg/kg	SC	Borchard et al. (1990)
Cimetidine	5–10 mg/kg q6–12h	PO	Allen (1993)
Dexamethasone	0.5–2 mg/kg, then decreasing dose q12h for 3–14 d	PO, SC	Harkness and Wagner (1995)
Diphenhydramine	12.5 mg/kg	IP	Borchard et al. (1990)
Doxapram	2–5 mg/kg	IP, IV	Harkness (1993)
Furosemide	1–4 mg/kg q4–6h	IM	Harrenstien (1994)
Glycopyrrolate	0.01–0.02 mg/kg	SC	Huerkamp (1995)
Human chorionic gonadotropin	100 IU per animal, repeat in 7–10 d	IM	Schaeffer (1997)
Kaopectate liquid	0.2 mL q6–8h per adult	PO	Johnson-Delaney (1996)
Lactobacilli	Administer during antibiotic treatment period, then 5–7 d beyond cessation	PO	Collins (1995)
Loperamide hydrochloride (Imodium A–D)	0.1 mg/kg q8h for 3 d, then q24h for 2 d	PO	Harkness and Wagner (1995)
Metoclopramide	0.5 mg/kg q8h	SC	Johnson-Delaney (1996)
Naloxone	0.01–0.1 mg/kg	SC, IP	Huerkamp (1995)
Oxytocin	0.2–3 IU/kg	SC, IM, IV	Anderson (1994)
Prednisone	0.5–2.2 mg/kg	SC, IM	Anderson (1994)
Vitamin B complex	0.02–0.2 mL/kg	SC, IM	Anderson (1994)
Vitamin C	0.2–0.4 mg/mL drinking water		Quesenberry (1994)
	20–200 mg/kg	SC, IM	Anderson (1994)
Vitamin E-selenium (Bo-Se)	0.1 mL/100–250 g	SC	Anderson (1994)
Vitamin K	1–10 mg/kg q24h for 4–6 d	IM	Harkness and Wagner (1995)
Yohimbine	0.5–1 mg/kg	IV	Harkness and Wagner (1995)

IM = intramuscular; IP = intraperitoneal; IV = intravenous; PO = per os; SC = subcutaneous.

BACTERIAL DISEASES

Antibiotic Toxicity

☞ Guinea pigs are highly sensitive to antibiotics, particularly those specific for gram-positive organisms. The normal intestinal flora of guinea pigs is predominantly gram-positive organisms such as streptococci and lactobacilli. Administration of antibiotics specific for gram-positive bacteria destroys the normal flora and permits an overgrowth of gram-negative organisms as well as clostridial organisms. Penicillins, including ampicillin and amoxicillin, lincomycin, clindamycin, erythromycin, bacitracin, and dihydrostreptomycin, all are capable of inducing toxicity and should be avoided. The offending antibiotics can cause toxicity when administered orally, parenterally, and even topically. *Clostridium difficile* appears to play the primary role in the enterotoxemia that follows antibiotic treatment. *Escherichia coli* has also been observed to produce a bacteremia in treated animals. The cecal mucosa is edematous and frequently hemorrhagic at necropsy. Tetracycline, cephaloridine, chloramphenicol, and the sulfonamides are among the less hazardous antimicrobials. All antibiotics should be administered with caution, using the minimal effective dosage.

Pneumonia and Respiratory Diseases

Bordetella bronchiseptica and *Streptococcus pneumoniae* are the most important bacteria that cause respiratory disease in guinea pigs. *Klebsiella pneumoniae, Pasteurella multocida, Streptococcus zooepidemicus, Citrobacter freundii,* and *Pseudomonas aeruginosa* have also been implicated. *Bordetella* and *Streptococcus* may exist as latent respiratory infections until the animal is stressed. Disease and mortality occur most often during winter months. Younger animals and pregnant sows are at risk for disease. Affected animals may have no clinical signs or may exhibit dyspnea, nasal discharge, sneezing, and other nonspecific signs such as anorexia, ruffled fur, and weight loss or they may die suddenly. Pregnant sows may abort or produce stillborn offspring.

B. bronchiseptica typically produces gross lesions of rhinitis, tracheitis, and pulmonary consolidation. Purulent bronchitis and bronchopneumonia with large accumulations of neutrophils and intraluminal debris are typically seen on histopathology. Otitis media accompanied by head tilt may also occur with *Bordetella* infections. Chloramphenicol, sulfamethazine and trimethoprim-sulfa are antibiotics of choice; however, treatment is often unrewarding.

S. pneumoniae is the causative agent of diplococcal pneumonia. Fibrinous pleuritis, pericarditis, peritonitis, and marked consolidation of affected lung lobes are typical gross lesions. Otitis media, metritis, and other suppurative processes may also occur. Acute bronchopneumonia with fibrinous exudation and polymorphonuclear cell infiltration are typical microscopic changes. Treatment may be approached as with *Bordetella* infections. No cases of transmission from animals to humans have been documented; it should be noted, however, that *S. pneumoniae* can cause respiratory and meningeal disease in humans, particularly in the elderly and those immunocompromised.

Cervical Lymphadenitis

Cervical lymphadenitis, characterized by abscessation of the cervical lymph nodes, is commonly seen in guinea pigs. *Streptococcus zooepidemicus* of Lancefield's group C is the most common cause. *Streptobacillus moniliformis* and other *Streptococcus* spp., however, are sometimes implicated. The condition is commonly called lumps. Initially, the swollen lymph nodes are firm in consistency. As the disease progresses, the lymphatic tissue is replaced by thick, creamy, purulent exudate, resulting in prominent soft swellings in the ventral cervical region. The infection is spread by various routes, including bite wounds and abrasion of the oral mucosa by rough food. The animals generally do not appear to be sick or bothered by the abscessed lymph nodes. Sometimes an acute, fatal, septicemic disease or pneumonia may occur. Occasionally, otitis interna is seen. Treatment may include surgical incision; drainage and lavage of lesions with chlorhexidine or tincture of iodine; and systemic antibiotic therapy with chloramphenicol, enrofloxacin, ciprofloxacin, or trimethoprim-sulfa. Control is best accomplished by culling affected animals prior to rupture of lesions.

Salmonellosis

Salmonellosis is an infrequent but usually highly lethal disease in guinea pigs. *Salmonella typhimurium* and *Salmonella enteritidis* are the most common isolates. The most likely source of infection in a colony is the ingestion of contaminated water or food, especially fresh vegetables and fruit that have been inadequately washed before feeding.

Salmonellosis usually occurs as an acute to subacute fatal septicemia. Clinical signs may include anorexia, weight loss, light-colored soft feces, conjunctivitis, dyspnea, and abortion. Gross lesions may be absent at necropsy in peracute and acute cases. Massive splenomegaly frequently occurs along with yellow–white nodules in the spleen, liver, and other organs. Multifocal granulomatous hepatitis, splenitis, and lymphadenitis, with infiltration by histiocytic cells and polymorphs, are frequently seen. A definitive diagnosis depends on the presence of typical lesions on histopatholgy and on recovery of organisms from the spleen, blood, or feces.

Treatment is usually not recommended in an outbreak because of the danger of species and interspecies spread and zoonotic potential. The most prudent approach is to euthanize all affected and contact animals and disinfect the environment thoroughly.

Tyzzer's Disease

Spontaneous cases of Tyzzer's disease, caused by *Clostridium piliforme,* have been reported in guinea pigs. Immunocompromised, stressed, and young animals are at highest risk. Affected animals may have a rough haircoat, appear lethargic, have watery diarrhea, and die suddenly. Typical gross necropsy findings include a necrosis and inflammation of the ileum, cecum, and colon and multiple necrotic foci in the liver. Treatment with chloramphenicol or tetracycline may be attempted but is usually unrewarding.

Ulcerative Pododermatitis

Ulcerative pododermatitis, or bumblefoot, is frequently associated with *Staphylococcus* spp. infection. Predisposing factors include obesity and trauma to feet caused by rough, unsanitized flooring. Wire flooring is particularly troublesome. Guinea pigs have swollen, painful granulomatous lesions on the ventral surface of their forefeet. Affected animals should be moved to cages with solid floors and provided with soft, deep bedding. The feet can be treated with warm water soaks, topical antibiotics and/or povidone iodine, and bandaged. Amikacin can be used systemically; care should be taken to ensure the animal is well hydrated.

Mastitis

Bacterial mastitis is common in lactating sows. *Pasteurella* spp., *Klebsiella* spp., *Staphylococcus* spp., *Streptococcus* spp., and others have been implicated. The mammary glands become warm, enlarged, and hyperemic and may produce bloody milk. The young should be weaned immediately and appropriate antibiotic therapy instituted in the sow. Hot packs applied to the mammary glands are also helpful.

Conjunctivitis

Chlamydia psittaci is the causative agent of guinea pig inclusion conjunctivitis. Cyclic outbreaks of severe disease are common in enzootically infected colonies. Adult animals are frequently asymptomatic. Overt signs of disease are primarily seen in one to three week old guinea pigs. Transmission may be by direct contact or aerosol. Clinical signs include a reddened conjunctiva, serous to purulent exudate, and photophobia. Definitive diagnosis is made from microscopic exam of conjunctival scrapings and identification of cytoplasmic inclusion bodies in epithelial cells. The disease tends to be self-limiting, with lesions healing in 3 to 4 weeks. Ophthalmic ointments may be used to make the animal more comfortable. *C. psittaci* should be considered a potential human pathogen.

Other agents have been implicated to cause conjunctivitis in the guinea pig including *Streptococcus zooepidemicus,* coliforms, *Staphylococcus aureus,* and *Pasteurella multocida.* Concurrent infection with *C. psittaci* is a possibility.

Cystitis and Urolithiasis

Urinary tract infections occur particularly in older sows. Culture and sensitivity to determine appropriate antibiotic therapy is indicated. Occasionally, cystotomy is indicated for removal of a large urolith.

VIRAL DISEASES

Several viral agents such as Sendai, pneumonia virus of mice, and simian virus 5 have the ability to replicate briefly in the guinea pig. These agents do not cause apparent disease but can serve as a reservoir of virus for other rodents. Guinea pigs can develop lymphocytic choriomeningitis if inoculated with contaminated biologicals.

Cytomegalovirus

Cytomegalovirus (CMV) is a common pathogen of guinea pigs. It belongs to the herpesvirus family and is species specific. Infections rarely cause detectable clinical disease unless the animal is immunosuppressed or stressed. Sometimes the animal will exhibit swelling and tenderness of the salivary gland area. Transmission occurs through shedding of the virus in the saliva or urine or transplacentally. Cytomegalovirus produces characteristic large, intranuclear and intracytoplasmic inclusion bodies in the salivary glands. The virus may persist in the host for years as an inapparent or latent infection.

Cavian Leukemia and Lymphosarcoma

Cavian leukemia, caused by a type C oncornavirus, is widespread and usually transmitted transplacentally. The virus remains dormant in the animal until aging or stress triggers expression of disease. Affected animals exhibit lymphadenopathy, hepatomegaly, splenomegaly, rough haircoat, and an ascending paralysis. Anemia and leukocytosis are often found on blood exam.

Adenovirus

Cavian adenovirus has been associated with outbreaks of pneumonia. Clinical disease primarily occurs in the young or in animals that have been subjected to experimental manipulation.

PARASITIC DISEASES

Acariasis

Two species of mites, *Trixacarus caviae* and *Chirodiscoides caviae,* are the most common cause of acariasis in guinea pigs. *T. caviae* is a burrowing, sarcoptic mange mite that can produce alopecia, crusting, and severe pruritis that may lead to self-mutilation and debilitation. Severe infections can be fatal. Lesions are usually distributed on the neck, shoulders, lower abdomen, and inner thighs. The mite is often not readily detected by skin scrapings. *C. caviae,* a fur mite, causes few clinical signs. Lesions when present are concentrated in the lumbar region and lateral aspect of the hindquarters. Mites are spread by direct contact with the host, animal bedding, or hair and debris. Treatments include pyrethroid flea powder dusts, lime sulfur dips, and ivermectin.

Pediculosis

Gliricola porcelli and *Gyropus ovalis* are biting lice that cause occasional alopecia, rough haircoat, and mild pruritis. Lice are spread by direct contact with the host or by contaminated bedding. Treatments include pyrethroid flea powder dusts, lime sulfur dips, and ivermectin.

Protozoans

Eimeria caviae, the intestinal coccidia of guinea pigs, is usually nonpathogenic but occasionally causes colitis, diarrhea, and death. Recently weaned animals are primarily affected. The sporulation time is 3–10 days; thus, good sanitation will disrupt the life cycle of the parasite. Sulfonamides can be used to treat.

Cryptosporidium wrairi is a major cause of enteric disease in guinea pigs. Juvenile animals are most frequently affected. Clinical signs include lethargy, rough haircoat, diarrhea, weight loss, and emaciation. Affected animals often have a greasy-appearing haircoat. Transmission occurs through ingestion of oocysts in contaminated water, food, and fomites. At necropsy, the small and large intestines usually contain watery ingesta. Hyperemia of the small intestine and serosal edema of the cecum may be seen. Smears of fresh feces or mucosal scrapings examined with phase contrast microscopy are generally the best method of diagnosis.

There is no effective treatment; however, addition of sulfamethazine to the water supply has been reported to suppress outbreaks. The environment can be cleaned with 5% ammonia to destroy the oocysts. *Cryptosporidium* spp. are not species specific and are potentially zoonotic.

The cysts of *Balantidium caviae* are commonly found in the feces of guinea pigs, but the organism is relatively nonpathogenic. *Klossiella cobaye* is considered a nonpathogenic renal coccidian.

Nematode Infection

Paraspidodera uncinata are small worms that reside in the cecum of guinea pigs. Infections are usually considered insignificant; however, heavy infections can cause diarrhea and unthriftiness. Transmission is by ingestion of infective eggs. Sanitation is important in controlling infection. Piperazine or ivermectin are effective treatments.

NEOPLASIA

The prevalence of tumors in guinea pigs is very low even in aged animals. Cavian leukemia/lymphosarcoma is the most common, followed by trichofolliculomas and fibroadenomas. Genetic factors appear to play an important role in the incidence of neoplasia. Guinea pigs seem to be somewhat protected from neoplasia by Kurloff cells and the enzyme asparaginase, which has antitumor activity.

MISCELLANEOUS CONDITIONS

Alopecia

Hair pulling and barbering are common behaviors seen in guinea pigs. Animals may chew their own hair or that of a cagemate. The location of hair loss can usually provide a clue about whether it is self-inflicted or has resulted from barbering by a dominant cagemate. There is no specific treatment for barbering other than removing the offending animal from the group. Providing good quality hay may be of some benefit. Measures to reduce stress levels should also be considered.

Sows in advanced pregnancy and during lactation frequently exhibit a bilateral alopecia over the back and rump. Nutrition, genetic, and endocrine factors may be involved. Around the time of weaning, a thinning of hair occurs during the transition from baby fur to more mature hair.

Dermatophytosis

Trichophyton mentagrophytes is the most common cause of ringworm in the guinea pig. Clinical infections are uncommon; however, guinea pigs frequently harbor the organism asymptomatically. Stressed animals are susceptible. Irregular areas of alopecia usually arise on the face and spread to the trunk and limbs. The lesions may appear crusty or scaly. Microscopic exam of a skin scraping can be used in diagnosis. *T. mentagrophytes* does not fluoresce under ultraviolet light. Topical antifungal creams, griseofulvin in dimethyl sulfoxide applied topically, or griseofulvin administered orally can be used for treatment. *T. mentagrophytes* is infective to humans and other animals.

Trauma

The most commonly encountered traumatic injury in guinea pigs is fracture of the tibia. Animals, especially young, can catch their legs and fracture them when housed on wire flooring. With pet animals, fractures often result from being dropped by children. A simple lightweight splint can be made to provide support for the fracture.

Liver contusions with hemorrhage into the peritoneal cavity are occasionally seen in guinea pigs that are mishandled or dropped.

Malocclusion

☞ Tooth overgrowth in guinea pigs usually involves premolars and anterior molars. The condition is easily overlooked because the cheek teeth are difficult to see on clinical exam. Affected animals exhibit excessive salivation, halitosis, chronic weight loss, and tongue trauma. Malocclusion tends to be a lifelong problem and may require attention every few months. The offending teeth can be trimmed with pediatric rongeurs or a dental bur in a sedated or lightly anesthetized animal. Affected animals should not be bred, as there is a genetic predisposition to malocclusion.

Heat Stress

Guinea pigs are highly susceptible to heat stress. Heat stress may occur even in moderate temperatures if there is high humidity and/or if the area is poorly ventilated. Clinical signs include excessive salivation, rapid shallow breathing, hyperemia of extremities, and elevated body temperature. Rapid cooling with cool water or ice water, steroids, and supportive care may be attempted; however, treatment is often unrewarding.

Water Deprivation

Animals can die of water deprivation even when ample water seems to be available to them. This may occur when water is provided by a device with which the animal is unfamiliar; when water devices are placed too high or are inaccessible, particularly to weanlings; and when water is unpotable. Other reasons include automatic watering devices or sipper tubes that become inoperable from plugging with foreign objects or air locks, and territorialism by dominant individuals that prevents subordinate animals from drinking.

Scurvy

☞ The guinea pig requires an exogenous source of vitamin C owing to a genetic deficiency of the enzyme L-gulonolactone oxidase, which is involved in the conversion of L-gulonolactone to L-ascorbic acid. Vitamin C deficiency frequently occurs when guinea pigs are fed rabbit chow or outdated and/or improperly stored guinea pig chow. A commercially available guinea pig diet that has been stored in a cool, dry place should be provided and used within 90 days of the milling date. Guinea pig diet should provide 15–20 mg of vitamin C per kg of body weight for maintenance. Signs of scurvy usually appear within 2 weeks after guinea pigs have been deprived of vitamin C. Clinical signs include reluctance to move, unkempt appearance, swelling around the joints, and infrequently diarrhea. The most prominent gross lesions seen at necropsy are hemorrhages in the muscle and periosteum, particularly around the stifle joint and rib cage, and epiphyseal enlargement at the costochondral junction. Affected guinea pigs should receive 50 mg/kg per day of oral or parenteral ascorbic acid until recovery is evident.

Circumanal Sebaceous Accumulations

Excessive accumulations of sebaceous secretions occur in the folds of the circumanal and genital region in adult male guinea pigs. The sebaceous secretions can also form a plug that accumulates in the folds between the two halves of the scrotum. These folds must be cleansed periodically with soap and water to preclude infection and unpleasant odors.

Preputial Infection and Vaginitis

Male guinea pigs occasionally develop preputial infections caused by lodging of foreign material in the preputial folds. Breeding males housed on bedding may be affected when pieces of bedding adhere to the moist prepuce following copulation and are drawn into the preputial fornix. Treatment involves removing the bedding particles and cleansing the area.

Vaginitis in female guinea pigs is usually caused by entrapment of wood chips or other bedding material in the vagina, causing a foreign body reaction. The problem is corrected by washing the area carefully and swabbing away the bedding material. It may be desirable to place the animal on a different type of bedding until the area has healed.

Dystocia

The most common cause of dystocia is incomplete relaxation of the pubic symphysis due to fusion and ossification of the pubic symphysis. Normally, 2–24 hours before parturition the pubic symphysis of a pregnant sow becomes separated, allowing the birth canal to increase in diameter. If sows are not initially bred prior to 7 months of age, the pubic symphysis will often fuse and ossify. Dystocia can also result from an excessively large or malformed fetus, large litter, obesity, pregnancy toxemia, and uterine inertia. Uterine inertia may respond to oxytocin; however, if parturition has not begun within 15 minutes after administration, a cesarean section should be performed.

Pregnancy Toxemia (Ketosis)

There are two different patterns of disease associated with pregnancy toxemia in the guinea pig—the fasting or metabolic form and the circulatory or toxic form. The clinical signs are similar, and both forms usually occur in late pregnancy. Animals exhibit depression, acidosis, ketosis, proteinuria, and ketonuria. They produce clear urine with pH lowered from around 9 to 5–6.

The fasting or metabolic form, referred to as ketosis, occurs in obese sows during the last 2–3 weeks of pregnancy. Sows during their first or second pregnancy are more frequently affected. Stress factors such as changes in feeding routines or environment may precipitate the disease. Affected animals usually become comatose and die within 5–6 days after onset of symptoms. A similar condition may be observed in obese, aged males. A reduced carbohydrate intake with subsequent mobilization of fat as a source of energy apparently is involved. Lesions seen at necropsy include fatty liver, fatty kidneys, ample fat stores, and an empty stomach. Treatments that may be tried include lactated Ringer's solution, calcium gluconate, propylene glycol, 5% glucose, and corticosteroids; however, prognosis is poor. The incidence can be reduced in breeding sows by controlling food intake to prevent obesity and by breeding at a body weight of 450–500 g. Breeding sows should not be disturbed by changing diets, moving to new quarters, or other factors that might induce fasting.

In the circulatory or toxic form, a large gravid uterus compresses the aorta caudal to the renal vessels, which causes uteroplacental ischemia. Blood pressure is reduced in the uterine vessels, causing placental necrosis and hemorrhage, thrombocytopenia, ketosis, and death. The guinea pig has been identified as a possible animal model for preeclampsia in pregnant women.

Gastric Dilation, Cecal Torsion, Typhlitis

Gastric dilation, cecal torsion, and acute typhlitis occur sporadically in guinea pigs of all ages. Animals are usually found dead with no previous indication of disease.

Diabetes Mellitus

A spontaneous diabetes mellitus that occurs in animals 3–6 months of age has been reported. Affected animals are not clinically ill but have hyperglycemia, glycosuria, and rarely ketonuria. Exogenous insulin is not required for survival. An infectious agent is thought to be involved.

Soft Tissue Calcification

Soft tissue or metastatic calcification occurs most often in guinea pigs over 1 year of age. Affected animals may be unthrifty and exhibit muscle stiffness or lameness. Mineral deposition may be confined to the soft tissue around the elbows and ribs or may be more widespread to the lung, trachea, heart, aorta, liver, kidney, stomach, uterus, and sclera. This syndrome is thought to be attributable to a dietary imbalance of two or more minerals, e.g., low magnesium and high phosphorus. Multiple linear chalky deposits on affected organs can be seen grossly at necropsy.

Nutritional Muscular Dystrophy

A myopathy has been associated with vitamin E/selenium deficiency. Clinical signs may include depression, hind limb weakness, conjunctivitis, and reduced reproductive performance in sows. Affected animals usually have elevated serum creatine phosphokinase (CPK) levels. Treatment with vitamin E/selenium injections may be of benefit.

Aging

Multiple ovarian cysts, fatty infiltration of the pancreas, and segmental nephrosclerosis are frequently observed at necropsy of aged animals.

■ GENERAL REFERENCES

Sources consulted to compile the material in this chapter include *The Biology of the Guinea Pig,* edited by J.E. Wagner and P.J. Manning (1976, Academic Press, Inc., Orlando, FL 32887); *The Biology and Medicine of Rabbits and Rodents* by J.E. Harkness and J.E. Wagner, 4th edition (1995, Williams & Wilkins, 1400 North Providence Rd., Building II, Suite 5025, Media, PA 19063); *Laboratory Animal Medicine* by J.G. Fox, B.J. Cohen, and F.M. Loew (1984, Academic Press, Orlando, FL 32887); *The UFAW Handbook on the Care and Management of Laboratory Animals,* 6th edition, edited by T.B. Poole (1987, Churchill Livingstone Inc., 1560 Broadway, New York, NY 10036); and *Pathology of Laboratory Rodents and Rabbits* by D.H. Percy and S.W. Barthold (1993, Iowa State University Press, 2121 South State Avenue, Ames, IA 50014).

■ TECHNICAL REFERENCES

Allen, D.G., J.K. Pringle, and D.A. Smith. 1993. *Handbook of Veterinary Drugs.* Philadelphia: JB Lippincott.

Anderson, N.L. 1994. Basic husbandry and medicine of pocket pets. In *Saunders Manual of Small Animal Practice,* ed. S.J. Birchard and R.G. Sherding, pp. 1363–1389. Philadelphia: WB Saunders.

Borchard, R.E., C.D. Barnes, and L.G. Eltherington. 1990. *Drug Dosage in Laboratory Animals: A Handbook,* 3rd ed. Caldwell, NJ: The Telford Press.

Brown, J.N., P.R. Thorne, and A.L. Nuttall. 1989. Blood pressure and other physiological responses in awake and anesthetized guinea pigs. *Lab Anim Sci* 39: 142–148.

Burgmann, P. and D.H. Percy. 1993. Antimicrobial drug use in rodents and rabbits. In *Antimicrobial Therapy in Veterinary Medicine,* 2nd ed., ed. J.F. Prescott and J.D. Baggot, pp. 524–541. Ames: Iowa State University Press.

Collins, B.R. 1995. Antimicrobial drug use in rabbits, rodents, and other small mammals. In *Antimicrobial Therapy in Caged Birds and Exotic Pets,* pp. 3–10. Trenton, NJ: Veterinary Learning Systems.

Flecknell, P.A. 1987. *Laboratory Animal Anesthesia.* London: Academic.

Flecknell, P.A. 1997. Medetomidine and atipamezole: Potential uses in laboratory animals. *Lab Anim* 26(2): 21–25.

Gilroy, B.A. and J.S. Varga. 1980. Ketamine-diazepam and ketamine-xylazine combinations in guinea pigs. *Vet Med Small Anim Clin* 75(3): 508–509.

Harkness, J.E. 1993. *A Practitioner's Guide to Domestic Rodents.* Lakewood, CO: American Animal Hospital Association.

Harrenstien, L. 1994. Critical care of ferrets, rabbits, and rodents. *Semin Avian Exotic Pet Med* 3: 217–228.

Heard, D.J. 1993. Principles and techniques of anesthesia and analgesia for exotic practice. *Vet Clin North Am Small Anim Pract* 23: 1301–1327.

Huerkamp, M.J. 1995. Anesthesia and postoperative management of rabbits and pocket pets. In *Kirk's Current Therapy XII: Small Animal Practice,* ed. J.D. Bonagura, pp. 1322–1327. Philadelphia: WB Saunders.

Johnson-Delaney, C.A. 1996. *Exotic Companion Medicine Handbook for Veterinarians.* Lake Worth, FL: Wingers.

Leash, A.M., R.D. Beyer, and R.G. Wilber. 1973. Self-mutilation following Innovar-Vet injection in the guinea pig. *Lab Anim Sci* 23(5): 720–721.

McKellar, Q.A., D.M. Midgley, E.A. Galbraith, E.W. Scott, and A. Bradley. 1992. Clinical and pharmacological properties of ivermectin in rabbits and guinea pigs. *Vet Rec* 130: 71–73.

Mason, D.E. 1997. Anesthesia, analgesia, and sedation for small mammals. In *Ferrets, Rabbits, and Rodents: Clinical Medicine and Surgery,* ed. E. V. Hillyer and K. E. Quesenberry, pp. 378–391. Philadelphia: WB Saunders.

Nakatani, T., Y. Suzuki, K. Yoshida, and H. Sinohara. 1995. Molecular cloning and sequence analysis of cDNA encoding plasma alpha-1 antiproteinase from Syrian hamster: implications for the evolution of Rodentia. *Biochem Biophys Acta* 1263(3) Sept 19: 245–248.

Quesenberry, K.E. 1994. Guinea pigs. *Vet Clin North Am Small Anim Pract* 24: 67–87.

Richardson, V.C.G. 1992. *Diseases of Domestic Guinea Pigs.* Oxford: Blackwell Scientific.

Schaeffer, D.O. and T.M. Donnelly. 1997. Disease problems of guinea pigs and chinchillas. In *Ferrets, Rabbits, and Rodents: Clinical Medicine and Surgery,* ed. E. V. Hillyer and K. E. Quesenberry, pp. 260–281. Philadelphia: WB Saunders.

Timm, K.I., S.E. Jahn, and C.J. Sedgwick. 1987. The palatal ostium of the guinea pig. *Lab Anim Sci* 37(6): 801–802.

White, W.J. and K.J. Field. 1987. Anesthesia and surgery of laboratory animals. *Vet Clin North Am Small Anim Pract* 17(5): 989–1017.

Wixson, S.K. 1994. Rabbits and rodents: anesthesia and analgesia. In *Research Animal Anesthesia, Analgesia and Surgery,* ed. A.C. Smith and M.M. Swindle, pp. 59–92. Greenbelt, MD: Scientists Center for Animal Welfare.

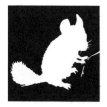

CHINCHILLAS

THE CHINCHILLA is a hystricomorph (hedgehoglike) rodent closely related to porcupines, guinea pigs, and agoutis. It belongs to the family Chinchillidae. The two most common species are *Chinchilla brevicaudata,* the short-tailed chinchilla, and *Chinchilla laniger,* the long-tailed chinchilla. Specific information in this chapter refers to *Chinchilla laniger.* Chinchillas were originally native to South America, where they inhabited the rocky slopes of the Andes Mountains in Peru, Bolivia, Chile, and Argentina. They were so extensively hunted for their pelts that they are now practically extinct in the wild. Fortunately, chinchillas have been successfully bred in captivity. Chinchillas resemble squirrels in appearance. Adults weigh from 400 to 600 g, with females being slightly larger than males. They are 2.5–35 cm (10–14 in.) in length. The standard color is a smoky blue–gray that ranges from very light to very dark. Selective breeding has produced a number of color mutations including beige, white, black, brown, silver, and violet.

Uses

Chinchillas are primarily raised for the fur trade. Recently, they have become more popular as pets. They are virtually odorless, easy to maintain, and have a charming, inquisitive temperament. Chinchillas are unsuitable pets for younger children, as they do not become as tame and trusting as a guinea pig.

The chinchilla is a popular animal for auditory studies. Their small size, ease of handling, presence of a cochlea that has three turns as does the human cochlea, and an auditory sensitivity similar to that of humans are positive attributes for auditory research. There is an absence of presbycusis in long-term studies and lack of susceptibility to naturally occurring middle ear infections. In addition, they have large bullae surrounded by thin bone that allows easy surgical access to the middle ear, cochlea, and surrounding structures.

Behavior

In their native environment, chinchillas live in groups in rock crevices or burrows at elevations above 800 m (2600 ft). They are social animals, with family groups of two to five sharing the same burrow. They rarely fight, although females can be quite aggressive toward strange males during breeding. Although they are normally nocturnal, chinchillas can be active during the day. They love to climb and jump. Most chinchillas like to be cuddled and carried. They are very dexterous, using their front paws as hands when eating. Chinchillas have different vocalizations but generally make very little noise. They will coo when content, bark when alarmed, spit and growl when very upset, and emit a babylike cry when they are frightened or injured. They do not hibernate.

Anatomic and Physiologic Features

Chinchilla biologic and reproductive data can be found in Table 6.1. Chinchillas have compact bodies covered with very soft, thick fur and have bushy tails. The palms and soles of their feet are devoid of fur. They have large eyes, large batlike ears, and long whiskers. Their coat grows in waves, starting at the head and moving back to the tail. The position of a pale bar line in the fur indicates the stage of growth of the fur. The pelt is most valuable when the bar line is at the end of the hair all over the body. The thymus gland is entirely intrathoracic. The dental formula is 2 (1/1, 0/0, 1/1, 3/3). The chinchilla's teeth are open rooted and grow throughout life. The incisors are yellowish in contrast to the molars, which are cream colored. The oral cavity is narrow and primarily filled by the tongue. The chinchilla has a palate like that of the guinea pig. The gastrointestinal tract is remarkably long. The jejunum nearly fills the entire abdomen, the cecum is large, and the proximal colon is highly sacculated, in contrast to the terminal colon, which is smooth. Typical of rodents, chinchillas are coprophagic.

Sexing chinchillas can be difficult, as the external genitalia of males and females appear similar. The female's prominent, cone-shaped clitoris may be mistaken for a penis at quick glance. Males have a longer anogenital distance and larger genital papilla. In the male, there is no true scrotum. The testicles are located in the inguinal canals or subcutaneously in the anal region. The female chinchilla is unique in that the vagina has a separate external opening between the rectum and urethral openings. The female has two uterine horns, each opening separately into the cervix, and three pairs of mammary glands.

Table 6.1. Chinchilla biologic and reproductive data	
Adult body weight	
Male	400–500 g
Female	400–600 g
Life span	10–18 y
Body temperature	37°–38° C (98.6°–100.4°F)
Heart rate	150 beats per minute
Respiratory rate	45–65 breaths per minute
Food consumption	21 g/d
Water consumption	—
Breeding onset	
Male	7–9 mo
Female	7–9 mo
Estrous cycle length	41 d
Gestation period	111 d
Postpartum estrus	Fertile
Litter size	2
Weaning age	6–8 wk
Breeding duration	3 y
Chromosome number (diploid)	64

Source: Adapted from Williams (1976), Hoefer (1994), and Merry (1990).

There are several distinctive characteristics of the hematologic and urinary profiles of chinchillas. Approximate blood values include a normal packed cell volume of 40%, eight million red blood cells, and 9500 white blood cells. The lymphocyte is the predominant white blood cell. A seasonal effect on hematologic values of laboratory-adapted chinchillas has been reported. The red blood cell count and hemoglobin levels are highest in the winter season. The white blood cell count is highest in the winter and early spring when reproductive processes increase. Urine is normally alkaline, with a pH of 8.5, and contains varying amounts of calcium carbonate crystals. The specific gravity often exceeds 1.045. White and red blood cells are normally not present in the urine, and casts are rare. The presence of a few squamous epithelial cells are normal, especially in females. Selected hematologic and biochemical values are listed in Appendix 1, Normal Values.

Breeding and Reproduction

Puberty occurs from 4 to 18 months of age, depending upon the time of the year the chinchilla is born. If young are born in the spring, puberty occurs in the fall and if born in the fall, puberty occurs approximately one year later. The chinchilla is seasonally polyestrous, with the main breeding season occurring between November and May. A harem system is generally used whereby one male has access to as many as five females. The females are very aggressive toward the male. A collared method is normally used to prevent the female from exiting her home cage and injuring the male. The estrous cycle lasts 41 days. The vagina is covered by the vaginal closure membrane except during estrus and parturition. Breeding occurs at night and is characterized by multiple intromissions. Ovulation is usually spontaneous. Detection of a vaginal plug either in the female or on the cage floor is a reliable indicator that mating has occurred. Vaginal plugs may be up to 3.75 cm (1.5 in.) long. Gestation is lengthy, 111 days. A postpartum estrus occurs 2–48 hours after parturition, and a postlactational estrus, 35–84 days after parturition.

The normal litter size is two, but may be as high as five. There is a disproportionate number of males born, with the ratio being 119 males to 110 females. The young are born precocious, fully furred, with teeth, and their eyes and ears open. The female chinchilla does not make a nest. If young appear chilled, it may be helpful to warm part of the cage flooring with a heating pad placed underneath it. Milk letdown is sometimes a problem. An injection of oxytocin can be given to help stimulate milk letdown. Young begin to eat solid food within 1 week of birth. The dust bath should be removed from cages with newborn litters so that the newborns will not get dust in their mouths and eyes. Generally, chinchillas are weaned when they are 6–8 weeks of age, but can be weaned as early as 3 weeks of age.

HUSBANDRY

Housing

☞ Chinchillas are active animals that enjoy climbing and jumping. Multilevel cages work well to accommodate their activity level. Chinchillas are usually housed individually in cages with wire-mesh or solid flooring. Solid-bottom cages with bedding material are better for group housing, harem mating, and females with young. White pine or hardwood chips are satisfactory bedding materials. Cedar chips or sawdust should not be used. If wire-mesh flooring is used, the mesh should be of small enough gauge, for example 15 mm × 15 mm, to prevent limb injuries. A cage that is 41 × 46 × 31 cm (16 × 18 × 12 in.) is big enough to house one chinchilla. A gnawing stone to wear down the teeth is available commercially and should be placed in the cage. Alternatively, fresh branches from willow, beech, hazelnut, or unsprayed fruit trees can also be used. Housing conditions ideally should include a temperature of

16°–21° C (61°–70°F), a humidity between 30% and 60%, 10–15 air changes per hour, and 12 hours of light per day. If they are kept in a dry, nondrafty environment, chinchillas can tolerate low temperatures just above freezing. It is important to avoid an environment with poor ventilation and high temperatures and humidity, as chinchillas are heat sensitive. Cages and feeding and watering receptacles should be cleaned weekly. They should be disinfected with chemicals, hot water 61.6°–82.2°C (143°–180°F), or a combination of both. Detergents and chemical disinfectants enhance the effectiveness of hot water, but they must be thoroughly rinsed from all caging surfaces with fresh water. Refer to Chapter 1, Mice, for a more detailed description of disinfection methods.

☞ Dust baths are an important part of the chinchilla's grooming habit and are necessary to maintain a good appearance. The dust baths help to absorb skin oils. Chinchillas should be provided with a pan filled with 2–3 cm of dust several times weekly. Sanitized chinchilla dust is available commercially. Silver sand and Fuller's earth at a 9:1 ratio can also be used. Playground sand or talc are not recommended. The pan should be removed after an hour or so after the chinchilla has rolled in the dust and fluffed its fur. It is important to keep the dust clean and free of feces.

Feeding and Watering

Chinchillas should be fed a commercial pelleted chinchilla chow that contains 16%–20% protein, 2%–5% fat, and approximately 18% fiber. The pellets should contain a minimum of 2700 cal/kg of diet. Guinea pig or rabbit chow is adequate. Adult chinchillas eat an average of 21 g of food per day. Thus, it is only necessary to feed a small amount of pellets, 1 to 2 tablespoons, each day. Chinchillas will spill food and overturn bowls, so it is best to use a self-feeder or counterweighted feeder attached to the cage. Good quality grass hay, such as timothy or alfalfa, which is free of mold and insecticides should be fed ad libitum. Cubed hay can be placed directly on the floor of the cage. Loose hay is best provided in a hay rack. The diet can be supplemented with small amounts of fresh apple or other fruit, oatmeal, raisins, carrots, and sunflower seeds. Excessive supplementation can result in obesity and digestive tract upsets and should be avoided. Dietary changes should be done slowly to avoid enteric problems. Chinchillas should be provided with fresh, potable water ad libitum by bottle or automatic watering system.

TECHNIQUES

Handling and Restraint

Chinchillas are easy to handle and respond best to a light touch and gentle approach. They are not aggressive biters, but will bite if agitated. To carry a chinchilla a short distance, lift it by the base of the tail and place the animal on the opposite forearm, up against the body with its head toward the elbow. To restrain a chinchilla, grasp the base of the tail with one hand and place the other hand over the shoulders and thorax. ☞ Figure 6.1 depicts this restraint technique. Care must be taken to avoid grasping or roughly handling the fur, for this can result in the loss of a patch of fur. This is called fur slip. Chinchillas should never be picked up by their ears.

Identification

Cage cards are most often used as a form of general identification. There are several permanent methods to identify chinchillas individually, including ear tagging or tattooing and placement of a microchip subcutaneously for quick electronic identification. Dyes or markers can be used as temporary identification methods.

Blood Collection

Table 6.2 lists approximate adult chinchilla blood volumes. Small amounts of blood can be collected from a toenail clip, foot puncture using a sterile needle, and peripheral veins such as the lateral saphenous, cephalic, or tail vein. The ear vein can also be used but is not recom-

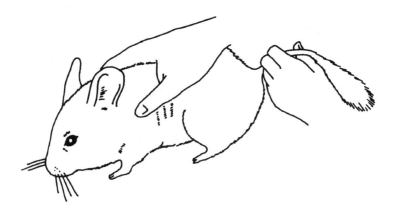

Figure 6.1. Restraint of the chinchilla.

Table 6.2. Adult chinchilla blood volumes

	Volume (mL)[a]
Total blood	20–32
Single sample	2–3
Exsanguination	8–12

Source: Adapted from Merry (1990).
[a]Values are approximate.

mended for repetitive sampling. Larger quantities of blood can be collected from the jugular vein. The orbital sinus, transverse (cranial) sinus, and cardiac puncture can also be used with anesthesia. Cardiac sampling involves a significant element of risk.

Urine Collection

Urine can be collected using a metabolic cage, gentle digital pressure on the bladder, or clean-catch method. Chinchillas that are annoyed will usually urinate, projecting their urine with accuracy for several feet.

Drug Administration

Palatable drugs can be incorporated into the food or water. If medications are unpalatable, 5 mL of sugar or syrup per liter can be added to the drinking water to improve the palatability. Liquids can be administered orally using an eyedropper or small syringe. Subcutaneous injections with a maximum volume of 8 mL per site can be given dorsally between the shoulders or in the flank area. Intramuscular injections can be given in the rear leg using the quadriceps or semitendinosus muscle. Smaller-gauge needles, such as 23 to 25 gauge, should be used for intramuscular injections, and no more than 0.3 mL of a solution should be administered in one site. The intraperitoneal route can also be used for volumes up to 10 mL. Intravenous injections are difficult but possible to do using the small peripheral vessels in the ears or legs.

Anesthesia, Surgery, and Postoperative Care

A variety of agents that can be used to tranquilize and anesthetize chinchillas are listed in Table 6.3. Food should be withheld from chinchillas for 6 hours prior to anesthesia. Atropine can be administered to dry mucous secretions 15 minutes before the induction of anesthesia. Several injectable agents can be used for anesthesia in chinchillas. Ketamine can be administered alone for short procedures and mixed with acetylpromazine or xylazine for longer and/or more painful procedures.

Table 6.3. Anesthetic agents and tranquilizers used in chinchillas

Drug	Dosage	Route	Reference
Inhalants			
Halothane	To effect	Inhalation	Hoefer (1994)
Isoflurane	To effect	Inhalation	Hoefer (1994)
Methoxyflurane	To effect	Inhalation	Hoefer (1994)
Injectables			
Alphadolone-alphaxalone	20–30 mg/kg	IM	Green (1982)
Diazepam	2.5 mg/kg	IP	Green (1982)
Fentanyl-droperidol	0.20 mL/kg	IM	Green (1982)
Ketamine	40 mg/kg	IM	Anderson (1994)
Ketamine	40 mg/kg	IM	Hoefer (1994)
+ acetylpromazine	0.5 mg/kg	IM	
Ketamine	20–40 mg/kg	IM	Hoefer (1994)
+ diazepam	1–2 mg/kg	IM	
Ketamine	20 mg/kg	IP, IM	Flecknell (1987)
+ diazepam	5 mg/kg	IP, IM	
Ketamine	20–40 mg/kg	IM	Clark (1984)
+ pentobarbital	30–40 mg/kg	IP	
Ketamine	30–40 mg/kg	IM	Anderson (1994)
+ xylazine	4–8 mg/kg		
Pentobarbital	30 mg/kg	IV	Hoefer (1994)
	40 mg/kg	IP	Hoefer (1994)
Tiletamine-zolazepam	20–40 mg/kg	IM	Hoefer (1994)

IM = intramuscular; IP = intraperitoneal; IV = intravenous.

A ketamine and pentobarbital combination can also be used. Pentobarbital is reported to be short acting in the chinchilla. Ophthalmic ointment should be used in the eyes of chinchillas anesthetized with ketamine or ketamine combinations, as their eyes will remain open and unblinking.

Inhalation anesthetic agents can be given via a chamber or face mask. Isoflurane is recommended, but halothane and methoxyflurane can also be used. A nose cone or face mask is generally used to maintain anesthesia, as chinchillas are very difficult to intubate. Care should be used during induction because some chinchillas hold their breath and then will take deep rapid breaths of the anesthetic agent. This can result in death if the concentration of anesthetic gases is high. The use of ophthalmic ointment is recommended to prevent drying of the ocular membranes by the anesthetic gases. Care should be taken to scavenge waste anesthetic gases for the safety of personnel in the area. A combination of reflexes should be used to monitor the depth of anesthesia.

Two of the most common surgical interventions performed in pet chinchillas include a simple castration and opening and drainage of an abscess. Males have open inguinal canals that require closure during castration. A number of surgical procedures involving the auditory system are commonly performed for research.

Surgery should be done in an aseptic manner. Postoperative care should include hydration, a method to prevent hypothermia, turning a nonambulatory animal every 30 minutes to prevent hypostatic pulmonary congestion, and stimulation to return to normal feeding. Analgesics should be administered when pain is observed or expected to occur. Table 6.4 lists analgesics that can be used in this species. Analgesic doses for the most part have not been studied in chinchillas; however, guinea pig doses can probably be used.

Table 6.4. Analgesia agents used in chincillas

Drug	Dosage	Route	Reference
Acetylsalicylic acid	100-200 mg/kg q6-8h	PO	Johnson-Delaney (1996)
Butorphanol	0.2 mg/kg	IM	Harkness (1993)
Meperidine	10-20 mg/kg q6h	IM, SC	Smith and Burgmann (1997)

IM = intramuscular; PO = per os; SC = subcutaneous.

Euthanasia

Chinchillas may be euthanized with inhalation anesthetic agent overdose, by injection of pentobarbital or other euthanasia solution given by the intravenous or intraperitoneal route, or with carbon dioxide (approximately 70%) in a prefilled chamber. Refer to Chapter 1, Mice, for a more detailed description of euthanasia methods.

THEREAPEUTIC AGENTS

Suggested chinchilla antimicrobial and antifungal drug dosages are listed in Table 6.5. Antiparasitic agents are listed in Table 6.6, and miscellaneous agents are listed in Table 6.7.

Table 6.5. Antimicrobial and antifungal agents used in chinchillas

Drug	Dosage	Route	Reference
Amikacin	2 mg/kg q8h	SC, IM, IV	Hoefer (1994)
Captan powder (Orthocide)	1 tsp/2 cups dust, add to dust box	Topical	Hoefer (1994)
Cephalosporin	25–100 mg/kg q6h	PO	Johnson-Delaney (1996)
Chloramphenicol	50 mg/kg q12h	PO	Collins (1995)
	50 mg/kg q12h	SC, IM	Hoefer (1994)
Ciprofloxacin	5–15 mg/kg q12h	PO	Smith and Burgmann (1997)
Doxycycline	2.5 mg/kg q12h	PO	Johnson-Delaney (1996)
Enrofloxacin	10 mg/kg q12h	SC, IM, PO	Hoefer (1994)
Gentamicin	2 mg/kg q8h	SC, IM, IV	Hoefer (1994)
Griseofulvin	25 mg/kg q24h for 30–60 d	PO	Jenkins (1992)
Lime sulfur dip	Dilute 1:40 with water, dip q7d for 6 wk	Topical	Anderson (1994)
Neomycin	15 mg/kg q24h	PO	Burgmann and Percy (1993)
Oxytetracycline	50 mg/kg q12h	PO	Collins (1995)
Sulfadimethoxine	25–50 mg/kg q24h for 10–14 d	PO	Smith and Burgmann (1997)
Sulfamerazine	1 mg/mL drinking water		Anderson (1994)
Sulfmethazine	1 mg/mL drinking water		Anderson (1994)
Tetracycline	0.3–2 mg/mL drinking water		Burgmann and Percy (1993)
	50 mg/kg q8–12h	PO	Burgmann and Percy (1993)
Trimethoprim-sulfa	30 mg/kg q12h	PO, IM	Hoefer (1994)
Tylosin	10 mg/kg q24h	PO, SC, IM	Collins (1995)

IM = intramuscular; IV = intravenous; PO = per os; SC = subcutaneous.

Table 6.6. Antiparasitic agents used in chinchillas

Drug	Dosage	Route	Reference
Carbaryl powder (5%)	Dust q7d for 3 wk	Topical	Anderson (1994)
Fenbendazole	20 mg/kg q24h for 5 d	PO	Johnson-Delaney (1996)
Ivermectin	0.2 mg/kg q7d for 3 wk	PO, SC	Anderson (1994)
Metronidazole	50–60 mg/kg q12h for 5 d	PO	Harkness (1993)
Piperazine citrate`	100 mg/kg q24h for 2 d	PO	Johnson-Delaney (1996)
Praziquantel	5–10 mg/kg, repeat in 10 d	PO, SC, IM	Smith and Burgmann (1997)
Pyrethrin powder	Dust q7d for 3 wk	Topical	Anderson (1994)
Thiabendazole	50–100 mg/kg q24h for 5 d	PO	Allen (1993)

IM - intramuscular; PO = per os; SC = subcutaneous.

Table 6.7. Miscellaneous agents used in chinchillas

Drug	Dosage	Route	Reference
Atropine	0.05 mg/kg	SC, IM	Merry (1990)
Calcium-EDTA	30 mg/kg q12h	SC	Hoefer (1994)
Cimetidine	5–10 mg/kg q6–12h	IM, PO, SC	Smith and Burgmann (1997)
Dexamethasone	0.6 mg/kg	IM	Anderson (1994)
Doxapram	5–10 mg/kg	IP, IV	Harkness (1993)
Furosemide	1–4 mg/kg q4–6h	IM	Harrenstien (1994)
Metoclopramide	0.5 mg/kg q8h	SC	Johnson-Delaney (1996)
Oxytocin	0.2–3 IU/kg	SC, IM, IV	Anderson (1994)
Prednisone	0.5–2.2 mg/kg	SC, IM	Anderson (1994)
Vitamin B complex	0.02–0.2 mL/kg	SC, IM	Anderson (1994)
Vitamin K	1–10 mg/kg	IM	Johnson and Delaney (1996)
Yohimbine	2.1 mg/kg	IP	Hargett et al. (1989)

EDTA = ethylenediaminetetracetic acid; IM = intramuscular; IP = intraperitoneal; IV = intravenous; SC = subcutaneous.

BACTERIAL DISEASES

Respiratory Disease

Pasteurella spp., *Bordetella* spp., *Streptococcus* spp., and *Pseudomonas aeruginosa* alone or in combination can cause respiratory disease in chinchillas. Symptoms may include anorexia, depression, nasal discharge, and dyspnea. Predisposing factors include overcrowding, high humidity, poor ventilation, and stress. Tetracycline is the antibiotic of choice except for *P. aeruginosa* infections when it is best to use gentamicin. Prognosis is poor if chronic respiratory disease is present.

Bite Wounds and Abscess Formation

Bite wounds with secondary abscess formation can be seen in chinchillas housed in group arrangements. *Streptococcus* spp. and *Staphylococcus* spp. are most commonly involved. The wounds and/or abscesses should be drained and surgically debrided. Antibiotic therapy based upon culture and sensitivity is indicated. Chloramphenicol is a good antibiotic to initiate therapy.

Enteritis

Enteritis is a common finding in chinchillas and can usually be traced to poor management. A number of conditions may be involved including colic, intussusception, diarrhea, mucoid enteritis, fecal impaction, and rectal prolapse. *Pseudomonas* spp., *Pasteurella* spp., *Proteus* spp., *Salmonella* spp., and *Escherichia coli* are frequently involved.

127

These organisms can also cause a septicemia with or without enteritis. Affected animals can be listless, dehydrated, produce soft or liquid feces, or have an absence of feces. Onset is often acute, which makes it difficult to treat. Predisposing factors include a sudden diet change, inappropriate or prolonged antibiotic use, overcrowding, stress, and diets too low in fiber and too high in fat and protein. Antibiotic therapy and fluid replacement are recommended for treatment. Gentamicin, sulfonamides, and neomycin are antibiotics of choice for enteritis.

Enterotoxemia

Clostridium perfringens, type D, has been reported to cause disease in chinchillas. The highest incidence occurs in young animals, 2–4 months of age. Animals may be found dead without signs of illness or may have diarrhea and appear to be experiencing abdominal pain. Enterotoxemia has been prevented by immunization with toxoid.

Antibiotic Toxicity

☞ Care should be taken when selecting antibiotics to use in chinchillas, as many agents can suppress normal gut flora. Antimicrobials that have a selective gram-positive spectrum, such as clindamycin, lincomycin, erythromycin, and ampicillin, should be avoided. Changes in enteric pH or normal gut flora can result in bacterial overgrowth and enterotoxemia. *Clostridium* spp. can produce enterotoxemia resulting in severe diarrhea and acute death. Broad spectrum antibiotics used for short periods of time are less likely to upset the normal gut flora.

Daily feeding of 5 mL of flavored yogurt to chinchillas undergoing antibiotic therapy has been reported to help replenish favorable gut flora. Providing an oral electrolyte solution such as those used for human infants may also be beneficial.

Pseudomonas Infections

Chinchillas appear to be very susceptible to *Pseudomonas aeruginosa.* They are most often infected by contaminated drinking water. Clinical symptoms may include conjunctivitis, otitis, pneumonia, dermal pustules, enteritis, mesenteric lymphadenopathy, metritis, and septicemia with acute death. Foci of necrosis are most commonly seen in the liver, kidney, and spleen at necropsy along with other general signs of septicemia. Gentamicin may be used to treat individual animals. Prevention includes chlorination of the drinking water to 10 ppm or acidifying the drinking water to a pH of 2.5–3.

Listeriosis

Chinchillas are highly susceptible to infection with *Listeria monocytogenes*. The disease can be sporadic in a colony or produce high mortality. All ages are affected, and encephalitic and enteric forms of the disease are seen. Clinical signs may include anorexia, malaise, diarrhea, depression, ataxia, circling, convulsions, and paralysis. The disease is usually peracute in chinchillas, with death occurring within 48–72 hours after onset of signs. Treatment with chloramphenicol or tetracycline can be attempted; however, it is generally unrewarding because affected animals die so rapidly. There has been some success with autogenous vaccines.

Pseudotuberculosis

Yersinia pseudotuberculosis can cause an acute or chronic contagious disease in chinchillas. The acute form is manifested as a septicemia. Anorexia, depression, progressive weight loss, intermittent diarrhea, or sudden death may be seen in the chronic form. Palpably enlarged mesenteric lymph nodes are a hallmark of this disease. Yellow–white foci of necrosis and caseous nodules are seen in the liver, spleen, mesenteric lymph nodes, and intestines. Treatment is usually ineffective.

Mastitis

Mastitis is fairly common and can be suspected if previously healthy neonates become restless, then lethargic. Mammary glands become hot and swollen. Treat with antibiotics based on culture and sensitivity. Sulfonamides may be helpful. Local hotpacking of the mammary glands is usually beneficial. Neonates should be fostered onto another female or hand-raised using puppy or kitten milk replacers.

Metritis

Proteus vulgaris, E. coli, Pseudomonas spp., *Staphylococcus* spp., and *Streptococcus* spp. are the most common organisms that cause metritis. Clinical signs include swelling and discoloration of the vulva, white to brown putrid exudate, and fever. Flushing the vagina and uterus with 2% boric acid solution or antibiotics two to three times per week is recommended.

VIRAL DISEASES

There are few reports of viral agents causing disease. Lymphocytic choriomeningitis virus has been reported to affect chinchillas. Chinchillas infected with human influenza A virus are a model for childhood otitis media.

PARASITIC DISEASES

Intestinal parasitism is generally uncommon. Infestation with coccidia, tapeworms, and nematodes are rare in well-managed facilities. Cystic subcutaneous masses caused by the intermediate stage of *Multiceps serialis* are occasionally seen. The dog is the definitive host of this parasite, whereas the chinchilla is the intermediate host. Transmission is by ingestion of contaminated feed. Parasitic cysts can be removed surgically. Infections with *Giardia* spp. can be serious and result in high mortality. Outbreaks of disease are frequently associated with poor sanitation. Affected animals usually have intermittent illness with sticky black feces. Metronidazole is the recommended treatment for giardiasis.

NEOPLASIA

Apparently, neoplasia is uncommon in the chinchilla as there are few reports.

MISCELLANEOUS CONDITIONS

Malocclusion

Malocclusion, or slobbers, as it is commonly called, can be seen with the incisors or cheek teeth and results in overgrowth and abnormal wear of the teeth. Chinchillas may have a selective appetite in the early stages that progresses to anorexia and excessive drooling. This causes the fur around the chin, chest, and forepaws to become wet, hence, the term "slobbers." Malocclusion of the incisors is easy to visualize; however, sedation and careful exam may be necessary to examine the cheek teeth. Treatment involves trimming the overgrown teeth with a dental bur or toenail trimmers under sedation. Routine trimming of the teeth is usually necessary, and affected animals should not be bred because there may be a hereditary predisposition to the condition. Placing a gnawing block in the cage is recommended.

Conjunctivitis

Conjunctivitis without clinical signs of respiratory infection is usually caused by irritation from the dust bath or dirty bedding. Treating with ophthalmic ointment, improving husbandry, and discontinuing dust baths for a few weeks are recommended.

Fur Chewing

Fur chewing is a serious problem of the chinchilla industry. The exact cause remains unknown; however, it appears to be a vice and seems to occur more in certain families. Loud noises, improper diet, hormonal imbalance, poor housing conditions, stress, and boredom have all been incriminated. Affected chinchillas are motley and have a lion's mane appearance, as they chew all of the fur within reach on their lower body to a short length. Hairballs are commonly found in the stomach at necropsy. Providing the animals with distractions such as pork fat and bacon rind for chewing toys sometimes works. Ranchers cull fur chewers from their stock.

Fur Slip

When chinchillas are handled roughly, become agitated during handling, or fight, the fur may come out in patches. The underlying skin appears clean and smooth. This release of fur occurs in response to the effect of adrenaline on the erector pili muscles. The fur may take up to 5 months to regrow.

Dermatophytosis

The most common cause of ringworm in the chinchilla is *Trichophyton mentagrophytes*. Lesions can occur anywhere on the body but typically appear as small, scaly areas of alopecia on the nose, ears, and feet. Ultraviolet light is not useful for diagnosis, as *Trichophyton* does not fluoresce. Griseofulvin given orally has been used successfully. To help prevent spread to cagemates, captan antifungal powder can be used in the dust box. Lime sulfur dips are also reported to be helpful.

Penile Hair Rings

Male chinchillas can accumulate a ring of twisted hair around the penis and under the prepuce. The condition can affect their breeding ability, as the ring of hair can cause irritation, infection, and damage to the penis. Treat by applying a sterile lubricant to the penis and prepuce and gently rolling the accumulated ring of hair off.

Heatstroke

Chinchillas are very prone to heatstroke, particularly if the humidity is high. Affected animals are usually found in a prostrate condition, panting, and have an elevated body temperature. Treatment involves cooling the animal's body with cold water until the temperature returns to normal and administering intravenous fluids. Care should be taken not to place cages near windows with direct sunlight.

■ GENERAL REFERENCES

Sources consulted to compile the material in this chapter include *Practical Guide to Laboratory Animals* by C.S.F. Williams (1976, Mosby-Year Book, Inc., 11830 Westline Industrial Drive, St. Louis, MO 63146); *Laboratory Animal Medicine* by J.G. Fox, B.J. Cohen, and F.M. Loew (1984, Academic Press, Inc., Orlando, FL 32887); An introduction to chinchillas by C.J. Merry, *Veterinary Technician* Vol 11, No 5 (1990, Veterinary Learning Systems, 425 Phillips Boulevard #100, Trenton, NJ 08618); and Chinchillas by H.L. Hoefer, *Veterinary Clinics of North America Small Animal Practice* 24: 103–110 (1994, W.B. Saunders Co., The Curtis Center, Independence Square West, Philadelphia, PA 19106-3399)

■ TECHNICAL REFERENCES

Allen, D.G., J.K. Pringle, and D.A. Smith. 1993. *Handbook of Veterinary Drugs.* Philadelphia: JB Lippincott.

Anderson, N.L. 1994. Basic husbandry and medicine of pocket pets. In *Saunders Manual of Small Animal Practice,* ed. S.J. Birchard and R.G. Sherding, pp. 1363–1389. Philadelphia: WB Saunders.

Boettcher, F.A., B.R. Bancroft, and R.J. Salvi. 1990. Blood collection from the transverse sinus in the chinchilla. *Lab Anim Sci* 40(2): 223–224.

Burgmann, P. and D.H. Percy. 1993. Antimicrobial drug use in rodents and rabbits. In *Antimicrobial Therapy in Veterinary Medicine,* 2nd ed., ed. J.F. Prescott and J.D. Baggot, pp. 524–541. Ames: Iowa State University Press.

Clark, J.D. 1984. Biology and diseases of other rodents. In *Laboratory Animal Medicine,* ed. J.G. Fox, B.J. Cohen, and F.M. Loew, pp. 183–206. Orlando: Academic.

Collins, B.R. 1995. Antimicrobial drug use in rabbits, rodents, and other small mammals. In *Antimicrobial Therapy in Caged Birds and Exotic Pets,* pp. 3–10. Trenton, NJ: Veterinary Learning Systems.

Flecknell, P.A. 1987. *Laboratory Animal Anesthesia.* London: Academic.

Green, C.J. 1982. *Animal Anesthesia: Laboratory Animal Handbooks 8, Laboratory Animals.* London: LTD.

Hargett, C.E., Jr., J.W. Record, M. Carrier, Jr., et al. 1989. Reversal of ketamine-xylazine anesthesia in the chinchilla by yohimbine. *Lab Anim* 18(7): 41–43.

Harkness, J.E. 1993. *A Practitioner's Guide to Domestic Rodents.* Lakewood, CO: American Animal Hospital Association.

Harrenstien. 1994. Critical care of ferrets, rabbits, and rodents. *Semin Avian Exotic Pet Med* 3: 217–228.

Huerkamp, M.J. 1995. Anesthesia and postoperative management of rabbits and pocket pets. In *Kirk's Current Veterinary Therapy XII: Small Animal Practice,* ed. J.D. Bonagura, pp. 1322–1327. Philadelphia: WB Saunders.

Jankubow, K., J. Gromadzka-Ostrowska, and B. Zalewska. 1984. Seasonal changes in the haematological indices in peripheral blood of chinchilla (*Chinchilla laniger*). *Comp Biochem Physiol* 78A(4): 845–853.

Jenkins, J.R. 1992. Husbandry and common diseases of the chinchilla (*Chinchilla laniger*). *J Small Exotic Anim Med* 2: 15–17.

Johnson-Delaney, C.A. 1996. *Exotic Companion Medicine Handbook for Veterinarians.* Lake Worth, FL: Wingers.

Smith, D.A. and P.M. Burgmann. 1997. Formulary. In *Ferrets, Rabbits, and Rodents: Clinical Medicine and Surgery,* ed. E.V. Hillyer and K.E. Quesenberry, pp. 392–403. Philadelphia: WB Saunders.

Timm, K.I., S.E. Jahn, and C.J. Sedgwick. 1987. The palatalostium of the guinea pig. *Lab Anim Sci* 37(6): 801–802.

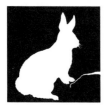

RABBITS

LABORATORY RABBITS belong to the order Lagomorpha and are collectively referred to as lagomorphs. The scientific name of the domestic rabbit is *Oryctolagus cuniculus,* which translates to "hare dug out of the earth." Hares belong to the genus *Lepus* and cottontails belong to the genus *Sylvilagus.* The three genera of rabbits cannot interbreed. Rabbit breeds can vary markedly in size, with a range of 1–9 kg (2.2–19.8 lb). There are numerous coat color variations, including albino, black, silver, and belted. The majority of laboratory rabbits are albino, having white coats and pink eyes. Dutch belted rabbits have a white coat with a black or brown belt around their abdomen and have dark eyes.

Breeds

Currently, the American Rabbit Breeders Association recognizes over 50 breeds of rabbits. Several of the more popular breeds include the New Zealand White (NZW), American Dutch, Californian, and Flemish Giant. The NZW is a medium-sized breed weighing between 3 and 5 kg (6.6–11.0 lb). It is the most popular breed for research purposes and is also used for meat production. The American Dutch is a small breed, weighing between 0.9 and 1.8 kg (2.0–4.0 lb). It is second in importance as a laboratory breed. The Californian breed is another large rabbit that is differentiated from the NZW by its dark ears, nose, and feet. It is primarily used for meat production. The Flemish Giant breed weighs between 6.5 and 9 kg (14.3–19.8 lb) and is occasionally used for research. Other breeds kept mainly for pets and show include the American Chinchilla, Satin, Rex, Silver Martin, American Checkered Giant, Polish, and Lop.

Uses

Rabbits are growing in popularity both as pets and for hobby breeding. They are clean, attractive, relatively easy to handle, and can grow to enjoy the attention given them as pets. They seldom bite but can inflict deep scratches if not held properly.

Rabbits are used in substantial numbers for research and drug testing. Their size, ease of handling, and the relative ease of blood collection due to their large ear vessels make them suitable for many types of experiments. They are frequently used in immunology studies because they are capable of producing large amounts of polyclonal antibodies. Although domestic rabbit meat cannot be produced as economically as poultry, millions of pounds per year are consumed in the United States.

Behavior

Rabbits are not generally aggressive toward people. They tend to be curious but easily frightened. When frightened, some rabbits may show aggression in the form of foot stomping and snorting. Some rabbits may even bite, although this is rare. Rabbits will produce a high-pitched scream when fearful or in pain. Sexually mature rabbits are territorial and will usually fight if housed together. Immature females age 3 months or younger that are housed together may establish stable groups; however, trauma, pseudopregnancies, and infertility can occur in group-housed rabbits. Rabbits can be effectively litter-box trained, as they typically choose one area of their cage for defecation and urination. They can also be harness and leash trained.

Depending on environmental conditions, wild rabbits are either nocturnal or diurnal. They usually feed at dawn and dusk and hide in their burrows during the heat of the day. Rabbits housed indoors in controlled environments tend to have alternating periods of wakefulness and rest throughout the day and night. Rabbits build nests out of their own fur for their young.

Anatomic and Physiologic Features

Rabbit biologic and reproductive data can be found in Table 7.1. The rabbit has a compact body and heavily muscled back and rear legs. Their lightweight skeleton comprises only 7% of their total body weight. The combination of strong muscles and fragile skeleton makes them susceptible to fracture of their lumbar vertebrae. They have long ears and a short tail and are covered with very fine, soft fur.

Domestic rabbits resemble rodents in many respects. The principal anatomic feature differentiating them is that rabbits have two pairs of upper incisor teeth, whereas rodents have only one pair. The additional pair, known as the peg teeth, are smaller and located directly behind the front pair. The purpose of these short cylindrical teeth is not clear. The

Table 7.1. Biologic and reproductive data for rabbits	
Adult body weight	
Male	2–5 kg
Female	2–6 kg
Life span	5–6 y (up to 15 y)
Body temperature	38.5°–40° C (101.3°–104° F)
Heart rate	130–325 beats per minute
Respiratory rate	30–60 breaths per minute
Food consumption	5 g/100 g/d
Water consumption	5–10 mL/100 g/d
Breeding onset	
Male	6–10 mo
Female	4–9 mo
Estrous cycle length	Induced ovulator
Gestation period	29–35 d
Postpartum estrus	None
Litter size	4–10
Weaning age	4–6 wk
Breeding duration	1–3 y
Chromosome number (diploid)	44

Source: Adapted from Harkness and Wagner (1995).

rabbit dental formula is 2 (2/1 incisors, 0/0 canines, 3/2 premolars, and 3/3 molars). All of the teeth are open rooted and continuously grow. The incisors may grow up to 10 cm (4 in.) in 1 year. The esophagus of the rabbit is unique in that it has three muscle layers that are striated throughout the entire length.

Rabbits, like rats and horses, cannot vomit. Their stomachs are thin walled and at necropsy, will often be ruptured. There are two lymphoid organs associated with the gastrointestinal system of the rabbit, the sacculus rotundus at the ileocecal junction, and the appendix or vermiform process at the tip of the cecum. The sacculus rotundus is considered to be analogous to the bursa of Fabricius in birds. These two lymphoid organs contain more than 50% of the total lymphoid tissue of the rabbit, accounting for the relatively small size of the spleen. For hindgut fermentation of their herbivorous diet, rabbits have a capacious cecum approximately 10 times the size of the stomach. There are two types of feces produced by rabbits: firm, dry daytime fecal pellets and soft, moist nighttime feces, which are also called cecotrophs. The cecotrophs are covered with mucus to protect them from the acid pH of the stomach and have a high content of water, nitrogen, electrolytes, and B vitamins. Healthy rabbits never have empty stomachs because of the practice of coprophagy.

Each of the eyes of the rabbit has an approximately 190° field of vision, but they also work together to have a small amount of binocular vision. Rabbits and rodents have harderian lacrimal glands behind their eyes. The blood flow through the large ears of the rabbit is the primary means of body temperature regulation. The right atrioventricular valve of the heart is bicuspid instead of tricuspid as occurs in other mammals. Rabbits are the only known mammal in which the renal tubules can be dissected free from the kidney with an intact basement membrane.

The genital tract of the doe, like that of most domestic animals, is bicornuate but differs in that there is a double cervix. The two horns of the uterus open into the vagina through separate cervices. The uterine horns are curled and lie in the caudal abdomen dorsal to the urinary bladder. The female has four to five pairs of mammary glands. The males do not have nipples. In the mature male, the scrotal pouches can be located anterior and lateral to the penis. Inguinal canals remain open for life. The testes generally descend around 12 weeks of age. Lateral to the external genitalia are the paired, hairless inguinal spaces, which usually contain white-to-brown secretions from the inguinal glands. Someone unfamiliar with rabbit anatomy could conceivably mistake an inguinal space for the anus.

Mature females rabbits often have a prominent dewlap under their chin. Mature male rabbits normally have larger heads than females. Differentiating males from females can be accomplished readily in adults by gently pressing the skin back from the genital opening. The female has a short slitlike opening, and pressing the skin back exposes the mucosal surface of the vulva. In the male, this procedure will cause the penis to be everted. In the newborn, when pressure is applied against the genital orifice, the penis will evert equally all the way around, whereas the vulva protrudes only laterally and ventrally. The posterior end of the vulva does not evert because it is closely attached near the anus.

There are several distinct characteristics of the hematologic, clinical chemistry, and urinary profiles of rabbits. Rabbit neutrophils have intracytoplasmic eosinophilic granules that cause them to resemble eosinophils. They are called pseudoeosinophils or heterophils. True eosinophils have larger, darker granules than heterophils. Lymphocytes are the predominant leukocyte. Basophils are more common than in other mammals, making up 2%–7% of the leukocyte population. Serum calcium can fluctuate with diet and may be as high as 15 mg/dL. Rabbit urine has an alkaline pH of approximately 8.2 and a specific gravity ranging between 1.003 and 1.036. It may appear cloudy owing to the high quantities of triple phosphate and calcium carbonate crystals and, to the inexperienced observer, may be mistaken for a purulent discharge.

Dietary porphyrins will occasionally cause the urine color to vary from dark red to orange. Rabbits differ from most other mammals in that calcium and magnesium ions are excreted primarily in the urine rather than in the bile. Hematologic and biochemical parameters for the rabbit are listed in Appendix 1, Normal Values.

Breeding and Reproduction

Onset of puberty varies with breed. Smaller breeds generally mature earlier, and larger breeds mature later. Does are initially bred between 4 and 6 months at a weight of 3–4 kg. Males are first used for breeding at approximately 6 months. Rabbits do not have a definite estrous cycle. They have 7–10 days of receptivity followed by a short period, 1–2 days, during which they are not receptive to the male. They are induced ovulators like the cat and the ferret.

During breeding, agonistic behavior prevails, with chasing, squealing, tail flagging, enurination, and combat. In the wild, courtship chasing between adults is an early form of sexual activity. When breeding rabbits, the female should be taken to the male's cage. If the female is receptive, copulation will take place soon after introduction of the male. The buck elevates his hindquarters, walks stiff legged, and lays his tail flat across his back. This maneuver supplies a visual stimulus to the doe. Additionally, inguinal gland secretions serve as an olfactory stimulus. The buck may turn his hindquarters and eject a small amount of urine, called enurination, toward a doe or at another male, followed by some form of circling about the cage. On occasion, a doe will refuse to mate with one buck but will readily accept another. She also may accept a buck once but refuse him a second time. Females may attempt to castrate males, so rabbits should be paired for only short periods and observed closely. After ejaculation, the male falls off the female to either side or backward because both feet are off the ground simultaneously at the time of ejaculation.

Ovulation occurs about 10 hours after mating. Approximately 25% of matings are anovulatory. Ovulation can also be induced by administration of human chorionic gonadotropins or other luteinizing hormones if a producer wishes to employ artificial insemination. Pseudopregnancies are a common occurrence in rabbits and are caused by sterile matings, mounting by other does, or stimulation by a nearby male. Pseudopregnancy lasts between 15 and 17 days.

The gestation period ranges from 29 to 35 days, with an average of 31 days. Pregnancy can be detected by radiographs after day 11 and by palpation on days 14–16. Females will begin building a fur nest 3–4 days before parturition. Parturition or kindling is usually rapid but can last 1–2 days. Dystocia is uncommon.

Litters usually consist of six to seven rabbits. The young, officially called kits but commonly referred to as bunnies, normally nurse only once a day, either early in the morning or late in the evening. Owners may grow concerned by this "poor mothering" by the doe. The young are born blind, deaf, hairless, and helpless. Their ears open at 8 days, their eyes open at 10 days, and they begin to eat solid food at about 16–17 days of age. They may be weaned at 4–6 weeks of age.

Orphaned rabbits can be fed orphaned puppy formula with a syringe, doll-size bottle, or by gastric intubation. Milk should be offered three times a day, giving up to 5 mL/d the 1st week, 15 mL/d the second week, and 25 mL/d the third week. Newborn rabbits do not require colostrum because all passive immunity is acquired through the placenta.

HUSBANDRY

Housing

In the research laboratory, rabbits are normally housed in front-opening, stainless steel cages that have mesh or grid floors with excreta trays beneath. Most commercial producers house rabbits in wire-mesh hanging cages. Adult rabbits (>5.4 kg) must be provided with at least 0.46 m² (5.0 ft²) of floor space per rabbit and 36 cm (14 in.) of cage height to enable normal posture. If a litter box is used, pelleted paper or pelleted grass products are recommended. Do not use clay litter or shavings. Litter products should be nontoxic and digestible if eaten. Near the end of gestation, nest boxes should be placed in cages for the birth of the young.

For indoor housing of rabbits, heat is not required because they can tolerate cold temperatures very well. Rabbits can be housed outdoors provided that they are protected from extremes in environmental conditions. The recommended temperature range for rabbits housed in research facilities is 16°–22°C (61°–72°F) with a relative humidity between 30% and 70%. If the ambient temperature exceeds 29.5°C (85°F), auxiliary ventilation is required. Ventilation must be adequate to maintain health and minimize draft and odors, and 10–15 air changes per hour are recommended. In the laboratory, the light cycle is usually controlled by a timing device that provides 12–14 hours of light per day.

Excreta trays should be cleaned as often as needed to control odor and ammonia levels. Daily cleaning is optimal. The carbonate and phosphate crystals from urine precipitate to build up a scale on cages. Urine scale is best removed by soaking or rinsing in an acid solution. Cages, water bottles, and feed hoppers should be disinfected with chemicals, hot water 61.6°–82.2°C (143°–180°F), or a combination of both. Detergents and chemical disinfectants enhance the effectiveness of hot water, but they must be thoroughly rinsed from all caging surfaces with fresh water. Refer to Chapter 1, Mice, for a more detailed description of disinfection methods.

Feeding and Watering

Rabbits should be fed a firm, dry pelleted commercial feed that contains at least 15% protein and 10% crude fiber. Higher fiber diets that contain approximately 22.5% fiber are used to reduce obesity and prevent hairball formation. Food consumption will vary with age, ambient temperature, and water availability. Once daily feeding of 5 g/100 g of body weight per day will maintain an adult, medium-sized rabbit. Rabbits require an average of 8.82 kJ/kg of diet for daily maintenance and 10.5 kJ/kg during growth, gestation, or lactation. Food pellets should be placed in self-feeding J-type hoppers attached to the front of the cage rather than in an open bowl, which becomes easily contaminated. Offering a limited amount of high-fiber, low-calcium grass hay can help to maintain the health of the rabbit's gastrointestinal system.

The average water consumption of a rabbit is 10 mL/100 g of body weight per day, which is approximately twice the amount of food consumed on a weight basis. Water consumption increases with ambient temperature, whereas food intake decreases. Water bottles are readily accepted by rabbits and are preferable to water bowls. Automatic watering systems are much more efficient for both production colonies and research environment.

Rabbits are naturally coprophagic. They take cecotrophs directly from the anus and swallow them intact. The soft pellets contain twice the protein and half the fiber of the hard fecal pellets. Coprophagy improves the utilization of nitrogen, provides an abundance of certain B vitamins, and conserves water.

TECHNIQUES

Handling and Restraint

Rabbits should be handled gently but firmly. They are prone to kick their hindlimbs, which can cause deep scratches in their handlers. A rabbit should be picked up by obtaining a firm grip on the loose skin over the scruff of the neck with one hand while using the other hand to support the animal's hindquarters and to control back leg movement. Figure 7.1 demonstrates this restraint technique. If the hindlimbs are not supported, the rabbit may break its back in struggling. The ears should never be used for picking up a rabbit.

To carry a rabbit, it should be placed on the forearm with its head concealed in the bend of the elbow. Rabbits feel insecure and will slip and slide on stainless steel examining tables. Placing the animal on a towel or wrapping it in a towel will make the rabbit calmer and easier to handle. Many types of restraint boxes are commercially available. These restraint devices primarily serve to control the body of the rabbit while the head or ears are being manipulated. A cat-restraint bag may also be used for rabbits. When examining the underside of a rabbit, a gentle downward stroking on the abdomen will usually have a calming affect.

Repeated gentle stroking of a rabbit's abdomen when placed on its back in a V-trough can immobilize or hypnotize a rabbit. The eyes of the rabbit may have to be covered initially. The response is variable from rabbit to rabbit, but when it works, the rabbit relaxes and its respiratory

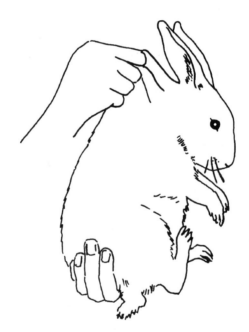

Figure 7.1. Restraint of the rabbit.

rate slows from the normal 50 to about 20 breaths per minute. This technique can be helpful for obtaining a radiograph or clipping toenails or teeth, but it does not generally allow more invasive procedures.

Identification

Cage cards should be used as a form of general identification. Individual identification methods include ear tags, ear tattoos, or placement of a subcutaneous microchip that is electronically encoded. Fur dyes can serve as a temporary method of identification.

Blood Collection

The marginal ear, cephalic, and lateral saphenous veins can be accessed to obtain small amounts of blood. These veins easily collapse with too much negative pressure. The auricular artery runs down the center of the ear pinna and is the best site for collection of larger blood samples. The position of the auricular vessels is shown in Figure 7.2. Warming the ear with a heat lamp or warm water and gently stroking the base of the ear will stimulate blood flow. Topical application of an irritant such as wintergreen oil or xylene can induce vasodilation. It is important to wash off any remaining topical irritant to avoid undue skin irritation. Administering 1 mg of acetylpromazine per medium-sized rabbit intravenously will also cause vasodilation. Another alternative is to inject a local anesthetic such as 2% xylocaine, subcutaneously, close

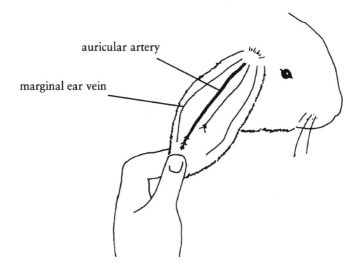

Figure 7.2. Blood vessels of the rabbit ear.

143

to the vessel to be bled. The jugular vein is another good site for blood collection that is often overlooked. The rabbit's head and front legs must be restrained securely to extend the neck, just as a cat or small dog would be restrained, to expose the jugular veins.

Cardiac punctures can be used to collect larger quantities of blood on an anesthetized or sedated rabbit but have a 10% mortality rate. This technique is best done as a terminal procedure due to its higher risk of mortality. Approximate blood volumes for adult rabbits are listed in Table 7.2.

Urine Collection

Urine can be collected as a clean catch sample, by gentle expression of the bladder of an anesthetized rabbit or by cystocentesis using a small-gauge needle. Metabolic cages and urethral catheterization are two alternative ways of collecting urine from rabbits.

Drug Administration

Palatable drugs may be administered to rabbits by incorporating them in the food or water. Small volumes of liquid medications can be administered by placing the tip of a syringe in the corner of the mouth and slowly injecting the liquid. Addition of sugar or syrup to the medication may increase palatability. Oral administration of unpalatable liquids may be accomplished using a stomach tube passed through a nostril or the mouth. If passed through the mouth, a mouth gag must be used and can be fashioned from a syringe casing, wooden dowel, or tongue depressor having a hole for passage of the tube. Stainless steel feeding needles (13 gauge, 16 in.) can also be used to administer drugs orally.

Subcutaneous injections should be administered under the loose skin between the shoulder blades. The volume of fluid that can be given under the skin ranges from 30 to 100 mL per site and depends on the size of the rabbit. Intramuscular injections with a maximum volume of 1–1.5 mL can be given in the large lumbar (epaxial) muscles running alongside the spinal column and in the large quadriceps and thigh mus-

Table 7.2. Adult rabbit blood volumes	
	Volume (mL)[a]
Total blood	160–480
Single sample	20–40
Exsanguination	60–160

Source: Adapted from Harkness and Wagner (1995).
[a]Values are approximate.

cles of the hindlimbs. Care must be taken to avoid the sciatic nerve, which runs behind the femur as depicted in Figure 7.3. Intravenous injections are most frequently given in the marginal ear vein. There have been recent reports describing the intranasal administration of certain anesthetic and tranquilizing agents.

To give an intradermal injection, the skin should be held tautly and the needle slowly advanced with the bevel facing up. The point of the needle should enter just under the layers of the epidermis and into the dermis. Intradermal injections are frequently used in immunology studies. Purified antigens that are suspended in a liquid medium and mixed with an antigenic stimulant, such as Freund's complete adjuvant, are then injected in small volumes, usually 0.1 mL or less, so that the skin forms a small, raised bleb. Both the intradermal site and the water/oil adjuvant act to allow slow release of the antigen. Peak titers are usually seen at 2 weeks. Booster injections of antigens with Freund's incomplete adjuvant or similar adjuvant are given to stimulate a stronger antibody response.

Anesthesia, Surgery, and Postoperative Care

Agents commonly used for anesthesia and tranquilization in rabbits are listed in Table 7.3. Although rabbits cannot vomit, withholding food for 2–6 hours before surgery will allow for a more accurate body weight. Atropine esterase, which hydrolyzes atropine, is present in the serum of about one third of the domestic rabbit population. As a result of the

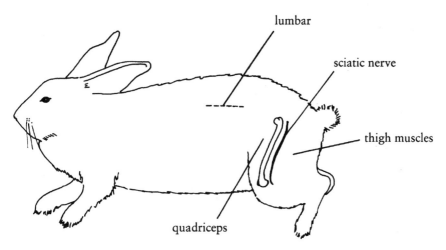

Figure 7.3. Intramuscular injection sites in the rabbit. (Adapted from Timm and Jahn 1980, Practical Methodology of the Rabbit. In *Practical Methodology* [slide series], ©Regents University of California)

presence of atropine esterase, these animals are refractory to administration of atropine. Rabbits can be challenging to anesthetize because they may have variable responses to anesthetics, are easily stressed and difficult to intubate, and many of their reflexes are unreliable indicators of the depth of anesthesia. With the correct technique and experience, most of these obstacles are easily overcome.

Table 7.3. Anesthetic agents and tranquilizers used in rabbits

Drug	Dosage	Route	Reference
Inhalants			
Halothane	0.5%–4% to effect	Inhalation	Gillett (1994)
Isoflurane	1.5%–5% to effect	Inhalation	Gillett (1994)
Methoxyflurane	0.5%–3% to effect	Inhalation	Wixson (1994)
Injectables			
Acetylpromazine	1–5 mg/kg	IM, SC	Gillett (1994)
Diazepam	5–10 mg/kg	IM	Gillett (1994)
	1–5 mg/kg	IV	Gillett (1994)
Fentanyl-droperidol	0.15–0.44 mg/kg	IM	Wixson (1994)
Ketamine	40 mg/kg	IM	Jenkins (1993)
+ acetylpromazine	0.5–1 mg/kg	IM	
Ketamine	25 mg/kg	IM	Flecknell (1987)
+ diazepam	5 mg/kg	IM	
Ketamine	25 mg/kg	IM	Flecknell (1997)
+ medetomidine	0.5 mg/kg	IM	
Ketamine	10 mg/kg	IV	Flecknell (1987)
+ xylazine	3 mg/kg	IV	
Ketamine	30–40 mg/kg	IM	Gillett (1994)
+ xylazine	3–5 mg/kg	IM	
Ketamine	10 mg/kg	Intranasal	Robertson and Eberhart
+xylazine	3 mg/kg	Intranasal	(1994)
Ketamine	35 mg/kg	IM	Lipman et al. (1990)
+ xylazine	5 mg/kg	IM	
+ acetylpromazine	0.75 mg/kg	IM	
Ketamine	35 mg/kg	IM	Marini et al. (1992)
+ xylazine	5 mg/kg	IM	
+ butorphanol	0.1 mg/kg	IM	
Midazolam	2 mg/kg	IV	Flecknell (1987)
	2 mg/kg	Intranasal	Robertson and Eberhart (1994)
	4 mg/kg	IM, IP	Flecknell (1987)
Pentobarbital	30–50 mg/kg	IP, IV	Harkness and Wagner (1995)
Propofol	7.5–15 mg/kg	IV	Adam et al. (1990)
Thiopental (1%)	15–30 mg/kg	IV	Wixson (1994)
Tiletamine-zolazepam	Generally not recommended (except intranasal) because of nephrotoxicity		Doerning (1992)
Tiletamine-zolazepam	10 mg/kg (no renal compromise)	Intranasal	Robertson and Eberhart (1994)
Urethane	1000 mg/kg	IP, IV	Flecknell (1987)
Xylazine	1–3 mg/kg	IM	Flecknell (1987)

IM = intramuscular, IP = intraperitoneal; IV = intravenous; SC = subcutaneous.

There are a number of injectable agents that can provide adequate anesthesia for short procedures. Fentanyl/droperidol combination or acetylpromazine can be administered subcutaneously or intramuscularly for light sedation. The ketamine/xylazine combination remains a popular anesthetic choice. The combination of ketamine and xylazine, however, can be unpredictable, and there is a reported 20%–40% "failure rate" with this regimen. Butorphanol can be added to ketamine/xylazine for better analgesia. Propofol has been used in rabbits and appears to be safe for very short term anesthetic maintenance. Long-term infusion of propofol has been reported to cause significant hypotension, hypoxemia, lipemia, and death in rabbits. Tiletamine hydrochloride has been associated with renal nephrotoxicity and is best avoided in rabbits. Caution should be exercised when using sodium pentobarbital or other barbiturates, as they have a narrow margin between surgical anesthesia and death. In addition, barbiturates provide variable analgesia and cause respiratory depression. The intranasal administration of certain anesthetic and tranquilizing agents has recently been described and appears to offer a quick and safe route for some agents. Absorption of the drugs is through the vessels of the cribriform plate and leads directly to the central nervous system. This route should be used with caution, as some agents have been shown to elicit variable responses in rabbits and may even cause acute respiratory failure and death.

Inhalant agents, such as isoflurane, halothane, and methoxyflurane, are safe and commonly used in rabbits. Although rabbits can be masked down, great care must be taken in restraining them to avoid possible struggle and fracture/luxation of the lumbar spine. Administration of halothane or isoflurane to rabbits via a face mask or anesthetic induction chamber is associated with apnea and a marked bradycardia. Premedicating a rabbit with acetylpromazine, droperidol/fentanyl, or other suitable sedative will allow for an easier and safer masking induction.

To intubate a rabbit, a long (40 mm), thin (size 0 or 1) laryngoscope blade can be used to allow visualization of the larynx. A stylet inside of the appropriately sized endotracheal tube (2–3 mm outside diameter in 1–3 kg rabbits; 3–6 mm outside diameter in larger rabbits) can be helpful in guiding the tube into the trachea. Rotating the tube as it passes over the epiglottis facilitates passage into the trachea. A topical spray of lidocaine can be used to anesthetize the epiglottis. Alternatively, blind intubation of rabbits can be used. It is a method that when properly performed is both faster and less traumatic than the laryngoscope method. The rabbit's head is held with the palm of the hand on the back of the skull and the thumb and index finger placed along the length of each mandible. The most important step is to extend the neck adequately, with the nose pointing straight up or even slightly back (hyperextended), so the path down the trachea is straight. Figure 7.4 shows the proper positioning of the head. The endotracheal tube is passed over the tongue until it is at the entrance to the larynx as evidenced by condensation in the tube when the rabbit exhales. During exhalation, the tube should be quickly and firmly passed forward while rotating it so that it enters the trachea. This method can be mastered with patience and practice.

The depth of anesthesia is best gauged by the rate and depth of respiration and the degree of jaw tension. Other indicators of the depth of anesthesia in decreasing order of reliability are the ear pinch, pedal reflex, corneal reflex, and palpebral reflex. The ear pinch is more sensitive and persists longer than the others. Clipping rabbit hair is difficult at best. Using a sharp 40 blade held flat against the skin, stretching the skin taut, and clipping slowly and carefully are important steps to avoid traumatizing the skin. The skin should be lightly scrubbed in preparation for surgery. Rabbits are adept at removing sutures; thus, it is best to use metal staples or clips when closing the incision. For optimal postoperative recoveries, surgeries should be performed with attention to maintaining body temperature, blood pressure, and aseptic technique.

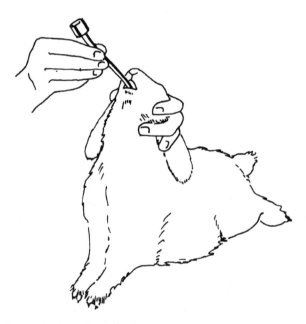

Figure 7.4. "Blind" endotracheal intubation of the rabbit. (Adapted from Harkness and Wagner 1995, *The Biology and Medicine of Rabbits and Rodents,* 4th edition, Philadelphia: Williams & Wilkins)

Surgical procedures that are occasionally performed on pet rabbits include ovariohysterectomies (OHEs), castrations, and gastrotomies. Rabbits have a very narrow linea alba and veins that tear easily. The incision for an OHE in a rabbit should be made lower on the abdomen, similar to an OHE approach in a cat. The bladder should be gently emptied prior to incising the abdominal wall. The bladder is thin walled, and if pressure is applied too vigorously, it may rupture. Additionally, care must be taken to ligate both cervices of the rabbit that enter into the vagina separately, especially in larger does. In the male, both inguinal canals remain open throughout life and must be sutured closed during a castration to avoid herniation of abdominal contents. Gastrotomies are indicated for rabbits with hair balls that do not respond to medical therapy. Rabbits are sometimes used in experimental studies that require surgical manipulations, including placement of indwelling vascular catheters, orthopedic surgeries, and gastrointestinal surgeries.

Postoperative analgesics should be administered for invasive procedures or when pain is suspected as evidenced by depression or anorexia. A list of analgesic agents for rabbits is found in Table 7.4. Opiates such as butorphanol and buprenorphine are frequently used. Butorphanol is

Table 7.4. Analgesic agents used in rabbits

Drug	Dosage	Route	Reference
Acetaminophen	200–500 mg/kg	PO	Gillett (1994)
	1–2 mg/mL drinking water		Huerkamp (1995)
Acetaminophen-codeine	1 mL elixir in 100 mL drinking water		Wixson (1994)
Acetylsalicylic acid	100 mg/kg q4h	PO	Flecknell (1991)
Buprenorphine	0.01–0.05 mg/kg q6–12h	SC, IP, IV	Harkness and Wagner (1995)
Butorphanol	0.1–0.5 mg/kg q2–4h	SC, IM, IV	Harkness and Wagner (1995)
Flunixin meglumine	1–2 mg/kg q12–24h	SC	Heard (1993)
Ibuprofen	10–20 mg/kg q4h	PO	Harkness and Wagner (1995)
Ketoprofen	1 mg/kg q8–12h	IM	Johnson-Delaney (1996)
Meperidine	5–10 mg/kg q2–3h	SC, IP	Harkness and Wagner (1995)
Syrup	0.2 mg/mL drinking water		Huerkamp (1995)
Morphine	2–5 mg/kg q2–4h	SC, IM	Flecknell (1991)
Nalbuphine	1–2 mg/kg q4–5h	IM, IV	Heard (1993)
Oxymorphone	0.2 mg/kg q2–4h	IM	Wixson (1994)
Pentazocine	5–10 mg/kg q2–4h	IM, IV	Heard (1993)

IM = intramuscular; IP = intraperitoneal; IV = intravenous; PO = per os; SC = subcutaneous.

indicated for mild postoperative pain whereas buprenorphine is indicated for acute and chronic visceral pain. Buprenorphine can cause marked sedation if given too early in the anesthetic recovery period. Stanozol can be used to stimulate the appetite of rabbits following surgery. Verapamil or ibuprofen can be used postoperatively to decrease adhesion formation.

Euthanasia

Rabbits are most frequently euthanized by an overdose of barbiturate or euthanizing solution given intravenously. This method is painless, fast, easily accomplished, and relatively inexpensive. Inhalant anesthetics and carbon dioxide gas (approximately 70%) can be used but are less favorable methods, as struggling and vocalizations usually occur. Rabbits that are used for polyclonal antibody production are usually exsanguinated under anesthesia for the terminal collection of blood and harvesting of the antibody-rich serum.

THERAPEUTIC AGENTS

Table 7.5 lists a variety of antimicrobial and antifungal agents that can be used in rabbits. Refer to Table 7.6 for a list of antiparasitics for use in rabbits and to Table 7.7 for miscellaneous drugs used in rabbits.

Table 7.5. Antimicrobial and antifungal agents used in rabbits			
Drug	Dosage	Route	Reference
Amikacin	2–5 mg/kg q8–12h	SC, IM	Harkness and Wagner (1995)
Ampicillin	22–44 mg/kg in divided doses	PO	Russell et al. (1981)
Cephaloridine	11–15 mg/kg q12h	IM	Gillett (1994)
Cephalothin	12.5 mg/kg q6h for 6 d	IM	Russell et al. (1981)
Chloramphenicol	30 mg/kg q12h	PO	Jenkins (1993)
	30 mg/kg q8–12h	SC, IM, IV	Jenkins (1993)
Chlortetracycline	50 mg/kg q24h	PO	Burgmann and Percy (1993)
Ciprofloxacin	5–20 mg/kg q12h	PO	Quesenberry (1994)
Doxycycline	2.5 mg/kg q12h	PO	Carpenter et al. (1995)
Enrofloxacin	5–10 mg/kg q12h	PO, IM, SC	Carpenter et al. (1995)
	200 mg/L drinking water for 14 d		Broome (1991)
Gentamicin	1.5–2.5 mg/kg q8h	SC, IM, IV	Quesenberry (1994)
	4 mg/kg q24h	SC, IM	Burgmann and Percy (1993)
Griseofulvin	25 mg/kg q24h for 30–45 days	PO	Jenkins (1995)
Neomycin	30 mg/kg q12h	PO	Burgmann and Percy (1993)
Oxytetracycline	50 mg/kg q12h	PO	Burgmann and Percy (1993)
	1 mg/mL drinking water		Burgmann and Percy (1993)
Penicillin G, benzathine	42,000–60,000 IU/kg q48h	SC, IM	Russell (1981)
Penicillin G, procaine	42,000–84,000 IU/kg q24h	SC, IM	Gillett (1994)
Sulfadimethoxine	10–15 mg/kg q12h	PO	Harkness and Wagner (1995)
Sulfamethazine	1 mg/mL drinking water		Burgmann and Percy (1993)
Sulfaquinoxaline	1 mg/mL drinking water		Burgmann and Percy (1993)
Tetracycline	50 mg/kg q8–12h	PO	Burgmann and Percy (1993)
	250–1000 mg/L drinking water		Gillett (1994)
Trimethoprim-sulfa	30 mg/kg q12h	PO, IM	Harkness and Wagner (1995)
Tylosin	10 mg/kg q12h	PO, SC, IM	Burgmann and Percy (1993)
Vancomycin	50 mg/kg q8h	IV	Nicolau et al. (1993)

IM = intramuscular; IV = intravenous; PO = per os; SC = subcutaneous.

Table 7.6. Antiparasitic agents used in rabbits

Drug	Dosage	Route	Reference
Amprolium (9.6%)	0.5 mL/500 mL drinking water for 10 d		Harkness and Wagner (1995)
Carbaryl powder (5%)	Twice weekly	Topical	Harkness and Wagner (1995)
Coban	50 ppm in feed		Harkness and Wagner (1995)
Decoquinate	62.5 ppm in feed		Harkness and Wagner (1995)
Diclazuril	1 ppm in feed		Harkness and Wagner (1995)
Fenbendazole	10 mg/kg, repeat in 2 wk prn	PO	Hillyer (1994)
	50 ppm in feed for 2–6 wk		Okerman (1994)
Ivermectin	0.4 mg/kg q7–14 d	PO, SC	Hillyer (1994)
Lasalocid	120 ppm in feed		Harkness and Wagner (1995)
Lime sulfur (2%–3%)	dip q7d for 4–6 wk		Jenkins (1995)
Mebendazole	50 mg/kg	PO	Harkness and Wagner (1995)
	1 g/kg of feed		Harkness and Wagner (1995)
Monensin	0.002%–0.004% in feed		Harkness and Wagner (1995)
Piperazine	200 mg/kg, repeat in 2–3 wk	PO	Hillyer (1994)
	2–5 mg/mL drinking water for 7 d		Hillyer (1994)
Praziquantel	5–10 mg/kg, repeat in 10 d	PO, SC, IM	Allen (1993)
Pyrantel pamoate	5–10 mg/kg, repeat in 2–3 wk	PO	Quesenberry (1994)
Pyrethrin (0.05%) shampoo	Shampoo weekly for 4–6 wk		Smith and Burgmann (1997)
Robenidine	50 ppm in feed		Peeters et al. (1983)
Sulfadimethoxine	50 mg/kg once, then 25 mg/kg q24h for 10–20 d	PO	Hillyer (1994)
Sulfadimethoxine-ormetoprim (Rofenaid)	62.5–250 ppm in feed		Harkness and Wagner (1995)
Sulfamethazine	100 mg/kg q24h	PO	Gillett (1994)
	0.77 g/L drinking water		Harkness and Wagner (1995)
	0.5%–1% in feed		Harkness and Wagner (1995)
Sulfaquinoxaline	0.04%–0.1% drinking water		Harkness and Wagner (1995)
	125–250 ppm in feed		Harkness and Wagner (1995)
Thiabendazole	25–50 mg/kg	PO	Gillett (1994)
Thiabendazole-dexamethasone-neomycin (Tresaderm)	3 drops in each ear q12h for 7–14 d		Carpenter et al. (1995)

IM = intramuscular; PO = per os; SC = subcutaneous.

Table 7.7. Miscellaneous agents used in rabbit

Drug	Dosage	Route	Reference
Atipamezole	1 mg/kg	SC, IP, IV	Flecknell (1997)
Atropine	0.1–3 mg/kg	SC	Harkness and Wagner (1995)
Barium	10–14 mL/kg	PO	Quesenberry (1994)
Bromelin enzyme	1–2 tablets q24h for 3–5 d	PO	Quesenberry (1994)
Calcium-EDTA	27 mg/kg q6h for 2–5 d (make at 10 mg/mL in 5% dextrose or saline)	SC	Johnson-Delaney (1996)
Cholestyramine	2 g per animal q24h for 18–21 d, gavage with 20 mL water	PO	Harkness and Wagner (1995)
Cimetidine	5–10 mg/kg q6–12h	PO	Allen (1993)
Cisapride (Propusid)	0.5 mg/kg q8–24h	PO	Smith and Burgmann (1997)
Dexamethasone	0.2–0.6 mg/kg	SC, IM, IV	Gillett (1994)
Dipyrone	6–12 mg/kg q8–12h	SC	Jenkins (1995)
Doxapram	2–5 mg/kg q15min	IV	Huerkamp (1995)
Furosemide	5–10 mg/kg q12h	IM	Allen (1993)
Glycopyrrolate	0.01–0.02 mg/kg	SC	Huerkamp (1995)
Hairball laxative, feline	1–2 mL per animal q24h for 3–5 d	PO	Quesenberry (1994)
Human chorionic gonadotropin	20–25 IU per animal	IV	Harkness and Wagner (1995)
Lactobacillus	1 notch daily of paste; or ¼–½ tsp powder, or per package label; mix into food	PO	Johnson-Delaney (1996)
Loperamide hydrochloride (Imodium A-D)	0.1 mg/kg q8h for 3 d, then q24h for 2 d	PO	Harkness and Wagner (1995)
Meclizine hydro-chloride (Antivert)	2–12 mg/kg q24h	PO	Harkness and Wagner (1995)
Metoclopramide	0.2–1 mg/kg q6–8h	PO, SC	Harkness and Wagner (1995)
Naloxone	0.01–0.1 mg/kg	IV, IM	Gillett (1994)
Oxytocin	0.1–3 IU/kg	SC, IM	Harkness and Wagner (1995)
Pancreatic enzyme concentrate (Viokase-V)	Mix 1 tsp with 3 Tbsp yogurt, let stand 15 min, then give 2–3 mL q12h	PO	Allen (1993)
Papain enzyme	1–2 tablets per animal q24h for 3–5 d	PO	Quesenberry (1994)
Pineapple juice (fresh)	10 mL per medium-sized animal q24h for 3–5 d	PO	Quesenberry (1994)
Polysulfated glycosamino-glycan	2.2 mg/kg q3d for 21–28 d, then q14d	IM, SC	Jenkins (1995)
Prednisolone	0.25–0.5 mg/kg q12h for 3 d, then q24h for 3 d, then q48h	PO	Quesenberry (1994)
Stanozolol	1–2 mg	PO	Harkness and Wagner (1995)
Verapamil (Calan)	0.2 mg/kg q8h for nine treatments	SC	Harkness and Wagner (1995)
Vitamin A	500–1000 IU/kg once	IM	Johnson-Delaney (1996)
Vitamin B complex	0.02–0.4 mL/kg q24h	IM	Johnson-Delaney (1996)
Vitamin E-selenium (Bo-Se)	0.25 mL per rabbit	IM	Johnson-Delaney (1996)
Vitamin K	1–10 mg/kg	IM	Johnson-Delaney (1996)
Yohimbine	0.2–1 mg/kg	IM, IV	Gillett (1994)

EDTA = ethylenediaminetetracetic acid; IM = intramuscular; IP = intraperitoneal; IV = intravenous; PO = per os; SC = subcutaneous.

BACTERIAL DISEASES

Bacterial Pneumonia and Respiratory Diseases

Pasteurellosis is the single most common and troublesome disease of domestic rabbits. It is caused by *Pasteurella multocida*. Many rabbits harbor the organism in the upper respiratory tract without showing clinical signs. From this nidus, the organism may spread along the nasolacrimal ducts, eustachian tubes, down the trachea, hematogenously, and venereally. Following stress, a variety of syndromes may develop, including rhinitis, conjunctivitis, bronchopneumonia, otitis media and interna, genital infections, abscesses, and/or septicemia. There are a variety of *P. multocida* isolates that appear to differ in virulence. Some forms are associated with a rapidly fatal septicemia, whereas other strains induce a slowly progressive rhinitis.

Rhinitis or snuffles, the upper respiratory form of pasteurellosis, is characterized by sneezing and the presence of a mucopurulent nasal exudate. Exudate is often seen on the inner aspect of the forelegs as rabbits use their forelimbs to wipe their noses. Turbinate atrophy may be a sequelae with some strains of *P. multocida*. Animals may live for many months with snuffles, or the disease may progress to one of the other clinical forms.

The pulmonary form of pasteurellosis appears as an acute bronchopneumonia with variable consolidation of the lungs. Cyanosis is often a prominent feature of pneumonia in rabbits. At times, rabbits will die of acute bronchopneumonia without observable clinical signs.

A subacute to chronic suppurative conjunctivitis with epiphora may be a clinical manifestation of *P. multocida* infection. It is usually seen in conjunction with snuffles. The infection results in loss of fur around the medial canthus of the eye. Suppurative otitis media and otitis interna are common manifestations of this organism. With otitis interna, there are balance problems and torticollis, commonly called head tilt or wry neck. The head tilt may be so severe that the head is nearly upside down.

Reproductive tract infections in rabbits include pyometra in the doe and orchitis in the buck. Large subcutaneous abscesses may also be seen with *P. multocida* infections. The pyometra/abscess contents tend to be yellow–white and have a very thick, creamy consistency that is difficult to aspirate. Incising the abscess and removing the thick purulent material may be necessary to initiate successful treatment of the infection.

The organism is usually sensitive to a number of antibiotics, and remission is common. Infection is usually reestablished, however, after discontinuation of treatment because the organism is harbored in the nasal passages and tympanic bullae. Antibiotics often used in treating pasteurellosis include chlortetracycline, oxytetracycline, enrofloxacin, penicillin, ampicillin, and chloramphenicol. A degree of caution should be exercised in using antibiotics for prolonged periods in rabbits because of their susceptibility to developing a fatal diarrhea. Cesarean derivation of breeding stock and maintenance of animals in isolation have proven to be a successful means of eliminating pasteurellosis. This is expensive and probably only practical for research colonies. Breeders generally direct their efforts toward avoiding spread of infection and minimizing the incidence of clinical disease by 1) quarantine of incoming animals; 2) elimination of environmental stressors, giving particular attention to adequate ventilation; 3) isolation or culling of affected animals; and 4) provision of medicated feed. The use of medicated feed is sometimes indicated but should not be used to compensate for poor husbandry practices. Bacterins and vaccines have proven to be of little value in preventing pasteurellosis.

Bordetella bronchiseptica has been recovered from the respiratory tracts of both normal and diseased rabbits. Thus, its status as a pathogen is not well established. It may facilitate *P. multocida* infections of the lower respiratory tract and should be regarded as a potential pathogen in young rabbits 4–12 weeks of age.

The cilia-associated respiratory (CAR) bacillus isolates from rabbits have been recently characterized and found to be most closely related to *Helicobacter* spp. This is in contrast to the rat isolates, which are more closely related to gliding bacteria of the phylum *Flavobacterium*. The organisms appear to be opportunistic invaders of the respiratory tract and are found between the cilia of the respiratory epithelium. Naturally occurring infections are usually asymptomatic but may cause a slight nasal discharge. Histologically, there is slight hypertrophy and hyperplasia of the laryngeal, tracheal, and bronchial epithelium. Antimicrobial treatments for the CAR bacillus have not been evaluated for efficacy in rabbits.

Bacterial Enteritis and Miscellaneous Enteric Diseases

As a group, enteric diseases are second only to pasteurellosis as a health problem in domestic rabbits. Of the common diseases encountered, the enteric diseases are probably the least understood. In some cases, diarrhea is associated with a specific, well-defined agent, but in many cases, the cause of enteric disease is obscure. Specific enteric diseases include coccidiosis, enterotoxemia, Tyzzer's disease, and salmonellosis. Those of uncertain etiologies include colibacillosis and mucoid enteropathy.

Symptomatic treatment may be the best initial step in treating individual rabbits with acute diarrhea. The focus should be on maintaining hydration and body temperature, as well as changing the diet to one containing higher fiber and lower protein. It is important to keep the rabbit's anus free from fecal impaction and the hindquarters clean and dry. Analgesics may be indicated in depressed, anorexic rabbits.

Colibacillosis

Colibacillosis might appropriately be classified as a specific enteric disease; however, the role of the *Escherichia coli* organism is not completely understood. The type of *E. coli* that causes problems in rabbits is known as the enteropathogenic *E. coli* (EPEC). These organisms do not produce enterotoxins, and they do not invade the intestinal mucosa. Rather, the EPEC adhere to receptors on the enterocytes and probably release a *Shiga*-like cytotoxin. It is known that *E. coli* is either absent or present in low numbers in the gut of normal rabbits. In some cases of severe diarrhea, the organisms are isolated in large numbers. It is generally thought, however, that *E. coli* is a secondary agent rather than the primary cause of disease. Outbreaks of colibacillosis may be seen in sucklings or weanlings because of the prevalence of receptors, which allow EPEC attachment.

Clinical signs are nonspecific and may be attributed to any of the enteric pathogens. Gross findings include an edematous and hemorrhagic cecum. Histologically there may be villous atrophy, edema, congestion, and hemorrhage. Tentative diagnosis can be made by identification of nonhemolytic, facultatively anaerobic *E. coli* from a fecal culture on MacConkey's medium. A definitive diagnosis can be made with microscopy, serotyping, or biotyping.

Treatment is largely symptomatic. Systemic and parenteral antibiotics, intestinal protectants such as bismuth subsalicylate, fluids and electrolytes, and other supportive measures may be beneficial. Alteration of the diet to reduce the amount of concentrates fed to no more than 2–3 oz per day and providing added roughage, such as hay, is often more effective than are antibiotics in reducing mortality.

☞ ## Enterotoxemia

Clostridia perfringens, Clostridia difficile, and *Clostridia spiroforme* have all been implicated in this disease complex. It is now known that

C. spiroforme is the most common pathogen associated with enteritis in juvenile, 4- to 8-week-old rabbits. Clostridia are either absent or found in low numbers in the large intestine of rabbits. A disruption of the normal microflora of the gut appears to play an important role in the disease process. Clostridia may be isolated as the sole cause of enteric disease, but concurrent infections with *E. coli, C. piliforme,* or rotavirus are not uncommon. Changes in feed, weaning, antibiotic therapy, and concurrent infections may all be stressors that allow colonization of *C. spiroforme* and enterotoxin production. A depression in antibacterial resistance favors the increased growth of toxin-producing bacteria. The enterotoxins cause damage to the enterocytes, with functional impairment and subsequent diarrhea, dehydration, and death.

A hemorrhagic and edematous cecum is typically seen in these cases. Gram stains of a smear of cecal contents can be helpful in identifying curved or coiled gram-positive bacilli. Anaerobic cultures are also indicated for trying to obtain a presumptive diagnosis of *Clostridia*-mediated diarrhea. A definitive diagnosis requires the demonstration of the enterotoxin. Cytotoxicity assays and enzyme-linked immunosorbent assays are two in vitro tests that can identify *Clostridia* spp. exotoxins in the fecal material of rabbits. Treatment consists mainly of supportive therapy, as there is little evidence that enterotoxemia can be effectively treated with antibiotics.

Several antibiotics have been associated with outbreaks of enterotoxemia, including erythromycin, clindamycin, lincomycin, and streptomycin. Penicillin and its derivatives are routinely used in rabbits but have also been associated with enterotoxemia and must be used with caution. Antibiotics that are generally considered to be safe in rabbits include chloramphenicol, enrofloxacin, trimethoprim/sulfa, gentamicin, neomycin, vancomycin, and metronidazole. Preventive measures for animals receiving antibiotics include the oral administration of *Lactobacillus* spp. preparations to inhibit toxins or cholestyramine to absorb toxins.

☞ Mucoid Enteropathy

Mucoid enteropathy (ME) is a frequent disease problem in young rabbits 7–10 weeks old, although it can also be seen in adults. Whether it is a distinctive disease with a specific etiology is not clear. It may merely be a syndrome brought on by a combination of stress and dietary factors. Mucoid enteropathy may occur concurrently with other infectious enteric agents including coccidiosis, colibacillosis, clostridial enterotoxemia, and Tyzzer's disease.

Clinical signs include abdominal distention with sloshing sounds from the intestines, hunched posture, depression, polydypsia, anorexia, hypothermia 37°–38.5°C (99°–101°F), and constipation followed by profuse mucoid diarrhea.

Typical gross findings include the presence of clear gelatinous material in the colon or in more chronic cases, an impacted cecum. Histologically, the lesions consist primarily of hyperplasia and hypertrophy of the goblet cells on the intestinal mucosa with few inflammatory cells. Thus, it is properly classified as an enteropathy rather than an enteritis.

Treatment is usually ineffective, although intense fluid therapy given orally, subcutaneously, or intravenously; enemas; laxatives; and broad-spectrum antibiotics may help rabbits in the early stages of this disease. Preventive measures include decreasing food intake when shipped and for 48 hours postshipment.

Tyzzer's Disease

C. piliforme can cause an acute hemorrhagic typhlocolitis. Young rabbits between 7 and 12 weeks of age are most often affected. Tyzzer's disease is not recognized as a common health problem in rabbits. Rabbits may actually carry the organism asymptomatically and shed the organism in the feces. Stresses such as overcrowding, shipping, poor ventilation, and improper nutrition are precipitating factors that elicit an acute diarrheal disease. Profuse diarrhea and dehydration are characteristic clinical signs followed by death in 12–48 hours. Morbidity and mortality can be very high. At necropsy, focal necrosis of the liver and intestinal mucosa is seen.

A diagnosis can be made by identifying periodic acid-Schiff or silver positive intracytoplasmic filamentous bacilli in histologic sections of the liver, heart, or cecum. Alternatively, a Giemsa-stained impression smear of the hepatic lesions may reveal the typical bacilli. Per os inoculation of susceptible weanling gerbils with fecal material from the suspect animal is one of the most sensitive screens for *C. piliforme*.

Oxytetracycline is suggested for treatment; however, the prognosis for animals showing clinical signs of Tyzzer's disease is very unfavorable. Institution of sound husbandry practices and elimination of environmental stress factors are crucial in controlling an outbreak in a rabbit colony.

Salmonellosis

Salmonella spp. infections are a relatively uncommon cause of enteric disease in rabbits. Clinical signs, other than diarrhea that may be evident with salmonellosis, are abortion and septicemia with rapid death.

Although various antibiotics may be effective in eliminating clinical signs of salmonellosis, treatment of affected animals is not usually advisable owing to the zoonotic potential of this organism and the possibility of inapparent carriers.

Miscellaneous Bacterial Infections

Staphylococcus aureus infections may be seen in a number of forms, such as septicemia, dermatitis, and abscesses. It is one of the most common causes of conjunctivitis in rabbits. Staphylococcal mastitis often causes septicemia in the doe and multiple abscesses in nursing bunnies maintained in unsanitary conditions. Chloramphenicol, gentamicin, or tetracycline in conjunction with topical treatment is sometimes effective. Antibiotic treatment of staphylococcal infections, however, is frequently discouraging.

Mastitis occurs sporadically in lactating does and occasionally during pseudopregnancy. Mastitis is sometimes called blue breast because the skin over the mammary gland changes from pink to red then to bluish purple. Several microorganisms including *S. aureus, Pasteurella* spp. and *Streptococcus* spp. are causative agents. Causative organisms may be introduced by means of splinters from nest boxes, trauma from the teeth of nursing young, or unsanitary housing conditions. Treatment involves isolating the affected doe and treating her with appropriate antibiotics. Lancing and flushing abscesses may be necessary. The young should be removed from the doe but not foster nursed on another doe because of the probability of spreading the disease to a healthy animal.

Necrobacillosis or Schmorl's disease, caused by *Fusobacterium necrophorum,* is characterized by ulceration of the skin and by subcutaneous swelling about the face, neck, and oral cavity. Although the organism is commonly present in the digestive tract of rabbits, the incidence of disease is low. The infection is transmissible to humans. The recommended treatment for affected rabbits includes debridement, drainage of abscesses, provision of systemic antibiotics such as penicillin or tetracycline, and improved sanitation.

Tularemia, caused by *Francisella tularensis,* usually causes sudden death of affected animals. Typical lesions at necropsy are small foci of necrosis in the spleen and liver. The organism can be transmitted by direct contact, via aerosols or ingestion, or by bloodsucking arthropods. The disease is rare in domestic rabbits because of lack of exposure to the appropriate arthropod vectors. It can cause a potentially fatal zoonotic disease in humans. The disease is seen primarily in hunters and wildlife personnel. Hunters should wear gloves when skinning game.

Listeriosis, caused by *Listeria monocytogenes,* is a rare disease in rabbits. It usually causes abortions or nonspecific signs and death. The presence of a blood-tinged vaginal discharge following abortion suggests the possibility of listeriosis. Occasionally, central nervous system signs are seen. The importance of the organism is related to its zoonotic potential. Antibiotics of the tetracycline group and penicillin have been used in treating listeriosis.

Pseudomonas aeruginosa is not a common pathogen in rabbits but may produce skin infections with blue–green discoloration and involve other organs. Infections are treated by topical application of 3% hydrogen peroxide. Chlorination of drinking water should prevent the organism from colonizing the water.

Pseudotuberculosis is caused by *Yersinia pseudotuberculosis.* The disease is not commonly seen in domestic rabbits in the United States. The organism typically produces caseous nodules in various organs. Treatment of pseudotuberculosis in rabbits is not usually successful. The organism can infect humans.

☞ ## Spirochete Infections: Venereal Spirochetosis

Venereal spirochetosis, also known as rabbit syphilis, vent disease, and treponematosis, is caused by *Treponema cuniculi.* The organism is serologically and morphologically similar to *Treponema pallidum,* which causes syphilis in humans; however, *T. cuniculi* is nonpathogenic for humans. The disease is characterized by the presence of raised, crusted, occasionally hemorrhagic, ulcerative foci on the external genitalia, perineal region, and face. The disease may be confused clinically with hutch burn. At times, the lesions may resemble those caused by ear mites and sarcoptic mange. Many rabbits are serologically positive, but are asymptomatic.

The disease is transmitted by direct contact, usually venereally but occasionally by extragenital routes. Affected rabbits should be isolated during the acute disease. Treponematosis can be differentiated from other cutaneous diseases by dark-field examination of scrapings from the lesions. Three doses of benzathine penicillin G at 84,000 U/kg intramuscularly administered at weekly intervals is reportedly effective in eliminating the infection. Penicillin derivatives should be used with great caution because of the possibility of inducing a fatal enterotoxemia.

VIRAL DISEASES

Myxomatosis

Myxomatosis is caused by a poxvirus, the myxomavirus. The natural host in the United States is wild cottontails *(Sylvilagus)*, although it is also enzootic in wild *Oryctolagus* in the western United States. Severe disease with a high fatality rate is seen in naive *Oryctolagus*. Transmission is usually by mosquitoes but can be by direct contact. The initial clinical signs seen are gelatinous subcutaneous masses. Several days later, a mucopurulent conjunctivitis with generalized subcutaneous edema develops, which causes the rabbit's eyes to swell shut and the ears to droop. There is a vaccine used in Europe, which is not approved in the United States.

Fibromatosis

Fibromatosis is caused by another poxvirus, the Shope fibroma virus, which is antigenically related to the myxomavirus. The virus is enzootic in wild cottontails in the United States but can be seen in *Oryctolagus*. Transmission is usually by arthropod vectors that mechanically spread the virus. The lesions include subcutaneous masses that are firm rather than gelatinous. Most masses involve the feet and legs, but they can occur on the face and perineum. Masses may persist for several months but usually regress spontaneously. Generalized and fatal infections have been reported in newborns. There is no prevention or treatment available.

Papillomatosis (Cutaneous)

Papillomatosis is caused by a papovavirus and results in formation of horny warts, usually on the neck, shoulder, or abdomen. Lesions are primarily seen in cottontails. The virus is spread mechanically from infected hosts by arthropod carriers. About 35% will regress spontaneously within 6 months. Another 25% will progress to squamous cell carcinoma.

Papillomatosis (Oral)

Another papovavirus causes papillomas on the underside of the tongue and buccal cavity. The domestic rabbit, *Oryctolagus,* is the natural host. Lesions are usually seen in rabbits 2–18 months of age. Papillomas spontaneously regress within a few weeks.

Rotavirus

Rotavirus causes an enteritis with mild to severe diarrhea in 1- to 3-week-old rabbits. Outbreaks occur in naive colonies with high morbidity and mortality. Serologic surveys reveal that rotavirus is enzootic in many commercial rabbitries. Maternal antibodies play a large role in protecting against the disease. Diagnosis is based on clinical signs and histologic findings. The only treatment is supportive therapy.

Viral Hemorrhagic Disease

The etiologic agent of viral hemorrhagic disease has not been thoroughly classified but is believed to be a calicivirus. It is highly contagious and is spread by direct contact or aerosols. It has never been seen in the United States, but there is a high risk of introduction from rabbits in Asia and Europe. There was an outbreak of the disease in Mexico that was successfully eradicated.

The disease is seen in rabbits older than 2 months. The usual clinical sign is sudden death without premonitory signs. Morbidity and mortality range between 80% and 100%. Gross lesions include diffuse hemorrhage throughout the trachea, lungs, liver, spleen, kidneys, thymus, and peritoneum. There is an inactivated viral vaccine that can provide protection for 6 months and can be used to protect valuable colonies.

Cardiomyopathy

A cardiomyopathy caused by a coronavirus has been reported. The hearts of affected animals exhibit myocardial necrosis and degeneration with little inflammatory response.

Miscellaneous Viral Diseases

Rare reports of other viruses in rabbits include adenovirus, parvovirus, herpesvirus, and coronavirus. These viruses have only been identified to cause disease in very isolated cases and are not yet considered to be common pathogens of rabbits.

PARASITIC DISEASES

Ear Mites

Psoroptes cuniculi, the rabbit ear mite, is a nonburrowing mite that chews on the epidermal skin of the inner ear and causes an intense inflammatory response. A dry, brown crusty material accumulates on the

162

inner surface of the ear. This condition is very common in rabbits from conventional colonies.

Scratching of the ears and head shaking may be seen in rabbits as a result of the inflammation and pruritis associated with severe mite infestations. Crusty lesions may be seen on the back of the neck from scratching. Rarely, a secondary bacterial infection occurs, leading to otitis media or interna. The mites can easily be seen with the aid of an otoscope or by placing the crusts in mineral oil on a slide and examining with a microscope.

The most efficient treatment method involves giving two injections of ivermectin at 400 µg/kg subcutaneously at 7- to 14-day intervals. Other treatments include generous applications of mineral oil with miticides, or similar commercial products. Topical treatment must be repeated three or four times weekly to kill the newly hatched mites. In severe cases, the ear canal should be gently cleansed to remove accumulated debris prior to medicating with a miticide.

Fur Mites

Cheyletiella parasitovorax, the dandruff mite, causes thinning of the fur and scaly lesions. Because the mite does not burrow, it is easily killed by application of cat flea powders or shampoos containing permethrins to the rabbit and bedding at weekly intervals. Infestation resulting in dermatitis has been reported in humans, dogs, and cats.

Mange Mites

Although, rabbits are susceptible to *Notoedres cati* and *Sarcoptes scabiei,* these mites do not commonly cause infestation.

Fleas

Dog and cat fleas will occasionally infest rabbits. Treatment is the same as for cats, with permethrin dusts and shampoos. The environment must also be treated to eliminate the parasite.

Cuterebra

Cuterebra spp. larvae live in the subcutaneous tissue and appear as large lumps with perforated breathing holes, usually on the neck or upper extremities. They grow up to 1 in. long and are similar in appearance to ox warbles. Treatment consists of incising the skin and removing the larvae. Care must be taken to avoid crushing the larvae, which can result in acute shock and death in the rabbit.

Pinworms

The rabbit pinworm, *Passalurus ambiguus,* is a whitish hairlike worm that can be seen in the rabbit's cecal contents. Pinworms are considered not to be very pathogenic to rabbits and are not infective to humans. Diagnosis is made by identifying the typical egg in the feces. They can be treated with piperazine, fenbendazole, or thiabendazole. Ivermectin may be an effective treatment option, although thorough studies have not been performed.

Tapeworms

The rabbit tapeworm, *Cittotaenia ctenoides,* seldom causes clinical problems and can be controlled by proper sanitation. Larval forms of *Taenia pisiformis* may be found at necropsy in the abdominal cavity or liver of rabbits ingesting food or water contaminated by dog or cat feces. *Taenia serialis* larval cysts are occasionally seen in the subcutaneous tissues of rabbits and can sometimes be surgically removed. Rabbits are not usually treated for *Taenia* spp. infections; however, mebendazole has been reported to kill the larvae of *T. pisiformis.*

☞ Protozoa

Encephalitozoonosis is usually a latent disease of rabbits caused by the protozoan organism *Encephalitozoon cuniculi.* This agent commonly infects domestic rabbits and is occasionally found in rodents. The agent is shed in the urine and ingested. There is evidence that vertical transmission occurs in rabbits.

The organism causes lesions in the brain and kidney, but clinical signs are rare and usually reflect involvement of the central nervous system. Grossly, there is fibrosis and pitting of the renal cortex. Lesions in the brain require microscopic examination for detection. It is primarily important as a complicating factor in interpretation of experimental data.

A tentative clinical diagnosis can be made with positive serology and typical central nervous system signs, including ataxia, depression, posterior paresis, and head tilt. There is no known treatment. Colonies can be cleaned of this organism by serologic screening and selection of clean animals. Several clinical laboratories that provide serologic screening for *E. cuniculi* are listed in Chapter 10, Serologic Testing and Quality Control.

☞ Coccidiosis

Coccidiosis is common in conventional rabbit colonies. In rabbits, it has two forms: intestinal and hepatic. Intestinal infections are by far the most common. The intestinal form is caused by several species of *Eimeria* including *Eimeria magna, Eimeria perforans, Eimeria media,* and *Eimeria irresidua.* The hepatic form is caused by *Eimeria stiedae.*

Adult rabbits usually show no clinical signs from infection with *E. stiedae,* but heavy infections in young animals may cause weight loss, diarrhea, and a potbellied appearance. At necropsy, the liver is enlarged and contains irregularly shaped, slightly raised yellow–white foci. Microscopically, bile duct hyperplasia and inflammation can be seen.

In mild cases of intestinal coccidiosis, few if any clinical signs are evident. Weight gains may be poor. The fecal material may be formed but softer than normal and tends to stick to the mesh of the cage floor. When present, diarrhea may range from an intermittent to a profuse watery form with traces of blood. Mortality can be seen in the young. The life cycle is direct as in other species. Transmission occurs through the ingestion of sporulated infective oocysts. Sporulation can occur in as little as 2 days if the ambient temperature and humidity are optimal. Reingestion of the soft nighttime fecal pellets does not allow time for sporulation; therefore, infection by this route is unlikely. With both intestinal and hepatic coccidiosis, oocysts appear in the feces except in animals that die very soon after onset of illness. Oocysts remain infectious in the environment for several months. A yeast, *Saccharomycopsis guttulatus,* is commonly found in rabbit feces and should not be incorrectly identified as a coccidial oocyte.

Prevention and control of coccidiosis is achieved by 1) strict cleaning and disinfection procedures; 2) use of wire hanging cages, J-type feeders, and water bottles or automatic watering devices; 3) medicated feed or water; and 4) in some cases, culling of infected animals.

There is no effective treatment for elimination of *E. stiedae* from the liver, but medication can be helpful in preventing the initial infection. Among the drugs used for treating or preventing coccidiosis are sulfamethazine, sulfadimethoxine, sulfaquinoxaline, sulfadimethoxine/ormetoprim, amprolium, monensin, robenidine, decoquinate, and lasalocid.

NEOPLASIA

☞ ## Uterine Adenocarcinoma

The most common neoplasm of domestic rabbits is uterine adenocarcinoma. The incidence of uterine adenocarcinoma is very high in does 5 years of age and older. A doe's reproductive performance generally declines several months before the tumor can be detected clinically. Other clinical signs may include a bloody vulvar discharge or bloody urine. Metastasis to the lungs and other organs occasionally occurs. Because of the frequency of uterine neoplasia in mature does, an OHE should be considered for pets not used for breeding.

Lymphosarcoma

Lymphosarcoma is the most common neoplasm seen in juvenile and young adult domestic rabbits. Characteristic findings include hepatosplenomegaly, lymphadenopathy, and pale nodules in the kidneys. The effectiveness of chemotherapeutics has not been investigated.

Prolactin-Secreting Pituitary Adenomas

Acidophil adenomas have recently been described in aged, nulliparous NZW rabbits. The tumors secrete prolactin and are associated with mammary gland abnormalities, including enlarged, nonpainful teats that are frequently engorged with fluid. Pituitary tumors may be more common in the domestic rabbit than previously realized.

Miscellaneous Neoplasms

Embryonal nephromas and bile duct adenomas are the third and fourth most common tumors seen in rabbits, respectively. Reports of other neoplasms are occasionally seen in the literature.

MISCELLANEOUS CONDITIONS

Buphthalmia

Buphthalmia is a form of glaucoma that is one of the more common inherited diseases of domestic rabbits. With this disease, there is an increase in the size of the anterior chamber, resulting in corneal opacity and increased prominence of the eyeball. The condition comes on slowly and does not appear to be painful to the rabbits. No treatment is necessary, although enucleation is an alternative.

Dermatophytosis

Ringworm in rabbits is most frequently caused by *Trichophyton mentagrophytes*. Because *T. mentagrophytes* does not fluoresce under ultraviolet light, microscopic examination or culturing of hair or skin scrapings is usually required to establish a diagnosis. Lesions are pruritic, crusty, and hairless and in most cases first appear on the head, ears, or toes. Ringworm is rarely encountered in domestic rabbits except in animals housed under poor husbandry conditions. Lesions may be treated with topical antifungal creams applied twice daily or by administration of griseofulvin orally.

☞ Fracture or Luxation of the Lumbar Spine

Fractures of the caudal lumbar spine are common, particularly at the L7–S1 junction. A sudden onset of posterior paralysis in a rabbit strongly suggests a fracture or luxation of the lumbar spine. Usually, it is due to failure to support the hindquarters and commonly occurs in rabbits that are dropped. The prognosis after back injury depends on the location and severity of the cord lesion but is usually unfavorable. Therapeutic criteria are similar to those for dogs and cats and may include steroids, frequent rotation of the animal to prevent pressure sores, and twice-daily manual expression of the bladder. Occasionally, an animal will recover with cage rest, but in most cases posterior paralysis with urinary and fecal incontinence persists and euthanasia is recommended.

☞ Hair Balls (Gastric Trichobezoars)

Gastric hair balls should be suspected in rabbits that suddenly stop eating and drinking and pass no fecal material but otherwise appear alert and in good health. The presence of a hair ball can usually be detected by palpation. In some cases, a radiograph may be necessary to confirm the diagnosis. Hair balls are in most cases the result of excessive self-grooming, often attributed to boredom. Deficiencies of copper, magnesium, certain amino acids, and fiber have been suggested as contributing causes. The incidence may be high in recently purchased animals as a result of shedding presumably due to a change in diet and room temperature.

A dose of 10–15 mL of mineral oil administered by a stomach tube and followed by gentle gastric massage, rehydration, and metoclopramide may be effective. Another suggested therapeutic regimen includes fresh pineapple juice at 10 mL once daily or divided every 12 hours for 5 days. The pineapple juice contains the enzyme papain, which may help digest the hair in the stomach. Papain may also be purchased in nutrition stores. Offering fresh greens may stimulate the appetite and induce gut motility. Bromelin enzyme can be used as a treatment and preventive. Surgical removal of a hair ball may be indicated with a valuable animal. Most treatments are ineffective but medical treatment is usually preferred over surgical intervention, which is associated with a high mortality rate. Death following blockage of the stomach by a hair ball is usually attributable to ketosis.

A high-fiber (up to 20%) pelleted diet is one of the best ways to prevent hair balls. Providing roughage such as alfalfa hay, apples, or cabbage may also be beneficial in prevention of hair balls and may assist in the passage of masses of hair. Rabbits should be brushed during shedding season to remove loose hair.

Heatstroke

Rabbits are very susceptible to overheating. Young rabbits in nest boxes, as well as older, obese, or pregnant rabbits are particularly prone to heat prostration. Other predisposing factors include a high ambient temperature over 29.5°C (85°F), high humidity (70% or higher), poor ventilation, and crowding. Rabbits housed outdoors should be provided shade. Treatment is aimed at quickly reducing the body temperature and providing supportive care such as steroids and intravenous fluids. Prognosis is usually guarded to poor.

☞ Ketosis (Pregnancy Toxemia)

Ketosis occasionally occurs in rabbits and in most cases is seen in obese does a few days prior to parturition. It is analogous to ketosis in guinea pigs and sheep in terms of etiology, treatment, and prevention. See the discussion on ketosis in Chapter 5, Guinea Pigs.

☞ Malocclusion

Tooth overgrowth results when open-rooted teeth do not properly occlude and, therefore, are not worn away. Although all of the rabbit's teeth continuously grow, overgrowth is most commonly seen in the incisors. Overgrowth of the incisors can occur with mandibular prognathism, which has a genetic basis. The shorter upper jaw causes the lower incisors to grow anterior instead of posterior to the upper teeth. Other causes of malocclusion include trauma and tooth root infection. Overgrowth of the cheek teeth may be underdiagnosed because of the difficulty in viewing these teeth. Use of an otoscope in an awake rabbit or a vaginal speculum in a sedated rabbit will allow visualization of the cheek teeth. Rabbit teeth grow an average of 10–12 cm (4–5 in.) per year.

Overgrown incisors may be treated by trimming them with a motorized dental bur or Dremel drill. The use of nail clippers is best avoided, as it can cause tooth fractures if not properly used. Pointed or sharp edges may be smoothed with a nail file. Repeat trimmings are indicated on an as-needed basis, typically monthly. Culling of an affected animal and its offspring is the only successful means of eradication in a breeding group.

Moist Dermatitis

Two forms of moist dermatitis that occur in rabbits are sore dewlap and hutch burn. Various bacteria may be involved, but the underlying cause of these conditions is constant wetting of fur. The usual conditions that lead to sore dewlap are drooling from malocclusion or drinking from open pans or crocks. Treatment consists of removing the cause of wetness, clipping the fur from the affected area and applying a topical drying ointment.

Hutch burn is a superficial inflammatory condition of the anogenital area caused by prolonged contact of the skin with urine or soiling by diarrhea. Treatment involves eliminating the underlying cause, cleansing the lesion, and applying a topical drying ointment, such as zinc oxide, and perhaps a topical antibiotic ointment. Prevention is best achieved by adhering to generally accepted husbandry practices.

Muscular Dystrophy

Vitamin E deficiencies can result in nutritional muscular dystrophy. Clinical signs are neonatal mortality, infertility, keratitis, and muscular weakness in growing rabbits. Commercial diets usually provide adequate amounts of vitamin E.

Splay Leg

Splay leg is the term used to describe an abnormality in which a rabbit is unable to abduct one or more limbs. It is usually due to a recessive inherited trait. The most common form is subluxation of the hip. Affected animals sit with their legs splayed out sideways. There is no effective treatment, and prevention is accomplished by culling animals carrying this trait.

☞ ## Ulcerative Pododermatitis

Ulcerative pododermatitis is commonly called sore hock, but it actually involves the ventral metatarsal region rather than the hock. It usually occurs in heavy rabbits maintained on rounded wire-mesh floors rather than flat-bar floors. The condition may also occur in nervous rabbits that stomp their feet or in animals housed on solid floors that become urine soaked.

The lesion consists of a circumscribed ulcerated area of the skin that is covered by a dry crusty scab. Abscesses, caused by organisms such as *S. aureus,* may form under the scab. Affected individuals may lose weight and sit in a humped position or shift weight on their hind feet.

Treatment consists of providing soft, clean, dry bedding in a solid-bottom cage or providing a flat surface in a wire-mesh-bottom cage for the rabbit to sit on. Lesions may be treated by application of a topical ointment such as zinc oxide. A bandage affords protection against further trauma. If abscesses are present, broad-spectrum systemic antibiotics are indicated.

Urolithiasis

Urolithiasis is relatively common in pet rabbits. Calcium excretion by the kidney coupled with a high urinary pH of approximately 8.2 may predispose urinary solutes to precipitate. Clinical signs may be nonspecific including anorexia, lethargy and abdominal distention. Hematuria and stranguria are inconsistently seen.

Diagnosis can often be made by palpation of the bladder. Radiography is also helpful because calcium uroliths are radio dense. Surgical removal of the uroliths followed by diuresis with Ringer's solution for several days is the standard treatment for pet rabbits. Antibiotic therapy may be indicated if a positive culture is obtained. The role of diet has not been thoroughly investigated, but adding variety to the diet may be indicated for rabbits maintained exclusively on a pelleted ration.

■ GENERAL REFERENCES

Sources consulted to compile the material in this chapter include *The Biology and Medicine of Rabbits and Rodents* by J.E. Harkness and J.E. Wagner, 4th edition (1995, Williams & Wilkins, 1400 North Providence Rd., Building II, Suite 5025, Media, PA 19063); *Laboratory Animal Medicine,* edited by J.G. Fox, B.J. Cohen, and F. M. Loew (1984, Academic Press, Inc., Orlando, FL 32887); *The Biology of the Laboratory Rabbit,* edited by D.H. Ringler (1994, Academic Press, Inc., Orlando, FL 32887); *The UFAW Handbook on the Care and Management of Laboratory Animals,* 6th edition, edited by T.B. Poole

(1987, Churchill Livingstone Inc., 1560 Broadway, New York, NY 10036); and *Pathology of Laboratory Rodents and Rabbits,* by D.H. Percy and S.W. Barthold (1993, Iowa State University Press, 2121 South State Avenue, Ames, IA 50014).

■ TECHNICAL REFERENCES

Adam, H.K, J.B. Glen, and P.A. Hoyle. 1990. Pharmacokinetics in laboratory animals of ICI 35868, a new I.V. anesthetic agent. *Br J Anaesth* 52(8): 743–746.

Aeschbacher, G. and A.I. Webb. 1993. Propofol in rabbits. 1. Determination of an induction dose. *Lab Anim Sci* 43(4): 324–327.

Allen, D.G., J.K. Pringle, and D.A. Smith. 1993. *Handbook of Veterinary Drugs.* Philadelphia: JB Lippincott.

Broome, R.L. and D.L. Brooks. 1991. Efficacy of enrofloxacin in the treatment of respiratory pasteurellosis in rabbits. *Lab Anim Sci* 41(6): 572–576.

Burgmann, P., and D.H. Percy. 1993. Antimicrobial drug use in rodents and rabbits. In *Antimicrobial Therapy in Veterinary Medicine,* ed. J.F. Prescott and J.D. Baggot, pp. 524–541. Ames: Iowa State University Press.

Butt, M.T., R.E. Papendick, L.G. Carbone, and F.W. Quimby. 1994. A cytotoxicity assay for *Clostridium spiroforme* enterotoxin in cecal fluid of rabbits. *Lab Anim Sci* 44(1): 52–54.

Carpenter, J.W., T.Y. Mashima, E.J. Gentz, et al. 1995. Caring for rabbits: an overview and formulary. *Vet Med* (April): 340–364.

Cundiff, D.D., C.L. Besch-Williford, R.R. Hook, C.L. Franklin, and L.K. Riley. 1995. Characterization of cilia-associated respiratory bacillus in rabbits and analysis of the 16S rRNA gene sequence. *Lab Anim Sci* 45(1): 22–26.

Doerning, B.J., D.W. Brammer, C.E. Chrisp, and H.G. Rush. 1992. Nephrotoxicity of tiletamine in New Zealand White rabbits. *Lab Anim Sci* 42(3): 267–269.

Flecknell, P.A. 1987. *Laboratory Animal Anesthesia.* London: Academic.

Flecknell, P.A. 1991. Post-operative analgesia in rabbits and rodents. *Lab Anim* 20: 34–37.

Flecknell, P.A. 1997. Medetomidine and atipamezole: Potential uses in laboratory animals. *Lab Anim* 26(2): 21–25.

Flecknell, P.A., I.J. Cruz, J.H. Liles, and G. Whelan. 1996. Induction of anaesthesia with halothane and isoflurane in the rabbit: a comparison of the use of a face-mask or an anaesthetic chamber. *Lab Anim Sci* 30(1): 67–74.

Gillett, C.S. 1994. Selected drug dosages and clinical reference data. In *The Biology of the Laboratory Rabbit,* 2nd ed., ed. P.J. Manning, D.H. Ringler, and C.E. Newcomer, pp. 467–472. San Diego: Academic.

Heard, D.J. 1993. Principles and techniques of anesthesia and analgesia for exotic practice. *Vet Clin North Am Small Anim Pract* 23(6): 1301–1327.

Hillyer, E.V. 1994. Pet Rabbits. *Vet Clin North Am Small Anim Pract* 24(1): 25–65.

Huerkamp, M.J. 1995. Anesthesia and postoperative management of rabbits and pocket pets. In *Kirk's Current Therapy XII: Small Animal Practice,* ed. J.D. Bonagura, pp. 1322–1327. Philadelphia: WB Saunders.

Jenkins, J.R. 1993. Rabbits. In *A Practitioner's Guide to Rabbits and Ferrets,* ed. J.R. Jenkins and S.A. Brown. Lakewood, CO: American Animal Hospital Association.

Jenkins, J.R. 1995. Rabbit drug dosages. In *Exotic Animal Formulary,* ed. L. Bauck, T.H. Boyer, and S.A. Brown, pp. 13–17. Lakewood, CO: American Animal Hospital Association.

Johnson-Delaney, C.A. 1996. *Exotic Companion Medicine Handbook for Veterinarians.* Lake Worth, FL: Wingers.

Lipman, N.S., R.S. Marini, and S.E. Erdman. 1990. A comparison of ketamine/xylazine and ketamine/xylazine/acepromazine anesthesia in the rabbit. *Lab Anim Sci* 40(4): 395–398.

Lipman, N.S., Z. Zhi-bo, K.A. Andrutis, R.J. Hurley, J.G. Fox, and H.J. White. 1994. Prolactin-secreting pituitary adenomas with mammary dysplasia in New Zealand White rabbits. *Lab Anim Sci* 44(2): 114–120.

Marini, R.P., D.L. Avison, B.F. Corning, and N.S. Lipman. 1992. Ketamine/xylazine/butorphanol: a new anesthetic combination for rabbits. *Lab Anim Sci* 42(1): 57–62.

Mills, D.L., and R. Walshaw. Elective castrations and ovariohysterectomies in pet rabbits. *J Am Anim Hosp Assoc* 28: 491–498.

Nicolau, D.P., C.D. Freeman, C.H. Nightingale, and R. Quintiliani. 1993. Pharmacokinetics of minocycline and vancomycin in rabbits. *Lab Anim Sci* 43(3): 222–225.

Okerman, L. 1994. *Diseases of Domestic Rabbits,* 2nd ed. Oxford: Blackwell Scientific.

Peeters, J.E., R. Geeroms, H. Varewyck, I. Bouquet, P. Lampo, and P. Halen. 1983. Immunity and effect of clopidol/methyl benzoquate and robenidine before and after weaning on rabbit coccidiosis in the field. *Res Vet Sci* 35(2): 211–216.

Perkins, S.E., J.G. Fox, N.S. Taylor, D.L. Green, and N.S. Lipman. 1995. Detection of *Clostridium difficile* toxins from the small intestine and cecum of rabbits with naturally acquired enterotoxemia. *Lab Anim Sci* 45(4): 379–384.

Quesenberry, K.E. 1994. Rabbits. In *Saunders Manual of Small Animal Practice,* ed. S.J. Birchard and R.G. Sherding, pp. 1345–1362. Philadelphia: WB Saunders.

Robertson, S.A., and S. Eberhart. 1994. Efficacy of the intranasal route for administration of anesthetic agents to adult rabbits. *Lab Anim Sci* 44(2): 159–165.

Russell, R.J., D.K. Johnson, and J.A. Stunkard. 1981. *A Guide to Diagnosis, Treatment, and Husbandry of Pet Rabbits and Rodents.* Edwardsville, KS: Veterinary Medicine.

Smith, D.A. and P.M. Burgmann. 1997. Formulary. In *Ferrets, Rabbits, and Rodents: Clinical Medicine and Surgery,* ed. E.V. Hillyer and K.E. Quesenberry, pp. 392–403. Philadelphia: WB Saunders.

Steinleitner, A., H. Lambert, C. Kazensky, I. Sanchez, and C. Sueldo. 1990. Reduction of primary postoperative adhesion formation under calcium channel blockade in the rabbit. *J Surg Res* 48(1): 42–45.

Wixson, S.K. 1994. Rabbits and rodents: anesthesia and analgesia. In *Research Animal Anesthesia, Analgesia and Surgery,* ed. A.C. Smith and M.M. Swindle. Greenbelt, MD: Scientists Center for Animal Welfare.

172

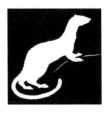

FERRETS

THE EUROPEAN FERRET belongs to the order Carnivora and the family Mustelidae. The scientific name of the domestic ferret is *Mustela putorius furo,* which appropriately translates into "stinky weasel thief." The domestic ferret is believed to be derived from the wild European polecat and is related to the skunk, weasel, otter, badger, and mink. The domestic ferret should not be confused with the native North American black-footed ferret, *Mustela nigripes.* There are two varieties of domestic ferret: the wild type, or fitch, and the albino. The wild type has a buff-colored coat with black mask, limbs, and tail. The albino is white with pink eyes. Male ferrets are called hobs, females are known as jills, and the young are referred to as kits. Adult male ferrets weigh 1–2 kg, whereas females are much smaller, weighing 600–900 g.

Uses

The ferret's popularity as a pet has continued to increase in recent years. Ferrets tend to have a friendly disposition, and their inquisitive nature makes them interesting pets. An objectionable feature of ferrets is their strong musky odor. Castration or ovariohysterectomy (OHE) will greatly diminish the smell by eliminating the hormones that stimulate production of the musky sebaceous secretions of the apocrine skin glands. Owing to a concern that escaped pet ferrets would become an established feral species, several states have laws that prohibit or regulate the keeping of ferrets as pets.

Although not used in large numbers for research, ferrets are valuable in a number of areas of study, including reproductive physiology, virus-induced neoplasms, bacterial infections, and viral diseases of humans and other animals. They have been particularly useful for studies of canine distemper, vesicular stomatitis, *Helicobacter pylori* gastritis, and human influenza. Ferrets have been used as an alternative carnivore for drug studies, replacing dogs and cats. Because they have a similar oropharyngeal anatomy to the human infant, ferrets are also commonly used for neonatal intubation practice.

Behavior

Ferrets are inquisitive, friendly, and playful by nature. They tend to be social and do well either housed alone or in sexually distinct groups. Sexually intact males, however, will fight with other males during the breeding season, and females with litters may show aggression in order to protect their kits. Ferrets love playmates and can get along with other ferrets, cats, and nonhunting breeds of dogs. Their carnivorous instincts, however, will cause them to hunt and kill small animals, especially rodents and birds. There are reports of ferrets attacking human infants; thus, they should never be left unsupervised with infants.

Ferrets will usually only bite when they are frightened, starving, or in pain. Nipping, however, is one their favorite ways of getting attention. This behavior must be discouraged from becoming a habit, as they can inflict deep punctures with their sharp pointed teeth. There are two differing opinions on how best to eliminate this behavior. One method is with a loud "No!" followed by a thump on the nose. Another method is to grasp the ferret firmly by its scruff and say a loud "No!" Some feel that hitting a ferret may actually cause them to be nervous and more likely to bite out of fear. Ferrets may express their anal scent glands when they are excited or angry. Frequent gentle handling will greatly decrease the likelihood of unpredictable behavior in ferrets.

Ferrets spend from 15 to 20 hours per day sleeping. They are nocturnal animals and like to burrow. They can be easily trained to use a litter box, like cats, as they prefer to urinate and defecate in one place. Ferrets learn quickly and can be trained to come to particular cues such as a bell or clicker. They easily adapt to a harness and lead. Their curious nature will often get them into trouble if allowed to roam freely in a house. They like to chew on objects such as electrical cords or anything made out of rubber or plastic. To avoid gastrointestinal obstructions, soft latex and rubber dog and cat toys should not be offered to ferrets. Appropriate toys include paper bags, hard rubber balls with bells inside of them, polyvinyl chloride pipes, and cat teasers. Ferrets also like to swim and may be provided with a shallow pan of water to play in.

Anatomic and Physiologic Features

Ferret biologic and reproductive data can be found in Table 8.1. Ferrets have long, thin bodies with short legs, a medium-length tail, and thick, soft fur. Large seasonal fluctuations in weight are due to the ac-

Table 8.1. Ferret biologic and reproductive values

Adult body weight	
Male	1–2 kg
Female	600–900 g
Life span	5–11 y
Body temperature	37.8°–40° C (100°–104° F)
Heart rate	200–400 beats per minute
Respiratory rate	33–36 breaths per minute
Food consumption	140–190 g/d
Water consumption	75–100 mL/d
Breeding onset	
Male	8–12 mo
Female	7–10 mo
Estrous cycle length	Continuous until intromission
Gestation period	41–43 d
Postpartum estrus	Occasional
Litter size	8
Weaning age	6–8 wk
Breeding duration	2–5 y
Chromosome number (diploid)	40

Source: Adapted from Fox (1988).

cumulation of subcutaneous fat during the autumn months and its subsequent loss in the spring and summer. They have apocrine skin glands that produce sebaceous secretions that are responsible for their distinct musky odor. The albino coat color becomes more yellow as the ferret matures because of sebaceous secretions from its skin. The ferret also has glands on either side of the anus, which are mistakenly blamed for the musky odor. Their normal rectal temperature is in the range of 38°–39°C (100°–102°F), but excitement may raise this to 40°C (104°F). They do not have well-developed sweat glands and as a result, are prone to heat exhaustion at temperatures approaching 32°C (90°F). They dissipate heat mainly through their respiratory system.

Their dental formula, 2 (3/3 incisors, 1/1 canines, 3/3 premolars, 1/2 molars), is unique among carnivores in having only 3 premolars rather than 4. Supernumerary teeth are common in adults. They have a simple stomach similar to that of humans. The intestinal tract is short, having a transit time of 3–4 hours. There is no cecum, appendix, taeniae coli, or ileocolonic sphincter.

Ferrets have a very long trachea and large-diameter airways, which give them lower airway resistance. Their lungs have two left lobes and four right lobes. Small, pale yellow, slightly elevated spots may be seen on the surface of the lungs at necropsy. These are foci of alveolar histiocytosis and are of no known clinical significance.

The reproductive systems of both males and females are similar to those of other carnivores, with a few exceptions. The female has a bicornuate uterus with only one cervical os. Females have four pairs of mammary glands. Males have open inguinal canals throughout their lives. During the nonbreeding season, August to November, spermatogenesis ceases, testicular size decreases, and the testes retract into the abdomen. Males reportedly do not have seminal vesicles but do have an os penis. Sexing of both adult and neonatal ferrets is accomplished without difficulty, as the penis is situated on the ventral abdomen and the anogenital distance is greater in the male. The female vulva is readily visible just ventral to the anus.

There are several distinct characteristics of the physiologic and laboratory profiles of ferrets. Hematocrit values, hemoglobin levels, erythrocyte counts, and reticulocyte counts tend to be somewhat higher in ferrets than in other species of laboratory animals. The average values for males are slightly higher than for females in all except reticulocyte counts. Female ferrets in estrus tend to have lower platelet and leukocyte counts. During the nonbreeding season, males have reduced plasma testosterone levels. The normal urine pH ranges between 6.5 and 7.5. Slight to moderate proteinuria is commonly found in ferrets. The naturally dark urine of the male may present difficulty in interpretation of urine chemistry tests when colorimetric methods are used. Hematologic and biochemical parameters for the ferret are listed in Appendix 1, Normal Values.

Breeding and Reproduction

Ferrets reach sexual maturity in the spring after their birth or at approximately 9–12 months of age. Females are seasonally polyestrous and are induced ovulators like the cat and the rabbit. Marked swelling of the vulva signals the start of estrus. The breeding season is light dependent, usually lasting from March to August. Artificial lighting can be used to induce the breeding season. Females that are not bred may remain in heat for up to 6 months. A protracted period of estrus is characterized by weight loss, increased susceptibility to uterine infections, and aplastic anemia. These features probably account for the common belief that unmated females will become depressed and die. Male sexual activity lasts from December to July, preceding female activity to allow for sperm maturation. The enlargement and descent of the testicles into the scrotum marks the period of sexual activity in the male.

Mating should occur 2 weeks after the onset of vulvar swelling. The female should be taken to the male's cage and observed for fighting. Mating in ferrets is frequently noisy and energetic with rolling, jumping, and the female submitting to being dragged around by the scruff of the neck. Copulation lasts from 1 to 3 hours. Part of this time is spent in achieving intromission because the males are poorly coordinated. Ovulation occurs 30–40 hours after mating. The females enlarged vulva will regress to normal size within 2 to 3 weeks after breeding if she is pregnant. If it doesn't regress, then she should be rebred. The average gestation length is 42 days. Fetuses can be palpated by 14 days. Nonfertile matings result in a pseudopregnancy, which also lasts 42 days. Females in estrus may be induced to ovulate by stimulation by other females or injections of human chorionic gonadotropin.

Litter size ranges from 2 to 17 kits. The young weigh 7–10 g on average and are born hairless and blind. Eyes and ears open at 21–37 days of age. Kits will begin eating solid food at about 3 weeks of age. They are weaned at 6–8 weeks, and reach their adult weight at about 4 months. Depending on the time of year, the female will return to estrus about 2 weeks after the young are weaned or the following March. Ferrets can produce two litters per year if bred early in the season.

HUSBANDRY

Housing

Ferrets can be housed in dog, cat, or rabbit cages that have been modified to ensure secure containment of these smaller animals. Ferrets are great escape artists, so their cages must be escape proof. Solid-bottom cages seem to be more suitable for their small feet than are slotted or wire-mesh flooring. If wire mesh must be used, a washable rug can be placed in the cage to help protect the ferrets' feet. They should be provided with enough room to move around freely. A 0.27 m^2 (3.0 ft^2) floor area with at least 36 cm (14 in.) of height for an adult ferret. Cages that have multiple floors are ideal for pet ferrets. A bedding material, such as wood chips or newspapers, can be used in solid-bottom cages. A waste pan can be placed under suspended cages with wire-grid floors. Ferrets seem to enjoy a den or nest box with a small entry hole, and they love to curl up in soft T-shirts or blankets.

Ferrets tolerate low temperatures without difficulty. A temperature range of 4°–18°C (39°–64°F) is generally optimal, but the young should not be kept at temperatures below 15°C (59°F). Ferrets are prone to heat exhaustion and should not be housed in direct sunlight. A humidity range between 40% and 65% and 10–15 air changes per hour are recommended. Ferrets housed without exposure to natural light should have timer-controlled artificial lighting that provides 12 hours of light per day. If reproduction is important, the artificial light should follow a specific schedule that mimics the natural pattern of day length change.

Ferrets habitually use one corner of the cage for defecation and urination. Daily removal of the soiled bedding and replacement with fresh bedding is ideal. In a research setting, cages and bottles are sanitized at least weekly. Cages, water bottles, and feed hoppers should be disinfected with chemicals, hot water 61.6°–82.2°C (143°–180°F), or a combination of both. Detergents and chemical disinfectants enhance the effectiveness of hot water, but they must be thoroughly rinsed from all caging surfaces with fresh water. Refer to Chapter 1, Mice, for a more detailed description of disinfection methods.

Feeding and Watering

Pelleted commercial chows, such as ferret, mink, and cat chows, containing at least 30%–35% protein and 18%–30% fat are adequate to maintain an adult ferret. Diets with 42% protein are suggested for growth. Young kits may need to have pellets softened in water. Ferrets eat on average 140–190 g per day. Food should be offered in heavy bowls that cannot be tipped over. They can be fed ad libitum and will generally eat 8–10 small meals throughout the day and night. Supplements are not necessary, but pet ferrets will enjoy an occasional snack, such as cooked egg or meat. Because ferrets cannot digest fiber well, fruits and vegetable snacks should be kept to a minimum and offered in very small increments. Chocolate and milk products should not be given, as they cause digestive tract upsets. All changes in diet should be introduced slowly and mixed with the original diet to allow adjustment. A fatty acid supplement, 0.25 mL per day, may be added to the diet if the coat becomes dry.

Ferrets consume about 75–100 mL of water per day. They should have fresh, potable water available ad libitum. A water bottle attached to the cage or heavy crock inside the cage works fine.

TECHNIQUES

Handling and Restraint

Frequent, gentle handling of ferrets will make them a more tractable pet or research animal. Ferrets can be picked up from behind with one hand placed under the chest and the other supporting their pelvis. They will often rest comfortably in the crook of one's elbow or may enjoy climbing into a roomy coat pocket.

Most ferrets are gentle and can be manually restrained without gloves. Gentle restraint is usually adequate for physical examinations. For more invasive procedures, a number of more secure restraints can be used. One way is to scruff the loose skin at the nape of the neck with one hand and suspend the ferret's body. This technique appears to relax and immobilize ferrets. The technique is shown in Figure 8.1. Most simple procedures, such as nail clipping, ear cleaning, and abdominal palpation can be performed on a ferret that is restrained in this manner. Another way is to place a hand across the shoulders with the thumb under the chin, the forefinger around the neck, and the other fingers around the

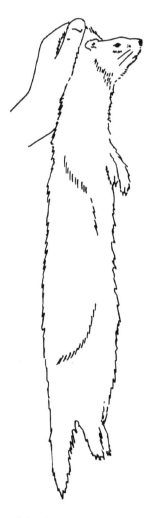

Figure 8.1. Restraint of the ferret.

chest behind the forelimbs. The other hand can be used to support the lower back. If a more secure hold is required, then the other hand is placed around the pelvis in front of the hindlimbs. Ferrets should not be stretched out as this may cause them to rigorously resist. Sick animals or females with young may bite and should be handled with caution.

Identification

Cage cards may be used as a general means of identifying caged ferrets. Permanent individual identification may be accomplished by ear tagging, ear punching, tattooing, or placement of a subcutaneous microchip.

Blood Collection

Approximate blood volumes for ferrets are listed in Table 8.2. Small amounts of blood, approximately 0.5 mL, can be obtained from a clipped toenail. Similarly, the lateral saphenous or cephalic veins can be accessed with a small-gauge needle and tuberculin syringe for collection of small amounts of blood. The superficial veins, however, are not readily discernible. Jugular veins and the caudal tail vein or artery are other alternative sites. The retroorbital sinus can also be used to obtain a small volume of blood in an anesthetized ferret. The technique is similar to that used in the mouse and is described in more detail in Chapter 1, Mice.

The jugular vein is the most accessible site for collection of larger blood volumes in ferrets. Restraint is similar to that used for a cat, with the forelimbs held over the end of a table and the chin restrained upward. The cranial vena cava and heart are two more sites that can be used to collect larger amounts of blood in an anesthetized ferret. Both of these sites carry a higher risk of hemorrhage and should be performed with caution.

Urine Collection

Urine may be collected from a metabolism cage or by cystocentesis. Excited ferrets will often void on the table.

Table 8.2. Adult ferret blood volumes	
	Volume (mL)[a]
Total blood	60–120
Single sample	6–12
Exsanguination	24–60

Source: Adapted from Hillyer and Brown (1994).
[a]Values are approximate.

Drug Administration

Oral dosing is easy to accomplish by placing a syringe at the corner of the ferret's mouth and slowly depositing the liquid on the back of the tongue. Unpalatable drugs can be given through a stomach tube using a mouth gag. Because ferrets lack a cough reflex, the proper placement of the stomach tube should always be verified by aspirating for stomach contents. A dose of 50 mL can be given orally to an adult ferret without adverse effects. Subcutaneous injections with a maximum volume of 5–10 mL per site can be made under the loose skin over the dorsal cervical area. Intramuscular injections having a maximum volume of 0.5 mL are given, as in the dog or cat, in the semimembranosus or quadriceps thigh muscles, and lumbar muscles. During the fall months of the year, allowance should be made for the thick layer of subcutaneous fat that requires a longer needle to deliver an injection. Ferrets can be distracted by placing a small dab of something sweet, such as Nutrical, on their belly and allowing them to lick it off while giving injections. Intraperitoneal injections with a maximum volume of 5–8 mL can be given just off of the midline in the lower abdominal quadrant. Care must be taken to aspirate before injecting the solution to ensure that the needle has not entered the bladder, bowel, or other organ. The cephalic or lateral saphenous veins can be used to deliver small volumes intravenously. Larger volumes should be administered through an indwelling catheter placed in the cephalic, saphenous, or jugular veins.

☞ Immunization

Ferrets must be routinely protected against canine distemper by vaccination with a modified live virus of chicken embryo origin. This vaccine has been found to be superior to the formalin-inactivated vaccine. Live vaccines of ferret origin or killed vaccines of canine origin are not recommended, as they are capable of causing the disease. If the dam has been immunized, the initial dose should be administered at 6–8 weeks of age. If kits are from susceptible, unvaccinated dams, they should be vaccinated between 4 and 6 weeks of age. Additional doses should be administered at 3- to 4-week intervals until the ferret is 16 weeks old. Booster injections should be given every year. Because distemper is almost invariably fatal, a ferret should be vaccinated at the time of its first visit to a veterinary hospital unless previously immunized or exhibiting signs of the disease. Anaphylactic reactions to repeated doses of vaccine have been reported; thus, as a precaution, it is prudent to have the ferret stay in the clinic for 15–20 minutes after the booster has been given. Diphenhydramine can be given prior to vaccination to prevent a repeat reaction.

A killed rabies vaccine labeled for use in ferrets is available and should be administered at 3 months of age and annually thereafter. A modified live rabies vaccine must not be used, as it has been implicated as causing an active case of rabies in a ferret.

Ferrets produced for research purposes are immunized against *Bordetella bronchiseptica* and *Pseudomonas aeruginosa*. *Bordetella bronchiseptica* bacterin is given at 6 weeks and boostered at 8 weeks of age. *Pseudomonas aeruginosa* bacterin is given to prevent acute hemorrhagic pneumonia around 11 weeks of age and appears to protect them for life.

Ferrets are not susceptible to canine hepatitis, canine parvovirus, mink virus enteritis, feline panleukopenia, feline rhinotracheitis, or feline calicivirus.

Anesthesia, Surgery, and Postoperative Care

Agents commonly used for anesthesia and tranquilization in ferrets are listed in Table 8.3. Ferrets should be fasted for at least 6 hours before surgery but should be allowed free access to water. There are a number of injectable agents that can provide adequate anesthesia for

Table 8.3. Anesthetic agents and tranquilizers used in ferrets

Drug	Dosage	Route	Reference
Inhalants			
Halothane	0.5%–3.5% to effect	Inhalation	Fox (1988)
Isoflurane	2%–5% to effect	Inhalation	Brown (1993)
Methoxyflurane	To effect	Inhalation	Fox (1988)
Injectables			
Acetylpromazine	0.2–0.5 mg/kg	SC, IM	Fox (1988)
Diazepam	1–2 mg/kg	IM	Fox (1988)
	1 mg per animal	IV	Hillyer and Brown (1994)
Fentanyl-droperidol	0.15 mL/kg	IM	Flecknell (1987)
Ketamine	30–60 mg/kg	IM	Fox (1988)
Ketamine	20–35 mg/kg	SC, IM	Hillyer and Brown (1994)
+ acetylpromazine	0.2–0.35 mg/kg	SC, IM	
Ketamine	25–35 mg/kg	IM	Brown (1993)
+ diazepam	2–3 mg/kg	IM	
Ketamine	8 mg/kg	IM	Flecknell (1997)
+ medetomidine	0.1 mg/kg	IM	
Ketamine	10–25 mg/kg	IM	Hillyer and Brown (1994)
+ xylazine	1–2 mg/kg	IM	
Pentobarbital	30–36 mg/kg	IP	Fox (1988)
Tiletamine-zolazepam	12–22 mg/kg	IM	Payton (1989)
Tiletamine-zolazepam	3 mg/kg	IM	Ko (1996)
+ ketamine	2.4 mg/kg	IM	
+ xylazine	0.6 mg/kg	IM	
Xylazine	1 mg/kg	SC, IM	Fox (1988)

IM = intramuscular; IP = intraperitoneal; IV = intravenous; SC = subcutaneous.

short procedures. Atropine or glycopyrrolate should be administered as a preanesthetic to reduce salivation and gastrointestinal secretions and to minimize cardiac arrhythmias. Ketamine-xylazine combination has been associated with a significant number of premature ventricular contractions and death. Ketamine-acetylpromazine combination seems to work well. Barbiturates are frequently given intraperitoneally in ferrets because venipuncture is difficult to achieve. Caution should be exercised when using sodium pentobarbital or other barbiturates, as they have a narrow margin between surgical anesthesia and death. Inhalant anesthetics can be used as a supplement to decrease the total amount of barbiturate needed.

Several inhalants, including isoflurane, halothane, and methoxyflurane, are safe and commonly used in ferrets. Ferrets can be masked down or placed in a small induction chamber. Premedicating a ferret with acetylpromazine or other suitable sedative will allow for an easier masking induction. They can then be maintained on a mask, but should be intubated with a noncuffed tube (1.5–3.0 outside diameter) for longer procedures. Because of their small size, a nonrebreathing system should be used. The depth of anesthesia can be monitored by rate and depth of respiration, heart rate, degree of jaw tension, and pedal and palpebral reflexes.

Pet ferrets are neutered at 6–8 months of age, although commercial breeders are neutering and descenting ferrets as early as 3–4 weeks of age. The same neutering procedures that are used in cats can be used in ferrets. Scrotal incisions with an open or closed technique can be used for castration. When performing an OHE, note the ovarian pedicles normally contain large amounts of fat. A neutered female is called a "sprite," and a neutered male is called a "gib." Neutering will reduce aggression in males and will diminish the musky scent released from the sebaceous skin glands by the action of estrogen and testosterone. An OHE will prevent aplastic anemia due to a prolonged state of estrus in the female. Surgical removal of the anal scent glands of ferrets is more tedious than anal sac removal in the dog. As in all animals, use of aseptic technique, prevention of hypothermia, and attention to hydration status will increase the number of successful postoperative outcomes. Postoperative analgesics should be administered for invasive procedures. A list of acceptable analgesic agents for ferrets is found in Table 8.4. Butorphanol is indicated to control mild postoperative discomfort. Buprenorphine works well to control acute or chronic visceral pain but causes more sedation.

Table 8.4. Analgesic agents used in ferrets			
Drug	Dosage	Route	Reference
Acetylsalicylic acid	0.5–22 mg/kg q8–24h	PO	Hillyer and Brown (1994)
Buprenorphine	0.01–0.03 mg/kg q8–12h	SC, IM, IV	Heard (1993)
Butorphanol	0.1–0.5 mg/kg q12h	IM	Brown (1995)
Flunixin meglumine	0.3 mg/kg q24h	PO, SC	Brown (1995)
Meperidine	5–10 mg/kg q2–4h	SC, IM, IV	Heard (1993)
Morphine	0.5–5 mg/kg q2–6h	SC, IM	Heard (1993)
Nalbuphine	0.5–1.5 mg/kg q2–3h	IM, IV	Heard (1993)
Oxymorphone	0.05–0.2 mg/kg q8–12h	IM, IV, SC	Heard (1993)
Pentazocine	5–10 mg/kg q4h	IM	Heard (1993)

IM = intramuscular; IV = intravenous; PO = per os; SC = subcutaneous.

Euthanasia

Acceptable methods of euthanasia include an overdose of a barbiturate or commercial euthanasia solution given either intravenously or intraperitoneally. Carbon dioxide (approximately 70%) in a prefilled chamber is also acceptable but may be associated with anxious behavior. Refer to Chapter 1, Mice, for more information on euthanasia guidelines.

THERAPEUTIC AGENTS

Antimicrobial and antifungal agents and recommended dosages for ferrets are listed in Table 8.5. Antiparasitic agents for use in ferrets can be found in Table 8.6 and miscellaneous drugs and dosages for ferrets are listed in Table 8.7.

Table 8.5. Antimicrobial and antifungal agents used in ferrets

Drug	Dosage	Route	Reference
Amikacin	10–15 mg/kg q12h	SC, IM	Brown (1993)
Amoxicillin	20 mg/kg q12h	PO, SC	Hillyer and Brown (1994)
Amoxicillin-clavulanate	13–25 mg/kg q8–12h	PO	Hillyer and Brown (1994)
Amphotericin B	0.4–0.8 mg/kg q7d (total dose 7–25 mg)	IV	Besch-Williford (1987)
Ampicillin	10–30 mg/kg q12h	SC	Brown (1995)
Cefadroxil	15–20 mg/kg q12h	PO	Brown (1995)
Cephalexin	15–30 mg/kg q8h	PO	Hillyer and Brown (1994)
Cephaloridine	10–15 mg/kg q24h for 5–7 d	SC, IM	Brown (1993)
Chloramphenicol	50 mg/kg q12h	PO, SC, IM, IV	Hillyer and Brown (1994)
Ciprofloxacin	10 mg/kg q12h	PO	Brown (1995)
Clindamycin	5.5–10 mg/kg q12h	PO	Brown (1995)
Cloxacillin	10 mg/kg q6h	PO, IV, IM	Johnson-Delaney (1996)
Enrofloxacin	5–10 mg/kg q12h	PO, SC, IM	Brown (1995)
Erythromycin	10 mg/kg q6h	PO	Besch-Williford (1987)
Gentamicin	5 mg/kg q12h	PO, IM	Brown (1993)
Griseofulvin	25 mg/kg q24h	PO	Hillyer and Brown (1994)
Ketaconazole	10–30 mg/kg q8h	PO	Besch-Williford (1987)
Lincomycin	11 mg/kg q8h	PO	Besch-Williford (1987)
Neomycin	10–20 mg/kg q6h	PO	Besch-Williford (1987)
Oxytetracycline	17–20 mg/kg q8h	PO	Besch-Williford (1987)
Penicillin, procaine	40,000–44,000 IU/kg q24h	IM	Brown (1993)
Sulfadimethoxine	30–50 mg/kg q12–24h	PO	Collins (1995)
Sulfamethazine	1 mg/mL drinking water		Collins (1995)
Tetracycline	25 mg/kg q12h	PO	Brown (1993)
Trimethoprim-sulfa	15–30 mg/kg q12h	PO, SC	Hillyer and Brown (1994)
Tylosin	10 mg/kg q8h	PO	Collins (1995)
	5–10 mg/kg q12h	IM, IV	Collins (1995)

IM = intramuscular; IV = intravenous; PO = per os; SC = subcutaneous.

Table 8.6. Antiparasitic agents used in ferrets

Drug	Dosage	Route	Reference
Carbaryl (5%)	Once weekly	Topical	Fox (1988)
Diethylcarbamazine	5–11 mg/kg q24h	PO	Hillyer and Brown (1994)
Ivermectin	0.4 mg/kg, repeat in 2–4 wk	PO, SC	Hillyer and Brown (1994)
	0.05 mg/kg/mo	PO	Hillyer and Brown (1994)
	0.5 mg/kg half dose in each ear, repeat in 2 wk	Topical	Hillyer and Brown (1994)
Lime sulfur	Dilute 1:40 with water, dip q7d for 6 wk	Topical	Fox (1988)
Metronidazole	15–20 mg/kg q12h for 2 wk	PO	Brown (1993)
Milbemycin oxime	1.15–2.3 mg/kg/mo	PO	Johnson-Delaney (1996)
Praziquantel	5–10 mg/kg, repeat in 2 wk	SC	Brown (1993)
Pyrantel pamoate	4.4 mg/kg once	PO	Besch-Williford (1987)
Pyrethrin powder	Once weekly for 3 wk	Topical	Fox (1988)

PO = per os; SC = subcutaneous.

Table 8.7. Miscellaneous agents used in ferrets

Drug	Dosage	Route	Reference
Aminophylline	4.4–6.6 mg/kg q12h	PO, IM	Hillyer and Brown (1994)
Apomorphine	5 mg/kg	SC	Besch-Williford (1987)
Atenolol	6.25 mg per animal q24h	PO	Brown (1995)
Atipamezole	1 mg/kg	SC, IP, IV	Flecknell (1997)
Atropine	0.04 mg/kg	SC, IM, IV	Hillyer and Brown (1994)
	5–10 mg/kg (organo-phosphate toxicity)	SC, IM	Brown (1995)
Barium (20%)	15 mL/kg	PO	Hillyer and Brown (1994)
Bismuth-subsalicylate (Pepto-Bismol)	0.25 mL/kg q4–6h	PO	Hillyer and Brown (1994)
Captopril	⅛ of 12.5 mg tablet per animal q48h, increase to q12–24h	PO	Hillyer and Brown (1994)
Chlorpheniramine	1–2 mg/kg q8–12h	PO	Hillyer and Brown (1994)
Cimetidine	10 mg/kg q8h	PO, IV	Hillyer and Brown (1994)
Cisapride (Propulsid)	0.5 mg/kg q24h, increase to 1 mg/kg if needed	PO	Johnson-Delaney (1966)
Dexamethasone	0.5–2 mg/kg	SC, IM, IV	Brown (1995)
Diazoxide	10 mg/kg/d divided q8–12h	PO	Hillyer and Brown (1994)
Digoxin	0.01 mg/kg q24h	PO	Brown (1995)
Diltiazem	3.75–7.5 mg per animal q12h	PO	Brown (1995)
Diphenhydramine	0.5–2 mg/kg q8–12h	PO, IM, IV	Brown (1995)
Doxapram	5–11 mg/kg	IV	Besch-Williford (1987)
Enalapril	0.5 mg/kg q48h	PO	Brown (1995)
Epoetin alfa	50–150 IU/kg	SC, IV	Brown (1995)
Famotidine (Pepcid)	0.25–0.5 mg/kg q24h	PO, IV	Brown (1995)
Ferric dextran	10 mg per average ferret prn	IM	Johnson-Delaney (1996)
Furosemide	2 mg/kg q8–12h	PO, SC, IM, IV	Hillyer and Brown (1994)
Glycoprrolate	0.01 mg/kg	IM	Heard (1993)
Gonadotropin-releasing hormone	20 µg/animal, repeat in 2 wk prn	SC, IM	Hillyer and Brown (1994)
Hairball laxative, feline	1–2 mL/animal q48h	PO	Brown (1993)
Heparin	200 IU/kg q12h for 5 d	SC, IM	Hillyer and Brown (1994)
Human chorionic gonadotropin	100 IU per animal, repeat in 1–2 wk prn	IM	Hillyer and Brown (1994)
Hydrocortisone sodium succinate	25–40 mg/kg	IV	Besch-Williford (1987)
Insulin, NPH	0.5–6 IU/kg or to effect	SC	Besch-Williford (1987)
Kaolin-pectin (Kaopectate)	1–2 mL/kg q2–6h prn	PO	Johnson-Delaney (1996)
Lactulose syrup	0.15–0.75 mg/kg q8–12h	PO	Brown (1995)
Megestrol acetate	Do not use, predisposes ferret to pyometra		Johnson-Delany (1996)
Mitotane	50 mg per animal q24h for 7 d, then q72h	PO	Hillyer and Brown (1994)
Nitroglycerin 2% ointment	⅟₁₆–⅛ per animal q12–24h		Brown (1993)
Oxytocin	0.2–3 IU/kg	SC, IM	Brown (1993)
Pentobarbital elixir	1–2 mg/kg q12h	PO	Brown (1995)

Table 8.7. (continued)			
Drug	Dosage	Route	Reference
Prednisone	0.6 mg/kg q24h, gradually taper dose	PO	Besch-Williford (1987)
Prednisolone sodium succinate	22 mg/kg	IV	Hillyer and Brown (1994)
Propanolol	0.2–1 mg/kg q8–12h	PO	Hillyer and Brown (1994)
Prostaglandin	0.1 mL per animal	IM	Brown (1993)
Stanozolol	0.5 mg/kg q12h	PO, SC	Brown (1993)
Sucralfate	⅛ of 1 g tablet per animal q6h	PO	Hillyer and Brown (1994)
Theophylline elixir	4.25 mg/kg q8–12h	PO	Johnson-Delaney (1996)
Thyroxin	0.2–0.4 mg/kg q12–24h	PO	Johnson-Delaney (1996)
Vitamin B complex	0.2–0.3 mL q24h	SC, IM	Johnson-Delaney (1966)
Yohimbine	0.5 mg/kg	IM	Sylvina (1990)

IM = intramuscular; IV = intravenous; IP = intraperitoneal; PO = per os; SC = subcutaneous.

BACTERIAL DISEASES

Proliferative Bowel Disease

Proliferative bowel disease, caused by a campylobacterlike organism, is an intestinal disorder that occurs in ferrets, hamsters, and pigs. In ferrets, it is characterized by protracted intermittent diarrhea of greater than 6 weeks' duration, weight loss, rectal prolapse, and dehydration. The disease is usually seen in young ferrets. Mucosal thickening and glandular epithelial hyperplasia of the colon are characteristic postmortem findings in ferrets, in contrast to the hamster and pig, in which it is primarily in the ileum. The intracellular campylobacterlike organism has been further characterized as a *Desulfovibrio* sp. Treatment with chloramphenicol at 50 mg/kg twice daily for 14–21 days and supportive parenteral fluids has resulted in remission of clinical signs and regression of lesions. Severe cases may occasionally result in death despite supportive care.

Gastritis

Helicobacter mustelae has recently been identified as the etiologic agent responsible for inducing gastritis and gastroduodenal ulcers in ferrets. The organism can infect young ferrets as early as 5–6 weeks of age and is highly prevalent in the adult population. Clinical signs include anorexia, weight loss, and lethargy. Teeth grinding, ptyalism, and melena are more indicative of gastric ulcers. Diagnosis is challenging but can be accomplished by mucosal biopsies and endoscopy. Treatment includes a 7- to 10-day regimen of amoxicillin and metronidazole combined with bismuth-subsalicylate, cimetidine, and sucralfate. Sucralfate requires an acidic pH to function properly; thus, the sucralfate dose should precede the cimetidine dose by at least 2 hours.

Botulism

Ferrets are highly susceptible to *Clostridium botulinum* type C. Botulism is very uncommon in laboratory or pet ferrets. It is primarily associated with large production colonies that have poor husbandry practices. Signs of muscular incoordination and stiffness appear in affected ferrets 12–96 hours after eating feed contaminated with clostridial spores. As the disease progresses, they may salivate and will hang limp when picked up. Death occurs in 1–7 days. Toxoids are available, and annual vaccinations are recommended for ferrets raised commercially. There is no successful treatment.

Tuberculosis

Ferrets are highly susceptible to certain avian, bovine, and human strains of *Mycobacterium* spp. The organism can be transmitted by inhalation, ingestion, or wound infection. The alimentary tract is the target organ of *Mycobacterium avium*. Tuberculosis may be suspected if a ferret has palpably enlarged mesenteric lymph nodes. A subcutaneous tuberculin test is not helpful in making a diagnosis. The current status of tuberculosis as a reemerging disease in people may lead to an increased incidence of the disease in pet ferrets. Infected ferrets should be euthanized due to the zoonotic potential.

Miscellaneous Bacterial Infections

Staphylococcus aureus and *Escherichia coli* are frequently associated with mastitis. Vaginitis is common in the female during estrus, especially when housed on hay or straw because the bedding may stick to the swollen vulva or enter the vagina and act as a nidus for a secondary bacterial infection. *Staphylococcus* spp. and *Streptococcus* spp. may cause abscesses arising from bite wounds during mating or from mouth injuries caused by bones in the diet. Treatment of localized infections should include drainage and local antibiotics.

Streptococcus zooepidemicus is often the causative organism in pneumonia and metritis.

VIRAL DISEASES

☞ ## Canine Distemper

Ferrets are highly susceptible to canine distemper virus, with mortality approaching 100%. Transmission is usually by aerosols or fomites. The incubation period is 7–9 days. The ferret initially loses its appetite and then develops a serous to mucopurulent ocular and nasal discharge. The eyelids stick together, and affected animals often develop a rash beneath the chin and in the inguinal region. Later, the foot pads swell and become hyperkeratotic. The anus commonly prolapses. The animal's condition deteriorates until it dies 2–3 weeks following exposure. Ferrets that survive the catarrhal phase may die in a neurotropic episode with hyperexcitability, excess salivation, muscular tremors, convulsions, and coma. This condition is called the screaming fits. Treatment is usually unsuccessful. Euthanasia is suggested as a practical alternative to symptomatic supportive therapy. Animal caretakers that have young puppies or work with unconditioned dogs should not be assigned to care for ferrets simultaneously.

☞ ## Human Influenza

Ferrets are susceptible to several strains of human influenza virus. Human influenza viruses are transmitted by aerosols, are highly infectious, and may cause initial signs similar to those of distemper. Within 48 hours of exposure, the ferret becomes listless and anorexic and has a sharp rise in rectal temperature. Sneezing attacks occur and may be accompanied by a mucoserous nasal discharge. Fever lasts for 1 day and returns on the 3rd day. Clinical disease may be present for 7–14 days. Recovery differentiates influenza from the early stages of distemper. Congestion may be relieved by use of antihistamines. Cough suppressants and antibiotics may also be helpful for symptomatic relief. Humans can be infectious for ferrets and the reverse is also true. Animal caretakers with upper respiratory infections should wear masks and gloves when handling ferrets.

☞ ## Aleutian Disease

Ferrets are susceptible to the parvovirus that causes Aleutian disease (AD) in mink. In contrast to the disease in mink, AD usually progresses slowly in ferrets. Clinical signs may include a slow wasting disease with black tarry stools, splenomegaly, episodic fevers, posterior paresis, tremors, and eventually death. Diagnosis is made by positive serology, hypergammaglobulinemia, and histologic findings. An increase in γ-globulins greater than 20% is considered diagnostic. Typical histopathologic lesions include lymphocytic and plasmacytic infiltrates in the meninges, liver, kidney, and spleen. There is no treatment or vaccine to prevent AD. Ferrets with clinical disease should be euthanized. Serum antibody titers can be checked by submitting samples to a diagnostic laboratory. See Chapter 10, Serologic Testing and Quality Control, for information.

Rabies

Ferrets are susceptible to rabies virus infections. There are a few reports of rabies in ferrets in the United States. Central nervous signs predominate with anxiety, lethargy, and posterior paresis. Ferrets should be vaccinated annually with a killed vaccine of chicken embryo origin. Ferrets that bite people may be subject to euthanasia and a rabies screen depending on the state regulations.

PARASITIC DISEASES

Sarcoptic Mange

Sarcoptes scabiei induces a dermatitis that most frequently involves the feet, causing them to become red, swollen, and ulcerated from irritation and chewing. In some cases, a more generalized alopecia and intense pruritis develop. Treatment consists of ivermectin at 0.4 mg/kg subcutaneously and repeating in 2 weeks. Soaking or shampooing the feet in warm water may help relieve pruritis. Antibiotics may be indicated if a secondary bacterial infection develops. Organophosphate compounds are not recommended.

Fleas

Ctenocephalides spp. fleas are common in ferrets, especially in multiple-animal households. If present, topical preparations used for elimination of fleas in cats are effective and safe.

Ear Mites

Otodectes cyanotis infection is a common problem in ferrets that causes wax accumulation in the ear canal. Treatment with ivermectin subcutaneously or topically, mineral oil with miticides, or similar commercial ear miticidal medication is effective.

Heartworms

Ferrets are susceptible to infection with *Dirofilaria immitis* and seemingly have little ability to tolerate the presence of adult parasites in the heart without lethal consequences. Ivermectin has been found to be effective against *D. immitis* larvae in ferrets and can be used as a preventive in heartworm endemic areas. Diethylcarbamazine has also been used as a preventive. There is one report of treatment of adult worms using thiacetarsamide.

Coccidiosis

The most common parasite identified in ferrets is coccidia, especially in young or stressed ferrets. Fecal examination should reveal the coccidial oocysts. Rectal prolapse can be a complicating factor of coccidial infections. Treatment with sulfadimethoxine is effective.

Miscellaneous Helminth Intestinal Parasites

Many types of intestinal parasites have been reported including *Toxascaris leonina*, *Toxocara cati*, *Ancylostoma* spp., *Dipylidium caninum*, *Mesocestoides* spp., and *Filaroides* spp. Identification of specific parasites is established by fecal examination. Treatments recommended for elimination of intestinal parasites are generally the same as for cats and dogs and include ivermectin and praziquantel.

NEOPLASIA

Pancreatic Beta Cell Tumors (Insulinomas)

Pancreatic beta cell tumors, also called insulinomas, are one of the most commonly reported neoplasms of ferrets. Clinical signs include episodes of weakness, lethargy, ptyalism, and vomiting. Diagnosis is based on clinical signs, blood glucose less than 60 mg/dL and possibly blood insulin greater than 350 pmol/L. Medical treatment involves using drugs such as prednisone and diazoxide that increase blood glucose concentration. Surgical treatment usually involves debulking the tumor. Prognosis depends on whether metastasis has occurred and on how aggressively treatment is pursued. Most cases are chronic and usually fatal, but proper treatment can prolong the life of the ferret.

Mast Cell Tumors

Ferrets frequently develop mast cell tumors. The masses intermittently appear and are associated with pruritis and alopecia. The tumors are described as being small, tan or erythematous, slightly raised, and circumscribed. A black, crusty exudate is often present around the mass. Most tumors are benign, in contrast to the more malignant mast cell tumors described in other species. Removal of the tumor by surgical excision is usually curative.

Lymphosarcoma

There is a high incidence of lymphosarcoma reported in ferrets. Young ferrets, less than 1 year of age, develop an acute disease with thymic enlargement. Older ferrets have a more chronic disease with lymphadenopathy. Clinical signs are nonspecific and include anorexia, weight loss, and lethargy. Prognosis depends on the time of diagnosis and response to therapy.

Miscellaneous Neoplasia

Other types of spontaneous neoplasms appear to be uncommon in ferrets. Ovarian leiomyomas, squamous cell carcinomas, adenocarcinomas, and malignant megakaryocytic myelosis have been reported.

MISCELLANEOUS CONDITIONS

☞ ## Aplastic Anemia

Female ferrets that are not bred and that undergo a protracted period of estrus will develop an aplastic anemia attributable to prolonged estrogenic exposure. This condition is not as common today, as most pet ferrets are spayed before being sold. Clinical examination of affected animals typically reveals pale mucous membranes, swollen vulva, alopecia, petechial hemorrhages, anorexia, and marked depression. Hematologic findings include severe anemia, thrombocytopenia, granulocytopenia, and hypocellularity of the bone marrow.

An OHE is the treatment of choice for ferrets that are diagnosed early enough and have normal blood parameters. If a ferret is anemic or thrombocytopenic, then one or two injections of 100 IU of human chorionic gonadotropin can be given to induce ovulation and return the ferret to anestrus. B vitamins and iron may help to correct the anemia and stabilize the patient. Once blood parameters have returned to normal, the ferret should be spayed. Prognosis is usually based on the severity of the anemia, with a packed cell volume (PCV) of less than 20% indicating a guarded prognosis and a PCV of less than 14% considered to be poor prognosis. Supportive care that includes the use of steroids, force feeding, and vitamin supplementation may improve the chances of survival. Because of the high incidence of this disease in unmated female ferrets and the poor response to even the most vigorous therapy, ovariohysterectomy is advisable before the first heat period of females not intended for breeding.

Cardiomyopathy

Both hypertrophic and dilative cardiomyopathies have been reported in ferrets. Usually middle-aged or older ferrets are affected. Clinical signs include respiratory distress, inappetence, and exercise intolerance. Diagnostic and therapeutic regimens are similar to those for cats. If diagnosed early and treated aggressively, ferrets can be stabilized for several months or years.

Dermatophytosis (Ringworm)

Dermatophytosis caused by *Microsporum canis* has been reported in young ferrets. Transmission is possible between pets and humans. Affected ferrets may be treated with antifungal baths and topical antifungal ointments, or griseofulvin administered per os.

Eclamptogenic Toxemia

Eclamptogenic toxemia occurs a few days before whelping. The exact etiology of the disease is unknown but is likely to be similar to that of the disease seen in guinea pigs. Precipitating factors include pregnancy, diet, and stress. The only characteristic postmortem change is a fatty yellow liver. See discussion on ketosis in Chapter 5, Guinea Pigs.

Eosinophilic Gastroenteritis

There have been several reports of eosinophilic gastroenteritis in ferrets. Clinical signs are nonspecific and include anorexia, weight loss, and diarrhea. Eosinophilia may be seen on a hemogram. Intestines and mesenteric lymph nodes may be palpably enlarged. Diagnosis is based on a complete blood count and gastric biopsy results. No etiologic agent has been identified in this syndrome. Ivermectin at a dose of 0.4 mg/kg subcutaneously and repeated in 2 weeks is recommended. Prednisone has been suggested as an alternative therapy.

Gastric Obstruction

Because of their propensity to chew on anything, ferrets will frequently ingest items that are too large to easily pass or are indigestible. Clinical signs may include scant feces, a palpable mass in the stomach, anorexia, and vomiting. Diagnosis and treatment are similar to what would be done for a cat or dog. Removal of items by use of an endoscope is possible in some cases. Surgery is sometimes necessary. Prevention should be focused at keeping soft rubber and other inappropriate "toys" out of the reach of the ferret. Ferrets should not be allowed to roam freely in a house without supervision.

☞ Hair Loss

Alopecia in ferrets is common and can be associated with a number of conditions including biotin deficiency, hyperadrenocorticism, ovarian tumor, estrus, seasonal molting, and high environmental temperature and humidity. A bilaterally symmetrical pattern of hair loss is seen with endocrine-based alopecia such as estrus, adrenocortical adenocarcinoma, and ovarian tumors. A random or patchy hair loss is seen with most other types of alopecia. Females usually molt following the first ovulation of the season and males molt in October or November. At times, ferrets may lose their hair for undetermined reasons.

☞ Hyperadrenocorticism

Hyperadrenocorticism is a common disorder of older ferrets and is usually associated with hyperplasia, adenoma, or adenocarcinoma of the cortex of the adrenal gland. There is an excess production of adrenal steroids, but cortisol is rarely increased. Thus, the typical signs associated with hyperadrenocorticism in dogs such as polyuria, polydypsia, polyphagia, pot-bellied appearance, and thin skin are rarely seen. Clinical signs in ferrets include alopecia, pruritis, swollen vulva in females, and increased sexual behavior in neutered ferrets. Alopecia may be confined to the tail or may involve the entire body. Surgical removal of the abnormal adrenal gland is usually curative. If both adrenals are enlarged, removal of the larger adrenal plus a subtotal adrenalectomy on the other gland is usually effective. A medical treatment regimen using lysodren has been described.

Infant Mortality

High infant mortality is a common problem for ferret breeders. Many of the deaths are attributable to females killing the young or to failure of lactation. Spontaneous congenital malformations including neuroschisis, gastroschisis, absence of limbs, and corneal dermoids are also relatively common.

Megaesophagus

This is an uncommon but frequently fatal disorder of unknown etiology in ferrets. Death is usually the result of aspiration pneumonia. Diagnosis and treatment regimens are similar to those for dogs.

Nursing Sickness

Postparturient females may be afflicted with nursing sickness. Signs include anorexia, weight loss, weakness, and muscular incoordination. The cause is thought to be a dietary salt insufficiency, and the problem may be corrected by addition of table salt to the feed.

Polycystic Kidneys

Renal cysts are common in ferrets. These are usually just an incidental finding on physical examination but may lead to renal failure if the polycystic disease is severe.

Splenomegaly

An enlarged spleen is a common physical exam finding in ferrets. Splenomegaly is a nonspecific finding and may be associated with several diseases. True hypersplenism is a rare finding. Hematology parameters are within normal limits in ferrets with benign splenomegaly. A fine needle aspirate of the spleen may be helpful in ruling out neoplasia. Surgical removal of the spleen may be necessary if the size of the spleen causes discomfort or anorexia.

Summer Enteritis

An enteritis of unknown cause occurs in warm weather. Whether this is a specific disease or a syndrome resulting from a variety of causes is unclear. The possibility that *Campylobacter* spp. may be the etiologic agent in at least some of these outbreaks should be considered. Signs in acute cases include anorexia, bloody diarrhea, and death within 3–4 days. In chronic cases of enteritis, diarrhea may be intermittent and the appetite normal. Apparently, the animal fails to digest its food, becomes emaciated, and dies within a month. Neomycin has been used successfully in treating the disease.

Urolithiasis

Urolithiasis is not uncommon in ferrets. There is a higher prevalence of the disease seen in males. Diagnosis and treatment are similar to those for other mammals with this disease. Surgery is usually the treatment of choice. Long-term dietary management has not been thoroughly investigated to establish whether it would prevent stone formation. Diets used to decrease stone formation in dogs and cats generally have lower protein levels than is recommended for ferrets.

Zinc Poisoning

Zinc poisoning has been reported in ferrets fed raw meat that has been placed directly on the floor of galvanized cages. Clinical signs of zinc toxicity include muscle tremors, lethargy, and uremia.

LESS COMMON MISCELLANEOUS CONDITIONS

Reports of anal gland impaction, dental tartar accumulation, intervertebral disk syndrome, and cataracts occasionally appear in the literature. Guidelines for diagnosis and treatment of these conditions have generally followed those established for domestic cats. Because of the limited systematic studies of ferret diseases, treatment is based largely on extrapolation from knowledge of similar diseases in dogs and cats.

■ GENERAL REFERENCES

Sources consulted to compile the material in this chapter include *Biology and Diseases of the Ferret,* by J.G. Fox (1988, Lea & Febiger, 600 Washington Square, Philadelphia, PA, 19106-4198); Ferrets by K. Rosenthal in *Veterinary Clinics of North America Small Animal Practice* Vol. 24 (1), edited by K.E. Quesenberry and E. V. Hillyer (1994, WB Saunders Co., The Curtis Center, Independence Square West, Philadelphia, PA 19106-3399); *Laboratory Animal Medicine,* edited by J.G. Fox, B.J. Cohen, and F. M. Loew (1984, Academic Press, Inc., Orlando, FL 32887); and *The UFAW Handbook on the Care and Management of Laboratory Animals,* 6th edition, edited by T.B. Poole (1987, Churchill Livingstone Inc., 1560 Broadway, New York, NY 10036).

■ TECHNICAL REFERENCES

Besch-Williford, C.L. 1987. Biology and medicine of the ferret. *Vet Clin North Am Small Anim Pract* 17(5): 1155–1183.

Brown, S.A. 1993. Ferrets. In *A Practitioner's Guide to Rabbits and Ferrets,* ed. J.R. Jenkins and S.A. Brown, pp. 43–111. Lakewood, CO: American Animal Hospital Association.

Brown, S.A. 1995. Ferret drug dosages. In *Exotic Animal Formulary,* ed. L. Bauck, T.H. Boyer, and S.A. Brown et al., pp. 5–11. Lakewood, CO: American Animal Hospital Association.

Collins, B.R. 1995. Antimicrobial drug use in rabbits, rodents, and other small mammals. In *Antimicrobial Therapy in Caged Birds and Exotic Pets,* pp. 3–10. Trenton, NJ: Veterinary Learning Systems.

Flecknell, P.A. 1987. *Laboratory Animal Anesthesia.* San Diego: Academic.

Flecknell, P.A. 1997. Medetomidine and atipamezole: Potential uses in laboratory animals. *Lab Anim* 26(2): 21–25.

Heard, D.J. 1993. Principles and techniques of anesthesia and analgesia for exotic practice. *Vet Clin North Am Small Anim Pract* 23(6): 1301–1327.

Hillyer, E.V. 1992. Ferret endocrinology. In *Current Therapy XI—Small Animal Practice*, ed. R.W. Kirk and J.D. Bonagura, pp. 1185–1188. Philadelphia: WB Saunders.

Hillyer, E.V. and S.A. Brown. 1994. Ferrets. In *Saunders Manual of Small Animal Practice*, pp. 1317–1344. Philadelphia: WB Saunders.

Johnson-Delaney, C.A. 1996. *Exotic Companion Medicine Handbook for Veterinarians*. Lake Worth, FL: Wingers.

Ko, J.C.H., L.S. Pablo, J.E. Bailey, and T.G. Heaton-Jones. 1996. Anesthetic effects of Telazol® and combinations of ketamine-xylazine and Telazol®-ketamine-xylazine in ferrets. *Contemp Topics* 35(2): 47–52.

Payton, A.J. and J.R. Pick. 1989. Evaluation of a combination of tiletamine and zolazepam as an anesthetic for ferrets. *Lab Anim Sci* 39(3): 243–246.

Sylvina, T.J., N.G. Berman, and J.G. Fox. 1990. Effects of yohimbine on bradycardia and duration of recumbency in ketamine/xylazine anesthetized ferrets. *Lab Anim Sci* 40(2): 178–182.

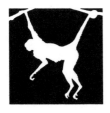

NONHUMAN PRIMATES

Nomenclature and classification of nonhuman primates are subject to periodic change. Nevertheless, individuals concerned with the medical care or research use of these animals should be able to recognize the more frequently seen species and categorize them correctly. Nonhuman primates can be differentiated by their unique biologic characteristics, environmental and nutritional requirements, and disease susceptibility. Other terms for nonhuman primates include subhuman primates, infrahuman primates, monkeys, simian primates, and apes. There is a huge range in size among different species of nonhuman primates with the smallest monkey weighing less than 100 g (0.22 lb) and the largest ape weighing more than 200 kg (440 lb).

Taxonomy

Nonhuman primates comprise three suborders: Prosimii, Tarsioidea, and Anthropoidea. The two main suborders are the prosimii, or early primates, and anthropoidea, or true primates. Tarsiers are classified in their own order because it has not been determined to which of the other two suborders they are more closely related. This chapter will concentrate mainly on several of the more important research and pet species of monkeys within the anthropoidean suborder.

Prosimians

Many species of prosimians resemble squirrels or rats more than true monkeys. Their natural diet consists primarily of insects, but some species prefer a fruit diet and some are carnivorous. Prosimian species include lemurs, indriids, aye-ayes, lorises, and galagos. All species of lemurs are classified as endangered. Few, if any, prosimian monkeys are presently used in biomedical research or kept as pets.

199

Anthropoidea (Simian Primates)

No single anatomic feature distinguishes simian primates from other animals. Some important characteristics are the presence of a simplex uterus, pectoral mammae, a pendulous penis, scrotal testes, a clavicle, and a hallux or big toe. The suborder Anthropoidea is divided into five families: New World (NW) monkeys, Old World (OW) monkeys, lesser apes, great apes, and humans.

NEW WORLD PRIMATES (FAMILY--CALLITRICHIDAE)

Marmosets and tamarins are separated from other species of NW primates by most taxonomists. They are the smallest and most primitive of the simian primates. They have soft silky hair and long nonprehensile tails. Representative species are common marmosets, pygmy marmosets, golden lion tamarins, and cotton-top tamarins. The common marmoset, *Callithrix jacchus,* is the callitrichid species that is most commonly used in research. The average weight is 300–350 g. The cotton-top tamarin, *Sanguinus oedipus,* is endangered and thus can only be used in research that benefits the species. The average weight is 450–550 g. Callitrichids have several unique characteristics. They possess claws rather than nails, have axillary rather than anterior mammary glands, and are biovulatory, thus, twinning is normal. Marmosets and tamarins are used in a variety of research applications including infectious disease, viral oncology, and behavioral and reproductive studies.

NEW WORLD PRIMATES (FAMILY—CEBIDAE)

Squirrel monkeys, *Saimiri sciureus,* have short, dense haircoats varying in color from orange to gray; a dark, round muzzle; and white hairless patches around their eyes. They have long prehensile tails and weigh 500–1000 g. Squirrel monkeys make popular research subjects because of their small size, tractable nature, and tendency to breed well in captivity. They are general-purpose experimental primates and are particularly important in atherosclerosis research. Squirrel monkeys are widely distributed throughout the rain forests of South America. There is an ongoing debate about the classification of the different types of squirrel monkeys. Animals from different geographic areas are generally distinguished by having a "gothic arch" (*S. sciureus)* or "Roman arch" (*Saimiri boliviensis*) in reference to the slightly differing color and shape characteristics of the hair around their eyes. Because there appears to be a wide variety of subspecies of squirrel monkeys with differing numbers of acrocentric chromosomes, it is suggested that monkeys used in biomedical research be karyotyped.

Owl monkeys, *Aotus trivirgatus,* are the only nocturnal anthropoid primates. They have short, dense haircoats varying in color from gray to red, a small dark muzzle, large owllike eyes, and white crescents of hair around each eye. They have long nonprehensile tails and weigh 900–1200 g. They are not as hardy, and do not adapt as well to the laboratory, as squirrel monkeys. Owl monkeys are one of the most important models for studies of human malaria. They are also of value in studies of viral oncology and are of special importance in vision research because of their unique eye structure. Owl monkeys are native to a wide area throughout the rain forests of South America. There may be as many as nine different species of owl monkeys; thus, captive monkeys used in biomedical research should be karyotyped before breeding.

Cebus monkeys, *Cebus* spp., are also called capuchins. They have medium-length, dense haircoats ranging from dark brownish black to white and long prehensile tails. Adults weigh on average 3–5 kg. *Cebus apella,* the black-capped capuchin, or organ grinder's monkey, is unique in having long, dark sideburns and tufts of dark hair arising from its brow. *C. apella* are occasionally used in research and have recently become popular as pets. Cebus monkeys are native to the rain forests of South and Central America.

Spider monkeys, *Ateles* spp., are aptly named because of their long, gangly arms and legs and thick, round bellies. These monkeys are unique in having hands with four fingers and no thumb and long prehensile tails. Adults weigh 5–7 kg. Spider monkeys are native to the rain forests of South and Central America. They are not used in research but are popular pet animals.

OLD WORLD MONKEYS (FAMILY—CERCOPITHECIDAE)

Rhesus monkeys, *Macaca mulatta,* are medium-sized monkeys that have short, reddish brown haircoats and medium-length tails. There is moderate sexual dimorphism, with males having larger bodies and weighing on average 6–11 kg, compared with females weighing 4–9 kg. Similarly, males develop large canines, whereas females do not. Rhesus tend to be one of the more aggressive macaque species. Rhesus are frequently used for vaccine testing, pharmacology and toxicology studies, and infectious disease research. Rhesus are found across a wide range of central Asia from Afghanistan to China. Because of destruction of their natural habitat as well as religious and political factors, the supply of rhesus monkeys from India is no longer available. All rhesus that are imported now come from domestic breeding programs.

Cynomolgus monkeys, *Macaca fascicularis,* are also referred to as crab-eating and long-tailed macaques. They are slightly smaller than rhesus and have long, nonprehensile tails and medium-length, olive hair-coats on their dorsum, with white to gray hairs on their ventrum and around their faces. The hair around their faces is longer and tends to form a small mane. Males have long, sharp canine teeth and are slightly larger than females. They tend to be less aggressive than rhesus monkeys. Cynomolgus are frequently used in drug testing and infectious disease research. They are found primarily in Southeast Asia. A population of M. *fascicularis* was introduced onto the island of Mauritius and are known to be free of herpes B virus and pathogenic retroviruses. They are now more readily available for importation than rhesus.

Of the baboons, *Papio anubis*, the olive baboon, and *Papio cynocephalus*, the yellow baboon, are the species most commonly used in biomedical research. They are large, weighing 15–30 kg. They have long haircoats, long nonprehensile tails, and a long prominent muzzle that gives them a dog-faced appearance. There is marked sexual dimorphism, with males exhibiting a shoulder mane; having longer, daggerlike canine teeth; and weighing 50% more than females. They are found over a wide range of Africa and tend to be agricultural pests. The baboon is a hearty primate that is especially desirable for surgery and reproductive physiology research.

African green monkeys, *Cercopithecus aethiops*, are small monkeys, with brownish green haircoats and long nonprehensile tails. They weigh 2–6 kg. Males are unusual in that they have brightly colored, blue scrotums. African greens are a species of guenon and are commonly referred to as vervets or grivets. They are occasionally used in biomedical research.

Mangabeys, *Cercocebus* spp., are slender animals with long legs and tails. *Cercocebus torquatus atys*, or sooty mangabeys, are susceptible to the organism that causes leprosy, *Mycobacterium leprae*, and may act as asymptomatic carriers of the simian immunodeficiency virus. They have been used in leprosy and autoimmune deficiency syndrome (AIDS) research, but their status as an endangered species now limits their use.

LESSER APES (FAMILY—HYLOBATIDAE)

Lesser apes include gibbons, *Hylobates* spp., and siamangs, *Symphalangus* spp. These animals have long arms and no tail. They are principally fruit and vegetable eaters. Both of these species are listed as endangered.

GREAT APES (FAMILY—PONGIDAE)

The chimpanzee, *Pan troglodytes*, is the highest form of nonhuman primate used in significant numbers in biomedical research. Adults grow quite large, with average weights of 40 kg for females and 50 kg for males. They are on the endangered species list, and none have been imported into the United States from the wild for several years. Some chimpanzees are available from established United States breeding colonies. They are used for testing hepatitis and AIDS vaccines and for psychobiology research.

Orangutans, *Pongo pygmaeus,* found in Borneo and Sumatra, appear to be approaching extinction. These animals are not used in biomedical research but are occasionally found in circus or animal acts.

Gorillas, *Gorilla gorilla,* are native to equatorial Africa. In the wild, the usual adult weight is 74–180 kg. These primates are endangered and used only rarely in studies that are not detrimental to their health, such as learning and behavioral research.

Uses

Although the number of pet monkeys has declined in recent years, some people continue to try to domesticate nonhuman primates. Ownership should be strongly discouraged for the following reasons: 1) they have a high potential to be carriers of zoonotic diseases including hepatitis, tuberculosis, shigellosis, salmonellosis, and herpes B virus; 2) they are virtually impossible to toilet train; 3) although most monkeys are cute and cuddly when young, many species become increasingly difficult to handle and even aggressive as they grow older; 4) most monkeys are destructive to property; 5) most monkeys have a tendency to bite; and 6) keeping primates as pets constitutes a drain on a limited wild population.

Nonhuman primates share anatomic and physiologic proximity to humans. Consequently, they serve a very important role in biomedical research. Historically, nonhuman primates have been important animals in the study of viral diseases including smallpox and polio. Today, they continue to be important models for the study of viral diseases, such as AIDS caused by the human immunodeficiency virus (HIV). Other areas of research include toxicology, behavior, learning, neurologic diseases (Parkinson's and Alzheimer's diseases), dentistry, reproduction, and infectious diseases.

The greatest number of nonhuman primates used in biomedical research are the macaque monkeys, primarily the rhesus and cynomolgus species. These two species of macaques constitute approximately 46% of the total number of nonhuman primates used in research. Baboons, African green monkeys, mangabeys, squirrel monkeys, owl monkeys, cebus monkeys, tamarins, and marmosets are used in moderate to small numbers. Chimpanzees are used in extremely limited numbers. Overall, monkeys constitute less than 5% of the total number of animals used in biomedical research each year.

Behavior

It is beyond the scope of this chapter to give a detailed description of the behavior of nonhuman primates, as it is extremely complex and diversified across the different species. This is merely a quick overview of some general behavioral patterns in nonhuman primates.

Nonhuman primates are extremely social animals. The most common social organization of nonhuman primates is that of a troop containing from 20 to 100 animals. Baboons and macaques have this type of organization. Within these troops, there is a definite hierarchical arrangement, with one male being the dominant or alpha male and one female being the dominant or alpha female. A small number of males comes next in the hierarchy, followed by a group of high-ranking females, and finally a group of low-ranking males, females, and younger animals. An animal's rank has a high correlation to the rank of its mother. The hierarchical position of a female in a troop normally remains quite stable, whereas the position of a male seems to be more transitory, with changes in leadership every 4–5 years. Depending on the stability of the hierarchy, fighting will frequently occur in social groupings. Subordinate monkeys will frequently lipsmack and present their hindquarters to the more dominant animals as a sign of submission. Looking directly into the eyes of a monkey is perceived as a threat and will often elicit aggressive behavior including yawns, which reveal their large canines, as well as threatening looks and postures. Nonhuman primates learn reproductive and social behaviors from the adults in their social groups. Thus, they must be reared in a reasonably normal social situation to develop normal behavioral patterns. Hand-reared and isolated animals frequently develop behavioral abnormalities and rarely mate.

Being highly social animals, monkeys usually do best when housed in social groups. There are several advantages to group housing, including environmental enrichment and development of normal reproductive and social behaviors. The main disadvantage to group housing is increased trauma from fighting. Many research and pet animals are housed singly, which can be very stressful and may induce abnormal stereotypic behaviors. The United States Department of Agriculture (USDA) regulations mandate that nonhuman primates used in research be provided with some form of environmental enrichment to promote psychological well-being.

Anatomic and Physiologic Features

Physical characteristics that serve to distinguish OW from NW monkeys are outlined in Table 9.1. General biologic and reproductive data are listed in Table 9.2. Most nonhuman primates used in research are so similar to humans morphologically that books on human anatomy and surgery can serve as excellent guides.

Rhesus monkeys and some other OW species have cheek pouches in which they stuff food to be chewed and swallowed later. Persons unfamiliar with this anatomic characteristic may think the monkey has a large tumor on the side of the face. In a number of species, including rhesus monkeys and baboons, males have large canine teeth. These are vicious weapons and are frequently shortened and blunted to reduce the danger from bites. Some species of OW primates have ischial callosities on their buttocks. These hard keratinized pads serve as protection for the bony prominence of the ischium.

There is a marked sexual dimorphism of body structure, weight, haircoat, and teeth size in some species of monkeys. Female monkeys have a simplex-type uterus, similar to the type found in humans. Most OW monkeys have monodiscoid or bidiscoid placentas. Determining the sex of nonhuman primates is usually simple, except in spider monkeys. The female spider monkey has pendulous labia that resemble a penis but may be recognized by the absence of a urethral opening. All OW primates have menstrual bleeding as a feature of their sexual cycle. This is absent in NW species. Twinning is extremely rare in OW monkeys; however, it is the norm in some species of NW monkeys.

Most mammals can synthesize vitamin C, but primates and guinea pigs require a dietary source. NW monkeys cannot utilize vitamin D_2 and must be provided with a source of vitamin D_3 in their diet. New World monkeys also require a higher percentage of protein in their diets than do OW monkeys.

Blood parameters vary to some extent from species to species and may also vary depending on the methods used for sampling. The type of

Table 9.1. Monkey physical characteristics: Old World vs. New World	
New World monkeys (Platyrrhines)	Old World monkeys (Catarrhines)
Prehensile tails are present in some species	No prehensile tails
No ischial callosities	Ischial callosities are present in some species
Broad-nosed	Narrow-nosed
Require vitamin D_3	Do not require vitamin D_3
Do not have cheek pouches	Cheek pouches are present in some species
Do not have opposable thumbs	Opposable thumbs are present in all species
Have three premolar teeth on each side	Have two premolar teeth on each side

environment a monkey lives in, such as group versus individual housing, may also affect certain blood values. It has been reported that baboon and chimpanzee hematologic and clinical chemistry values compare favorably with normal clinical values established for humans. Selected hematologic and biochemical values for several species of nonhuman primates are listed in Appendix 1, Normal Values.

Breeding and Reproduction

It is beyond the scope of this chapter to give a comprehensive description of breeding and the reproductive biology of nonhuman primates, as they are quite varied among the different species. General breeding and reproductive indices, as well as some peculiarities for some of the more common nonhuman primates are presented.

Puberty is marked in OW monkeys by the onset of menstrual cycling or menarche in the female and increased testicular size and spermatogenesis in the male. The average age of initiation of menarche in rhesus and cynomolgus macaques is between 2 and 3 years. The average age of sexual maturity of the female is between 2.5 and 3.5 years in these species, with the first birth usually occurring between 3 and 5 years. Males generally mature 1–2 years later than females.

Although most OW species are nonseasonally polyestrous with spontaneous ovulation, the rhesus macaque is a seasonal breeder, with most fertile cycles occurring in the winter months. The menstrual cycle lasts an average of 28–30 days in most species of OW monkeys. Baboons, rhesus, and chimpanzees have swelling and color changes of the perineal or sex skin that cycle with the hormonal changes. In rhesus monkeys, the sex skin has a corrugated appearance, whereas the sex skin of the baboon is smoother. Maximum turgescence and pinkish red color intensity are associated with the follicular phase of the menstrual cycle, estrus, and ovulation. Deturgescence and decreased color intensity occur rapidly after ovulation and is associated with the luteal phase of the menstrual cycle. Optimal mating time can be determined for individual monkeys who have regular cycle patterns by averaging three to four of their menstrual cycle lengths and mating them 3–4 days prior to deturgescence.

Many OW species, including the rhesus and cynomolgus macaques, as well as chimpanzees have a "placental sign" or vaginal bleeding. This occurs approximately the same time as menstruation would appear, but it is actually bleeding associated with implantation of the blastocyst. Gestation lengths for some of the more common species are listed in Table 9.2. Parturition in macaques frequently occurs in the late evening

Table 9.2. Biologic and reproductive data for select nonhuman primate species

	Rhesus	Cynomolgus	Baboon	Squirrel
Adult body weight				
Male	6–11 kg	6 kg	22–30 kg	500–1000 g
Female	4–9 kg	4 kg	11–15 kg	500–1000 g
Life span	30+ y	37 y	40–45 y	20 y
Body temperature	36°–40°C	36°–38°C	36°–39°C	33.5°–38.8°C
	(96.8°–104°F)	(96.8°–100.4°F)	(96.8°–102.2°F)	(92.3°–101.8°F)
Heart rate	150–333 beats per minute	107–215 beats per minute	80–200 beats per minute	225–350 beats per minute
Respiratory rate	10–25 breaths per minute	32–44 breaths per minute	29 breaths per minute	20–50 breaths per minute
Breeding onset				
Male	38 mo	42–60 mo	73 mo	60 mo
Female	34–43 mo	46 mo	51–73 mon	36–46 mo
Estrous cycle length	28 d	28 d	31–36 d	18 d
Gestation period	167 d	162 d	175–180 d	170 d
Weaning age	210–425 d	365–547 d	180–456 d	182 d
Chromosome number (diploid)	42	42	42	42

Source: Adapted from Johnson-Delaney (1994).

or early morning hours, with labor lasting 2–3 hours. Headfirst presentation of the fetus is normal. Infants begin nursing immediately after birth and nurse frequently throughout the day. Infant macaques and baboons may begin ingesting solid food around 2–3 months of age. Weaning is quite variable between the species and may occur anywhere between 6 and 8 months.

HUSBANDRY

Housing

The most suitable housing system for nonhuman primates depends on species, use, climatic conditions, and a number of other factors. In research laboratories, individual animals are usually housed in metal cages with slotted or grid floors. The Animal Welfare Act (AWA)-USDA regulations and the *Guide for the Care and Use of Laboratory Animals* give cage size specifications for nonhuman primates. Most macaque monkeys are less than 15 kg and can be comfortably housed in 0.56 m² (6.0 ft²) cages with at least 81.28 cm (32 in.) of height. A cage with a built-in squeeze design is desirable when animals are to receive frequent injections or blood collections. Cage pans are frequently used beneath individual cages to collect feces and urine. A wood chip bedding may be placed in the pans to help absorb some of the moisture. Alternatively, there may be a sloped metal floor beneath a row of cages that serves to divert the urine and feces into a sewage drain. Nonhuman primates are highly intelligent and frequently learn how to open cage doors and escape. To prevent escape of monkeys, a sufficiently secure lock, such as a padlock, should be placed on cage doors. There are a variety of ways to house breeding colonies, including indoor pens connected to outdoor runs, covered cylindrical enclosures referred to as "corn cribs," outdoor corrals with some form of protection from extreme weather conditions, and free range on islands.

As noted previously, the AWA-USDA regulations require that some form of environmental enrichment be provided to nonhuman primates used for research. It has been well documented that social interaction is the best form of enrichment. There are numerous cage designs which allow side-by-side or top and bottom cages to become one large social cage by simply pulling out dividing panels. If monkeys cannot be housed socially for scientific reasons, then other forms of environmental enrichment should be provided. For example, fruit, vegetables, seeds or food treats, foraging boards, mirrors, balls, swings, perches, televisions, radios, and more complex problem-solving devices such as puzzle feeders or video games can be used. It is best to offer a varied schedule of enrichments so that the monkeys will not become bored as quickly.

In housing nonhuman primates for research purposes, rigid control of room temperature, relative humidity, ventilation, and lighting are essential. A temperature range of 18°–29°C (64°–84°F), relative humidity range of 30%–70%, and 10–15 air changes per hour are recommended. Typically, 12–14 hours of light per day should be provided and can be controlled by automatic timers.

Nonhuman primate housing requires a minimum of once-daily cleaning. In certain situations, such as group housing in a gang cage, there is a sufficient amount of urine and feces produced to justify twice-daily cleaning. Generally, cage pans are removed, and the urine and feces are properly disposed of down a drain. If suspended pans are not used, then the feces and urine must be rinsed from beneath the cages and down the drain. Care must be taken to avoid getting the monkeys wet when this method is used. Floors should be thoroughly rinsed or mopped to remove any adherent debris. Pans can either be replaced with clean pans or washed thoroughly and replaced. Racks, cages, pans, water bottles, and feed hoppers should be sanitized at least once every 2 weeks with chemicals, hot water 61.6°–82.2°C (143°–180°F) or a combination of both. Refer to Chapter 1, Mice, for more specific information on disinfection of caging.

Feeding and Watering

Most commercially milled pelleted diets adequately meet the nutritional needs of nonhuman primates if properly stored and if fed within 90 days of milling to assure adequate vitamin C levels. The daily requirement of ascorbic acid is 1–4 mg/kg of body weight for maintenance. Commercial diets prepared for NW monkeys usually contain 25% protein and 9% fat, whereas OW monkey diets typically contain 15% protein and 5% fat. A 25% protein diet is recommended by some nutritionists for pregnant, lactating, or growing OW monkeys. Pet monkeys are often presented with protein deficiencies due to the high level of fruits and starches fed by owners. Protein-deficient monkeys are more susceptible to pneumonia, bacterial enteritis, and other illnesses.

Most pet owners and some laboratories supplement diets with fresh fruits and vegetables. Fresh fruit 3–4 times per week is probably advisable for NW monkeys. This practice is not necessary in OW species if the commercial chow is fresh and palatable.

Fresh, potable water should be provided ad libitum either through an automatic watering system or in water bottles attached to the cage.

Bottles are more labor intensive but provide a route for the administration of medications or dietary supplements. Automatic watering systems can malfunction and should be manually checked by the animal care staff daily to ensure the availability of water to each caged monkey. If a monkey stops eating, personnel should be trained to check the water source immediately.

TECHNIQUES

Handling and Restraint

One of the most striking features of primates is their great strength and agility. Chemical restraint is generally recommended for safe handling of all nonhuman primates. Individuals who handle monkeys must be adequately trained in order to minimize stress to the animal and to maximize safety for the handler. Personnel handling monkeys should wear protective clothing and personal protection devices, such as rubber gloves, face masks, and full-length arm protection (lab coat or sleeve protectors). Great care must be taken with macaque monkeys because of the potential for herpes B virus transmission from scratches or bites.

For primates weighing more than 2 kg, chemical restraint is strongly recommended. Administration of injections is greatly facilitated by restraint in a squeeze-back cage. Ketamine hydrochloride is the drug most frequently used for chemical restraint of nonhuman primates. Individual animals may have different responses to ketamine and may suddenly wake up. A second dose of ketamine should be available for quick response to these situations.

Manual restraint can be utilized for animals weighing less than 10 kg but should always be performed with at least two people. In addition to protective clothing, full-length leather gloves should be worn when handling unsedated monkeys. Leather gloves, however, are not impervious to sharp canine teeth. Manual restraint is usually accomplished by squeezing the monkey in its cage to immobilize it and then securing the upper arms of the monkey just above the elbows. The monkey can then be removed from its cage by pulling the arms behind the back so that its elbows touch. The second person is needed to release the squeeze mechanism, keep the cage door open, pry the monkey's fingers and toes off of the bars of the cage, and for obvious safety reasons. Monkeys restrained in this manner should be held away from the handler's body to avoid being grabbed or scratched by the monkeys feet. This restraint technique is shown in Figure 9.1.

Another option for restraint of awake monkeys includes the pole-

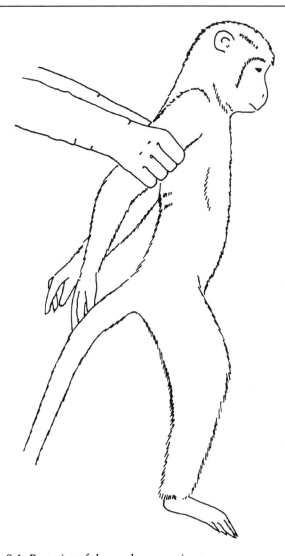

Figure 9.1. Restraint of the nonhuman primate.

and-collar method. This type of restraint is used primarily in a research setting. A small, loose-fitting, lightweight plastic or aluminum collar with two small handles is secured around the neck of the anesthetized monkey several days earlier to allow the monkey to acclimate to the collar. Two animal handlers grasp the collar handles with poles, assist the anesthetized monkey out of its cage, and place it in a restraint chair or on a restraint table where the neck collar is secured. Monkeys should be trained to this type of restraint with positive reinforcement and repetition. They usually adapt well to this routine. Animals placed in a restraint device should never be left unattended.

Restraint devices are specifically mentioned in the Animal Welfare Act regulations with the following specifications: 1) restraints are not to be considered a normal method of housing; 2) restraints must be approved by the institutional animal care and use committee; 3) restraint of animals should be kept to an absolute minimum amount of time; 4) restraints should not be used merely as a convenience but must be necessary to achieve research goals; and 5) restraints may require temporary or permanent removal of animals that become ill, injured, or behaviorally altered from the prolonged restraint.

Identification

Cage cards are used as a general means of identifying individually caged nonhuman primates. Other methods of individual identification include tattooing the chest or thigh, neck tags, ear tags, or placement of an electronic microchip. For group-housed monkeys, it is best to be able to identify them individually from a distance by means of a large identification tag placed around their neck. Temporary identification can be accomplished by using a unique hair-shaving pattern or marking the hair or skin with a marker or dye.

Blood Collection

Approximate blood volumes for several adult nonhuman primate species are listed in Table 9.3. Blood samples can easily be obtained from percutaneous venipuncture of the femoral vein or artery of monkeys. They are usually sedated for this procedure, and the femoral triangle must be cleaned with alcohol. If an arterial sample is taken, direct pressure must be applied for a minimum of 3–5 minutes to obtain adequate hemostasis.

Other collection sites include the cephalic and saphenous veins. When numerous blood samples are required, placement of an indwelling

Table 9.3. Adult nonhuman primate blood volumes

	Rhesus	Cynomolgus	Baboon	Squirrel
		Volume (mL)[a]		
Total blood	320–880	320–480	880–2400	40–120
Single sample	40–110	40–60	110–300	5–15
Exsanguination	120–330	120–180	190–330	15–45

Source: Adapted from Dysko and Hoskins (1995) and Johnson-Delaney (1994).
[a]Values are approximate.

catheter is preferable to multiple venipunctures. Catheters increase the efficiency and ease of blood sample collection, and reduce stress and pain to the animal. Monkeys can be trained to offer their arms or legs for blood collection with positive reinforcement, but this requires a considerable amount of time and dedicated staff. Surgical placement of vascular access ports and tether systems allow for long-term blood collection and chronic dosing.

Urine Collection

Urine can be collected by cystocentesis, placement of a urinary catheter, or free-catch. When using the free-catch method, the urine is collected by using a metabolism cage or a collection pan under the cage that has a wire grid to separate the urine and the feces.

Drug Administration

Drug administration routes for nonhuman primates are similar to those of most other large mammals. Oral dosing can be accomplished by placing the drug in a piece of fruit or on a piece of bread covered with peanut butter and jelly. Tablets can also be crushed or capsules opened to mix the drug in a favorite food. Many monkeys, however, are adept at picking out the drug or eating around it. Alternatively, there is at least one commercial vendor that will incorporate drugs into fruit-flavored tablets upon receipt of a prescription from a veterinarian. These tablets are well received by monkeys and ensure accurate enteral dosing. Unpalatable drugs can be given to a lightly sedated monkey through a nasogastric tube or orogastric tube using a mouth gag. The proper placement of the stomach tube should always be verified before administering drugs.

Subcutaneous injections can be made under the loose skin over the dorsal cervical area. Intramuscular injections are usually given in the thigh muscles, using care not to get too close to the back of the femur where the sciatic nerve courses. The triceps and gluteal muscles can also be used for intramuscular injections of larger monkeys.

The cephalic or saphenous veins can be used to deliver drugs intravenously. Larger volumes should be administered through an indwelling catheter. Surgical implantation of a vascular access port is another alternative for long-term dosing. The port is implanted subcutaneously, usually high on the back between the shoulder blades. Monkeys can be trained to present their port or be restrained via a pole-and-collar system for injections into the port. Alternatively, the vascular system can be accessed through a tether system. The tether system consists of a backpack pump or cage-top pump that allows for continuous infusion of drugs or saline. The vascular catheter exits through the skin on the back of the monkey and enters the backpack pump or goes through a swivel that protects the catheter as it courses up to the cage-top pump.

Anesthesia, Surgery, and Postoperative Care

Agents commonly used for anesthesia and tranquilization in nonhuman primates are listed in Table 9.4. Monkeys are usually anesthetized with an intramuscular injection of ketamine hydrochloride to remove them from their cage safely. Animals given ketamine are often adequately anesthetized for placement of a tracheal tube and can then be maintained by inhalation anesthesia. If a monkey is too light to be intubated on the initial dose of ketamine, a small intravenous bolus of ketamine or thiopental can be given to achieve intubation. Several inhalants including isoflurane and halothane are safe and commonly used in nonhuman primates. Monkeys should be premedicated with atropine or glycopyrrolate to minimize salivation and bradycardia.

Table 9.4. Anesthetic agents and tranquilizers used in nonhuman primates

Drug	Dose	Route	Reference
Inhalants			
Halothane	1%–4% to effect	Inhalation	Johnson et al. (1981)
Isoflurane	1%–2% induction, 0.5%–1.5% maintenance	Inhalation	Feeser (1992)
Injectables			
Acetylpromazine	0.5–1 mg/kg	IM, SC, PO	Johnson et al. (1981)
Chlorpromazine	1–6 mg/kg	IM, PO	Johnson et al. (1981)
Diazepam	0.25–0.5 mg/kg	IM, IV	Ialeggio (1989)
Fentanyl-droperidol	0.05–0.1 mL/kg	IM, IV	Johnson et al. (1981)
Ketamine	5–40 mg/kg	IM	Johnson-Delaney (1994)
Ketamine	4 mg/kg	IM	Feeser (1992)
+ acetylpromazine	0.4 mg/kg	IM	
Ketamine	10 mg/kg	IM	Woolfson et al. (1980)
+ diazepam	7.5 mg/kg	IM	
Ketamine	11 mg/kg	IM	White (1979)
+ xylazine	0.5–1.0 mg/kg	IM	
Meperidine	2–10 mg/kg for sedation	IM	Hughes (1981)
Pentobarbital	20–33 mg/kg	IV	Hughes (1981)
Propofol	5–10 mg/kg	IV	Sainsbury (1991)
Thiamylal sodium	25 mg/kg to effect	IV	Johnson et al. (1981)
Thiopental sodium	22–25 mg/kg	IV	Hughes (1981)
Tiletamine-zolazepam	2–6 mg/kg	IM	Ialeggio (1989)
Xylazine	6.0 mg/kg	IM	Clifford (1984)

IM = intramuscular; IV = intravenous; PO = per os; SC = subcutaneous.

Ketamine alone is not satisfactory for major surgery since it does not provide adequate analgesia. The ketamine/xylazine combination, however, can be used for minor short-term procedures. This injectable regimen usually provides about 30–45 minutes of anesthesia. Propofol given intravenously through an indwelling catheter provides a smooth induction of anesthesia and can be used to maintain anesthesia by intermittent bolus administration. Monkeys maintained on propofol should be intubated, as propofol may induce a short period of apnea. Monkeys recover from propofol smoothly and rapidly. The depth of anesthesia is best gauged by the rate and depth of respiration, heart rate, and degree of jaw tension. The palpebral and pedal reflexes may also be used. Intraoperatively, monkeys should have their body temperature maintained by use of a circulating heating blanket. Warm intravenous fluids are also helpful in preventing hypothermia. Placement of an indwelling catheter is important for long-term anesthesia that allows for administration of fluids and emergency drugs. Sterile technique is imperative.

Some of the routine surgeries performed on nonhuman primates include finger and tail amputations, laceration repair, and disarming of canine teeth. Use of a subcuticular suturing pattern is recommended when closing incisions. This method usually prevents monkeys from pulling sutures out and eliminates the need for suture removal. Current recommendations to disarm a monkey are to surgically cut and blunt the canine teeth, rather than extract the teeth. The most common approach consists of cutting the teeth to the level of the incisors, performing a pulpectomy with dental instruments, packing the root canal with dental paste, and capping the pulp cavity with a dental alloy. Postoperatively, monkeys can be placed in a recovery cage (or in their home cage if they are housed singly). A heat source such as a heat lamp should be provided to help prevent hypothermia. They should be observed frequently until they are sitting in an upright position. Monkeys with incisions should not be placed in a cage with other monkeys until their sutures are removed because cagemates frequently will groom the surgical site and remove the sutures. Analgesics should be given for invasive procedures that are known to cause pain in other mammals. Table 9.5 lists some analgesics that can be used in nonhuman primates. Buprenorphine is recommended for control of acute or chronic visceral pain but can cause sedation. Butorphanol is recommended for mild postoperative discomfort.

Table 9.5. Analgesic agents used in nonhuman primates

Drug	Dosage	Route	Reference
Acetaminophen	5–10 mg/kg q6h	PO	Johnson et al. (1981)
Acetylsalicylic acid	10–20 mg/kg q6h	PO	Johnson et al. (1981)
Buprenorphine	0.01 mg/kg q12h	IV, IM	Jenkins (1987)
Butorphanol	0.1–0.2 mg/kg q12–48h	IM	Heard (1993)
Flunixin meglumine	0.3–1 mg/kg q12–24h	SC, IV	Heard (1993)
Meperidine	2–4 mg/kg q4h	IM, IV	Rosenburg (1991)
	1–4 mg/kg q4–6h	IM	Fraser (1991)
Morphine	1–2 mg/kg q4h	IM, IV, PO, SC	Rosenburg (1991)
Naloxone	0.01–0.05 mg/kg	IV, IM	Flecknell (1987)
Naproxen	10 mg/kg q12h	PO	Junge (1992)
Oxymorphone	0.15 mg/kg OWM q4–6h	IM, IV, SC	Rosenburg (1991)
	0.075 NWM q4–6h	IM, IV, SC	Rosenburg (1991)
Pentazocine	1.5–3.0 mg/kg (not to exceed 60 mg)	IM, SC	Johnson et al. (1981)

IM = intramuscular; IV = intravenous; NWM = New World monkey; OWM = Old World monkey; PO = per os; SC = subcutaneous.

Euthanasia

After being sedated with an intramuscular injection of ketamine to remove them from their cage, nonhuman primates can be euthanized by an intravenous overdose of a barbiturate or commercial euthanasia solution. Other methods of euthanasia are permissible if the monkey is fully anesthetized, such as a bolus of potassium chloride or exsanguination and perfusion with a tissue fixative. Refer to Chapter 1, Mice, for more details about euthanasia guidelines in animals.

THERAPEUTIC AGENTS

Nonhuman primate antimicrobial and antifungal drug dosages are listed in Table 9.6. Antiparasitic agents are listed in Table 9.7, and miscellaneous drugs are listed in Table 9.8.

Table 9.6. Antimicrobial and antifungal agents used in nonhuman primates

Drug	Dosage	Route	Reference
Amikacin	2.3 mg/kg q24h	IM	Wissman (1992)
Amoxicillin	11 mg/kg q24h	IM, SC	Fraser (1991)
	11 mg/kg q12h	PO	
Amphotericin B	0.25–1 mg/kg q24h	IV	Johnson et al. (1981)
Ampicillin	20 mg/kg q8h	PO, IM, IV	Johnson et al. (1981)
Cefazolin	25 mg/kg q12h for 7–10 d	IM, IV	RPRC-WA (1987)
Cefotaxime	100–200 mg/kg q6–8h	IV	Pernikoff (1991)
Ceftazidime	50 mg/kg q8h	IM, IV	Feeser (1992)
Ceftizoxime	75–100 mg/kg q12h	IM	RPRC-WA (1987)

Table 9.6. (*continued*)

Drug	Dosage	Route	Reference
Ceftriaxone	50–100 mg/kg q12–24h	IM	Pernikoff (1991)
Cephalexin	20 mg/kg q12h	PO	Flecknell (1987)
Cephaloridine	20 mg/kg q12h	IM	Flecknell (1987)
Chloramphenicol	50–100 mg/kg q8h	IV, SC, PO	Johnson et al. (1981)
Ciprofloxacin	10–25 mg/kg q12h	PO	Kelly (1992)
Doxycycline	5 mg/kg divided q12h on day 1, then 2.5 mg/kg the following days	PO	Wolff (1990)
	2–5 mg/kg q12h	PO	Kelly (1992)
Enrofloxacin	5 mg/kg q24h for 10 d (to treat shigellosis)	PO, IM	Banish et al. (1993)
Erythromycin	75 mg/kg q12h for 10 d	PO	RPRC-WA (1987)
	5 mg/kg q12h for 7–14 d	IM	Fraser (1991)
Furazolidone	5 mg/kg q6h for 7 d	PO	RPRC-WA (1987)
Gentamicin	2–4 mg/kg q12h for 1–2 d then q24h	PO	Johnson et al. (1981)
	2–3 mg/kg q12h for 5–7 d	IM, IV	Johnson-Delaney (1994)
Griseofulvin	20 mg/kg q24h	PO	Johnson et al. (1981)
	200 mg/kg once q10d	PO	Johnson et al. (1981)
Isoniazid	15–25 mg/kg q12h (for chimps)	PO	Fineg (1966)
Isoniazid	5 mg/kg q24h	PO	de Stefani (1983)
+ rifampin	20 mg/kg q24h	PO	
Isoniazid	15mg/kg in grape juice q24h, dosages reduced by one-third after 6 wk	PO	Wolf (1988)
+ rifampin	22.5 mg/kg	PO	
+ ethambutol	22.5 mg/kg		
Kanamycin	7.5 mg/kg q12h	IM	Johnson et al. (1981)
Lincomycin	5–10 mg/kg q12h	IM	Weller (1992)
Methicillin	50 mg/kg q12h for 7 d	IM	RPRC-WA (1987)
Minocycline	15 mg/kg q12h for 7 d	PO	Junge (1992)
Neomycin	10–15 mg/kg	PO	Whitney (1977)
Nitrofurantoin	2–4 mg/kg q8h	IM, IV	Johnson et al. (1981)
Nystatin	200,000 units q6h continue for 48 h after clinical recovery	PO	Fraser et al. (1991)
Penicillin G, benzathine	40,000 IU/kg q3d	IM	Johnson et al. (1981)
Penicillin G, procaine	20,000 IU/kg q12h	IM	Johnson et al. (1981)
Piperacillin	100–150 mg/kg q12h for 7 d	IM, IV	RPRC-WA (1987)
	80–100 mg/kg q8h for 7–10 d	IM, IV	RPRC-WA (1987)
Rifampin	20 mg/kg q24h	PO	de Stefani (1983)
Sulfasalazine	30 mg/kg q12h	PO	Isaza et al. (1992)
Sulfisoxazole	50 mg/kg q24h	PO	Johnson et al. (1981)
Tetracycline	20–25 mg/kg q8–12h for 7–10 d	PO	Johnson-Delaney (1994)
	25 mg/kg q12h	IM, IV	RPRC-WA (1987)
Trimethoprim-sulfadiazine	24 mg/kg q12h	PO	Fraser et al. (1991)
	27 mg/kg q12h	SC	Fraser et al. (1991)
Trimethoprim-sulfamethoxazole	15 mg/kg q12h	PO	Isaza (1992)

IM = intramscular; IV = intravenous; PO = per os; SC = subcutaneous.

Table 9.7. Antiparasitic agents used in nonhuman primates

Drug	Dosage	Route	Reference
Albendazole	25 mg/kg q12h for 5 d	PO	Wolff (1990)
Bunamidine	25 mg/kg	PO	Weller (1992)
Chloroquine	10 mg/kg followed by 5 mg/kg 6 h later, then 5 mg/kg/d for 2 d	PO, IM	Wolff (1990)
+ primaquine	0.3 mg/kg/d for 14 d	PO	
Diethylcarbamazine	6–20 mg/kg q24h for 6–15 d	PO	Wolff (1990)
	20–40 mg/kg for 7–21 d	PO	Hollihn (1988)
Diiodohydroxyquin (iodoquinol)	30 mg/kg for 10 d	PO	Weller (1992)
Diiodohydroxyquin	630 mg per chimp q8h	PO	Weller (1992)
+ oxytetracycline	250 mg per chimp q8h	PO	
Fenbendazole	50 mg/kg q24h for 3–14 d, repeat in 3 wk	PO	Feeser (1992)
Ivermectin	0.2 mg /kg	PO, IM, SC	Fraser (1991)
Levamisole	10 mg/kg	PO	Wolf (1993)
Mebendazole	15 mg/kg for 3 d	PO	Wolff (1990)
	22 mg/kg/d for 3 d, repeat in 3 wk	PO	Fraser (1991)
Metronidazole	35–50 mg/kg divided q12h for 10 d	PO	Wolff (1990)
Paromomycin	10–20 mg/kg q12h for 5–10 d	PO	Marks (1994)
Piperazine	65 mg/kg q24h for 10 d	PO	Russell (1981)
Praziquantel	40 mg/kg for one dose	PO, IM	Wolff (1990)
Primaquine	0.3 mg/kg/d for 14 d; treat concurrently with chloroquine	PO	Wolff (1990)
Pyrantel pamoate	11 mg/kg for one dose	PO	Wolff (1990)
Pyrvinium pamoate	5 mg/kg q6mo	PO	Johnson-Delaney (1994)
Quinacrine	2 mg/kg q8h for 7 d	PO	Swenson (1993)
Sulfadimethoxine	50 mg/kg/d for the 1st day, then 25 mg/kg/d	PO	Wolff (1990)
Sulfasalazine	30 mg/kg q12h for 21 d	PO	Isaza (1992)
Thiabendazole	75–100 mg/kg, repeat in 3 wk	PO	Fraser (1991)
	50 mg/kg/d for 2 d (for *Strongyloides*)	PO	Wolff (1990)
Trimethoprim-sulfamethoxazole	30 mg/kg q6h for 14 d	PO	Swenson (1993)
	15 mg/kg q12h for 14 d (flavored pediatric suspension)	PO	Isaza (1992)

IM = intramuscular; PO = per os; SC = subcutaneous.

Table 9.8. Miscellaneous agents used in nonhuman primates

Drug	Dosage	Route	Reference
Acetylcysteine (Mucomist)	50–60 mL/h for 30–60 min q12h	Inhalation	Johnson et al. (1981)
Aminophylline	25–100 mg/animal q12h	PO	Johnson et al. (1981)
	10 mg/kg	IV	Feeser (1992)

Table 9.8. (*Continued*)

Drug	Dosage	Route	Reference
Ascorbic acid	4–10 mg/kg/d	PO	Krasnow (1987)
Atropine	0.04 mg/kg	IM, IV, SC	Melby (1976)
Biotin	20 µg per animal q24h	PO	Krasnow (1987)
Bismuth subsalicy-late (Pepto-Bismol)	1 mL/kg q6–8h as needed	PO	Johnson-Delaney (1994)
Chlorpheniramine	0.5 mg/kg/d in divided doses	PO	Johnson et al. (1981)
Cisapride (Propulsid)	0.2 mg/kg q12h with meals	PO	Hotchkiss (1995)
Dexamethasone	≤ 2 mg/kg	IV, IM, PO	Johnson et al. (1981)
Diphenoxylate-atropine sulfate (Lomotil)	1 mL per animal q8h	PO	Holmes (1984)
Diphenhydramine	5 mg/kg	IM	Feeser (1992)
Doxapram	2 mg/kg	IV	Flecknell (1987)
Ephedrine	12 mg q4h	PO	Johnson et al. (1981)
Folic acid	0.04–0.2 mg/kg q24h	PO	Krasnow (1987)
Furosemide	2 mg/kg	PO	Johnson et al. (1981)
Glycopyrrolate	13–17 mg/kg	IM	Sanders (1991)
Hyperimmune human serum	0.33 mL/kg	IM	Whitney (1977)
Insulin, NPH	0.25–0.5 units/kg/d initially and adjust accordingly	SC	Johnson-Delaney (1994)
Kaolin and pectin	0.5–1.0 mL/kg q2–6h	PO	Johnson et al. (1981)
Lactated Ringer's solution	20–40 mL/kg	IV, IP, SC	Johnson et al. (1981)
Metoclopramide	0.4 mg/kg q12h	PO	Hotchkiss (1995)
Multivitamins (Children's chewables)	1 tablet q24h	PO	Russell (1981)
Neomycin-methoscopol-amine bromide	20 mg/kg q6h	PO	Johnson et al. (1981)
Niacin	10–35 mg/wk	PO	Krasnow (1987)
Pantothenic acid	3 mg/kg/d	PO	Krasnow (1987)
Phenylephrine	one spray in each nostril q6h	Intranasal	Johnson et al. (1981)
Prednisolone sodium succinate	10 mg/kg	IV	Feeser (1992)
Prednisone	0.5–1 mg/kg q12h for 3–5 d, then q24h for 3–5 d, then q48h for 10 d, then half the dose q48h	PO	Isaza (1992)
Pyridoxine hydrochloride	3.5 mg/kg of diet, feed continuously while on Isoniazid therapy	PO	Koehn (1966)
Tetanus antitoxin	1500 units	IV	Merck (1979)
Tetanus toxoid	0.5 mL at 5–7 mo and 13–15 mo of age, then booster q5y	IM	Paul-Murphy (1994)
Trimeprazine	1–2 mg q6h	PO	Johnson et al. (1981)
Vitamin C	25 mg/kg/d	PO	Martin (1986)
Vitamin D3	2000 IU/kg in diet	PO	Whitney (1979)

IM = intramuscular; IP = intraperitoneal; IV = intravenous; PO = per os; SC = subcutaneous.

☞ ZOONOTIC DISEASES

One of the primary concerns in managing nonhuman primates is the protection of personnel from zoonotic diseases. All animals must be regarded as potential sources of zoonotic disease. Generally, the more closely related phylogenetically a species is to humans, the greater the danger for zoonotic disease transmission.

Some of the important bacterial diseases transmissible to humans are tuberculosis, shigellosis, salmonellosis, melioidosis, and staphylococcal or streptococcal infections. Among the important viral diseases transmissible to humans from nonhuman primates are herpes B, viral hepatitis, poxviruses, yellow fever, SV-40, poliomyelitis, rabies, and measles.

The more important parasites transmissible from nonhuman primates to humans include protozoan and helminth parasites such as *Entamoeba histolytica* and *Enterobius vermicularis*. Malaria can also be transmitted if a vector is available. Many parasites of OW monkeys are transmissible to humans. Parasites of NW monkeys are more closely related to those of dogs and rodents and are generally not transmissible to humans.

PHYSICAL EXAMINATION

Nonhuman primates should be placed in quarantine and receive a thorough physical examination soon after their arrival at a new facility. Pet monkeys should receive annual physical examinations. The examination of a nonhuman primate is performed in a manner similar to that for other species, with attention given to evidence of diarrhea, nasal or ocular discharge, dyspnea, condition of the skin and haircoat, alertness, and nutritional state. Two areas that should receive particular attention in primates are the lymph nodes and the mouth. Any enlargement or drainage of superficial lymph nodes should be noted, as it is suggestive of tuberculosis. In examining the mouth of a monkey, check for dental caries and broken teeth. Ulcers in the mouth of a macaque may be suggestive of herpes B virus. Hemorrhage of the gums and gingivitis are characteristic of vitamin C deficiencies. Shigellosis is sometimes also associated with gingivitis.

BACTERIAL DISEASES

The most common health problems of nonhuman primates are bacterial enteritis and bacterial pneumonia. These diseases may be latent in monkeys living in an unstressed state, but active disease may be precipitated by the stress of transportation, change in diet, or a new environment.

☞ ## Pneumonia and Respiratory Diseases

Nonhuman primates are susceptible to the human, bovine, and avian strains of *Mycobacterium*. The human strain, *Mycobacterium tuberculosis,* is by far the most frequent cause of simian tuberculosis. Although not the most common disease of nonhuman primates, it is potentially the most devastating that is likely to be encountered.

All species are capable of contracting tuberculosis, but the disease is more prevalent in OW monkeys than in NW monkeys. Young macaques are the most susceptible group. Disease frequently spreads rapidly throughout a colony. Older macaques, baboons, and apes have a disease more similar to that in humans with a slower progression. Experimentally induced tuberculosis has been observed to progress from initial infection to death anywhere from 6 weeks to 12 months. The primary route of transmission is through the respiratory tract. Other routes include intestinal tract invasion and cutaneous infection by bites or tattoo needles. Laboratory workers have an additional exposure to blood, sputum, excreta, cerebrospinal fluid, and exudates from lesions or tissues of infected animals. Simian tuberculosis poses a significant health hazard for humans.

The clinical signs of tuberculosis are usually not striking until the disease is in an advanced stage. The most commonly recognized signs are lethargy and weight loss. Other clinical signs are pneumonia, diarrhea, skin ulceration, and suppuration of lymph nodes. In some cases, no signs of illness are observed prior to sudden death of the animal.

Yellowish caseous nodules in the lungs and hilar lymph nodes are characteristic gross findings at necropsy. The liver, spleen, and lymph nodes of the abdominal, inguinal, and axillary areas are also frequently involved. Histologically, a classic presentation consists of tubercles with a central zone of caseation necrosis infiltrated with neutrophils and lymphocytes surrounded by a zone of epithelioid cells. Multinucleated giant cells of Langhans' type may be seen. Mineralization and fibrosis of the tubercles are rare in nonhuman primates.

Diseases from which tuberculosis must be distinguished include lung mites, pulmonary nocardiosis, pseudotuberculosis, systemic mycoses, and neoplasms. The most important tool for detecting tuberculosis is the intradermal tuberculin test. Other diagnostic tests include chest radiographs and cultures of sputum, blood, or feces. None of these alone are dependable or efficient diagnostic techniques. Radiography is of value in detecting advanced anergic cases; however, the lesions of nonhuman primate tuberculosis are often difficult to detect because calcium deposits within lymph nodes are rare and the heart blocks visualization of lesions around the hilar lymph nodes. Other factors that limit the value of thoracic radiographs are the small size of early lesions, lack of encapsulation, and the incidence of granulomas in many organs other than the lungs.

The most effective means of control is quarantine, testing, and elimination of reactors. The tuberculin skin test is the most practical and reliable method for detecting tuberculosis and is a vital part of the initial examination. The procedure most commonly employed is the injection of 0.1 mL undiluted mammalian tuberculin, containing 1500 or more tuberculin units, intradermally into the upper eyelid with a 25- to 27-gauge, 0.13-cm (0.5-in.) needle. A separate needle should be used for each monkey. Proper restraint or drug immobilization of the animal is essential to avoid injury to the eyelid. The eyelid is the preferred site because it facilitates reading of the test without recapturing the animal. Tests are read at 24, 48, and 72 hours. A positive reaction may range from mild, with only reddening, to severe, with marked reddening, edema, and occasionally ulceration. Isoniazid may be used to treat or prevent tuberculosis in extremely valuable animals such as great apes. Its effectiveness may be enhanced by combining with streptomycin or other drugs. Disadvantages of isoniazid are that it may 1) induce resistant strains, 2) mask the disease, 3) produce a pyridoxine deficiency, and 4) alter experimental results.

Streptococcus (Diplococcus) pneumoniae is a common cause of fibrinopurulent pneumonia in OW primates. Fibrinopurulent meningitis and arthritis are sequelae that are occasionally seen with *S. pneumoniae* infections. *Bordetella bronchiseptica* has been reported to cause a high incidence of fibrinopurulent hemorrhagic bronchopneumonia in NW monkeys. *B. bronchiseptica* is less of a problem in OW monkeys. Other organisms often associated with pneumonia in primates include *Klebsiella pneumoniae, Pasteurella multocida, Haemophilus influenzae, Staphylococcus aureus,* and other *Streptococcus* spp.

Clinical signs of pneumonia are generally nonspecific and include fever, rapid pulse, sneezing, coughing, mucopurulent nasal discharge, lethargy, anorexia, and dyspnea. In severe cases, cyanosis and prostration may be evident. With *S. pneumoniae,* meningitis with accompanying central nervous system signs is a frequent complication. The disease course may be several days to weeks.

Necropsy findings include lungs that are typically consolidated and red to gray. A fibrinous pleuritis, pericarditis, and occasionally empyema are characteristic of infections with *S. pneumoniae*. Meningitis appears grossly as a diffuse gray opacity of the meninges with an accumulation of yellow–white viscous material in the sulci.

Culture and sensitivities are important in selection of the most effective antibiotic. Penicillin, cephalosporins, enrofloxacin, tetracycline, and chloramphenicol are some antibiotics commonly used to treat bacterial pneumonia. Supportive treatment includes maintaining the ambient temperature at a comfortable level and providing nutritional supplements and fluids if animals refuse food and water. Bronchial dilators and decongestants are often useful.

Branhamella catarrhalis is the causative agent for "bloody nose syndrome" in cynomolgus macaques. Low humidity is believed to be a predisposing factor. Clinical signs include epistaxis and periorbital edema. Diagnosis is by isolation of the diplococcal organism and response to penicillin antibiotics.

☞ Bacterial Gastroenteritis

Three of the most common types of bacterial gastroenteritis in primates are shigellosis, campylobacteriosis, and salmonellosis. Clinically apparent shigellosis is most frequently due to *Shigella flexneri*. Transmission is by the fecal–oral route. Shigellosis can be transmitted to caretakers or other personnel, who may then become carriers of the organism. Although adults seldom become clinically ill, the disease can be severe or even fatal in children. Infections in monkeys and humans range from asymptomatic carriers to acute fulminant dysentery.

Clinical signs of shigellosis are depression, diarrhea that contains variable amounts of blood and mucus, weakness, emaciation, and dehydration. Abdominal pain is often evident, and the affected primate may bend forward in a sitting position with its hands folded across its abdomen. Typically, as the disease progresses, the animal becomes semicomatose and lies prostrate in its cage. Death may occur from 24 hours to 2 weeks after onset of illness.

Campylobacter jejuni is the organism most frequently isolated from active cases of campylobacteriosis diarrheal disease. This agent is primarily found in OW monkeys. Asymptomatic carriers are common, and transmission is fecal–oral. Clinical signs include liquid diarrhea, with or without blood, and severe dehydration. Diagnosis requires fecal culture on special media in 5% carbon dioxide.

Although less common than *Shigella* spp. and *Campylobacter* spp. infections, gastroenteritis from *Salmonella* spp. infections also occurs in nonhuman primates. Contaminated feed and contact with infected animals are the principal sources of infection with *Salmonella* spp. The clinical features of *Salmonella* spp. infection are similar to those of *Shigella* spp. infection except that vomiting is more common and the course of the disease is often less acute.

The gross lesions of shigellosis and salmonellosis are not readily distinguishable, and the two may exist as a mixed infection. In fatal cases of shigellosis, the colon is usually distended and contains mucus and occasionally blood. The mucosa is thickened, reddened, and may be ulcerated, and the surface covered by an exudate composed of fibrin and necrotic cells. Typical gross findings with salmonellosis are pasty-to-liquid intestinal contents, a swollen and reddened intestinal mucosa, and splenic congestion. *Salmonella* spp. infections frequently involve the ileum, whereas ileal involvement is infrequent with shigellosis.

It is often difficult to recover *Shigella* spp. organisms from rectal swabs, thus, a negative culture is not conclusive. In culturing for intestinal pathogens, the swab should be inserted into the rectum and the surface of the mucosa scraped. The bacteria are very sensitive to drying; thus, swabs must be protected before presentation to the laboratory. Ideally, plates are streaked directly from rectal swabs immediately following specimen collection.

Culture and sensitivities are important in selection of the proper antibiotic. Antibiotics commonly used in treating bacterial gastroenteritis include enrofloxacin, chloramphenicol, neomycin, trimethoprim, and furazolidone. The combination of trimethoprim and a sulfonamide is effective in treating both the active disease and the carrier state of *Shigella* spp. infections.

Supportive measures are very important in treatment of gastroenteritis in primates. Antisecretory drugs such as diphenoxylate hydrochloride, kaolin and pectin, or other intestinal absorbents are usually indicated for treatment of diarrhea. Fluid and electrolyte replacement is essential in cases of severe diarrhea. New World primates in particular need relatively large amounts of fluids. Lactated Ringer's or Ringer's solution have higher sodium contents and should be used for initial fluid replacement. Fluid replacement is preferentially given IV but may be given subcutaneously. For long-term fluid maintenance, solutions with lower sodium levels such as 2.5% dextrose/0.45% saline are generally recommended. Desiccated lactobacillus acidophilus is useful in treating chronic cases of diarrhea in nonhuman primates. If NW primates become weak and begin sitting on their buttocks, steps should be taken to prevent formation of decubitus ulcers that may develop because they lack ischial callosities.

Tetanus

Tetanus is caused by the neurotoxin produced by *Clostridium tetani*. Both OW and NW monkeys, as well as apes, are susceptible to infections with this organism. Clinical signs include tonic muscle spasms, lockjaw, opisthotonos, seizures, and respiratory paralysis. Vaccines are recommended for monkeys that are housed outdoors with an increased risk of becoming infected. An aluminum salt–absorbed toxoid vaccine should be used and administered to mimic a human vaccination schedule. Tetanus antitoxin can be effective in treating cases of tetanus.

Helicobacteriosis

Several species of OW monkeys, especially rhesus, harbor *Helicobacter pylori* in their stomachs. *Helicobacter* spp. have been identified as causative agents for gastritis and gastric ulcers in humans and many other species. There are usually no clinical signs in nonhuman primates except occasional vomiting. Diagnosis is based on gastric biopsy and culture results. Treatment is similar to that of humans including a 7- to 10-day regimen of amoxicillin and metronidazole combined antibiotic therapy with bismuth-subsalicylate, cimetidine, and sucralfate aimed at treating the ulcers. Sucralfate requires an acidic pH to function properly; thus, the sucralfate dose should precede the cimetidine dose by at least 2 hours.

Pseudotuberculosis

Pseudotuberculosis is caused by *Yersinia pseudotuberculosis* or *Yersinia enterocolitica*. The disease has been reported in both OW and NW monkeys. Wild rodents and birds are reservoir hosts, and transmission is by ingestion of contaminated feed. Acute yersiniosis typically occurs as an enteritis primarily affecting the jejunum and ileum. Clinical signs may include diarrhea, depression, and dehydration, or simply acute death. In its chronic form, septicemia results in necropurulent lesions in the liver, spleen, and other organs and may be confused grossly with tuberculosis. Microscopically, a lesion in the liver or lung consists of a central area of necrosis with neutrophils and clumps of bacteria surrounded by a zone of macrophages. Yersiniosis is a zoonotic disease.

Melioidosis

Melioidosis is caused by *Pseudomonas pseudomallei*, which is a saprophyte in Southeast Asia. The disease has been reported in OW monkeys and apes. The organism can remain clinically latent for years. The clinical course of melioidosis may be acute and fulminant or chronic. Multiple abscesses are seen as swellings in several locations. Gross findings in the lung typically consist of focal lesions up to 3 cm in diameter surrounded by a red halo. Humans are susceptible to the disease, but direct transmission from nonhuman primates has not been reported.

VIRAL DISEASES

☞ ### Herpesviruses

Although a large number of herpesviruses have been isolated from different species of nonhuman primates, the pathogenic effects of many of these isolates have not been established. A number of specific herpesviruses do produce highly fatal systemic diseases. In most herpes infections, there are two types of hosts: a reservoir or natural host in which the virus exists as a subclinical or latent infection and an aberrant or accidental host of a different species in which the infection is usually fatal.

Herpes simplex virus is the cause of fever blisters in humans. In this disease, humans are the reservoir hosts and certain species of nonhuman primates, primarily marmosets and owl monkeys, are fatally infected. Lesions in affected monkeys are similar to those seen with *Herpesvirus tamarinus* infections in these NW species.

The tamarin is the natural host for *H. tamarinus,* also known as herpes T. It can exist as a latent infection in squirrel, cebus, and spider monkeys. Host species may show oral vesicles or ulcers, similar to those of herpes simplex virus in humans and herpes B virus in macaques. Fatal infections most commonly occur in owl monkeys and marmosets. Lesions in fatally infected monkeys include facial swelling with self-mutilation; ulceration of the lips, tongue, and gastrointestinal tract; and hepatic necrosis.

The natural host of *Herpesvirus saimiri* is the squirrel monkey and infection in this species is asymptomatic. If the virus is inoculated into owl monkeys, marmosets, African green, howler, or spider monkeys, it induces a malignant lymphoma and lymphocytic leukemia.

Herpesvirus ateles is asymptomatic in its natural host, the spider monkey. It is similar to *H. saimiri* in that it causes a malignant lymphoma and lymphocytic leukemia in owl monkeys and marmosets.

H. simiae, also known as herpes B and Cercopithecine herpesvirus 1, is an important zoonotic disease of monkeys. Macaque primates, particularly rhesus and cynomolgus monkeys, are the natural hosts for herpes B. Humans are one of the aberrant hosts of this virus. Transmission to humans is usually through bites and scratches from infected monkeys. Monkeys may have conjunctivitis, vesicles/ulcers on the oral or genital mucosa, or may be asymptomatic. Obtaining macaques from herpes B–negative colonies is suggested. Persons in close contact with macaques should, however, be instructed to treat all macaques as potentially infectious carriers and to wear appropriate protective clothing to prevent exposure. Universal precautions should be followed in handling all equipment that may be contaminated with monkey blood (i.e., don't recap needles), urine, or saliva, as well as all blood, urine, or tissue samples obtained from macaques.

People that have been or will be exposed to macaques should be educated about the clinical manifestations of herpes B infection in humans. In humans, the disease is seen as an encephalomyelitis. Although the incidence of disease in humans is very low, infected humans have about a 70% case-fatality rate. Persons who are exposed either directly or indirectly to herpes B virus through bites, scratches, saliva or body fluids, needlesticks, fresh tissues, or fomites (e.g., cages), should immediately wash the site with copious amounts of water and a concentrated solution of soap or disinfectant, such as povidone-iodine or chlorhexidine, for a minimum of 15 minutes. Exposed persons should be examined by a physician who is knowledgeable about herpes B infection in humans. Guidelines for the prevention and treatment of B virus infections have recently been developed by an expert panel of virologists and/or physicians and are published. Paired sera should be obtained from the human and monkey on the day of exposure, as well as approximately 3 weeks later. Culture of the buccal mucosa and conjunctiva of each eye of the monkey and of the wound of the exposed individual should be submitted to a laboratory that performs this specialized procedure (see Chapter 10, Serologic Testing and Quality Control). Clinical signs may include vesicles, pain and itching at the exposure site, lymphadenopathy, fever, numbness, muscle weakness or paralysis in the exposed extremity, conjunctivitis, neck stiffness, sinusitis, headache, nausea, vomiting, altered mentation, and other central nervous system signs. Early treatment of humans with acyclovir, before they show central nervous system signs, has resulted in halting the disease progression but does not appear to eliminate the virus.

Simian agent 8 (SA8) is related to *H. simiae*. It is endemic in baboons and will infect African green monkeys. Transmission is primarily by venereal spread. Clinically, mild to severe vesicular or ulcerative lesions are seen involving the genitalia and oral cavity. The scrotum may be reddened and have weeping, crusty vesicles. Inguinal lymphadenopathy may occur. Lesions will often resolve spontaneously, but secondary bacterial infections may require antibiotic therapy. SA8 does not appear to be capable of infecting humans.

Simian varicella virus is a group of closely related herpesviruses that are antigenically related to human varicella-zoster but are not zoonotic to humans. Transmission is primarily by the respiratory route and is often latent in monkeys. Different viral serotypes have been involved in clinical disease of patas monkeys, African green monkeys, and macaques. Clinical signs involve a herpetic rash, depression, and respiratory difficulty with variable morbidity and mortality.

Measles

Measles (rubeola), caused by a human paramyxovirus, commonly produces a mild infection in macaques and most other species of OW primates. The NW species appear to be somewhat more resistant to infections. Clinical signs most frequently seen are the presence of a nasal and ocular discharge, conjunctivitis, facial edema, blepharitis, a papular skin rash, and sometimes giant cell pneumonia. In marmosets and owl monkeys, measles causes a fatal gastroenterocolitis with severe diarrhea rather than a pneumonia. Active infection with measles interferes with the antigenic response to the tuberculin test and may cause a false negative tuberculin test result.

Human measles vaccine is reported to be effective in protecting monkeys from the disease. The most important preventive measure is avoiding exposure to infected humans, the usual source of monkey infections.

☞ Poxviruses

Five different poxviruses are known to infect nonhuman primates: monkeypox, smallpox, benign epidermal monkeypox (BEMP), yaba, and molluscum contagiosum. All five viruses can infect humans. In most cases, only epidermal changes are seen in monkeys and humans.

Monkeypox is closely related to smallpox and vaccinia viruses. The disease in monkeys is characterized by 1- to 4-mm, circular papules on the skin, particularly the palms of the hands, which undergo vesiculation and ulceration. The disease in humans is similar to smallpox with clinical signs of fatigue, fever, and muscular and back pain. Papules develop and progress to vesicles, pustules, and scabs in approximately 10 days. Immunization with vaccinia protects both human and nonhuman primates against monkeypox.

BEMP is caused by the tanapox virus, which is antigenically related to yaba poxvirus. Outbreaks of disease have primarily been reported in macaques. Monkeys infected with BEMP develop skin lesions that are circular, with umbilication and an adherent scab in the center. Papules initially appear similar to monkeypox lesions but do not progress to pustules. Histologically, there is hyperplasia of the epithelium of the skin and epidermal necrosis with little damage to the underlying dermis. A notable characteristic of this disease is that there are usually only a few epidermal lesions seen on each infected animal or human. The lesions usually regress spontaneously in 2–4 weeks.

Yaba poxvirus is an oncogenic virus originally isolated from a subcutaneous histiocytoma in rhesus monkeys at Yaba, Nigeria. Outbreaks of disease have been reported in rhesus and baboons. Transmission is usually by a mosquito vector. The disease in both monkeys and humans is characterized by the presence of nodular subcutaneous lesions, primarily on the extremities, that progress to a maximum size of 2–5 cm in 3 weeks. The skin over these tumors has a tendency to ulcerate. Histologically, the tumors consist of proliferations of histiocytes, frequently with eosinophilic intracytoplasmic inclusions. Spontaneous regression generally occurs by 6–8 weeks.

Molluscum contagiosum is a poxvirus disease primarily of humans. Transmission is usually by direct contact. It has been reported in chimpanzees in which the lesions appear as waxy papular cutaneous elevations, especially on the eyelid and groin. Histologically, there are large, basophilic intracytoplasmic inclusion bodies called molluscum bodies.

Treatment of pox lesions, if indicated, should be directed at prevention of self-mutilation and secondary infection through the use of sedatives, antipruritic drugs, steroids, and antibiotics.

☞ Hepatitis Viruses

Hepatitis A virus (HAV), a picornavirus, causes a disease that was formerly known as infectious hepatitis. Naturally occurring infections have been reported in several nonhuman primate species including rhesus, cynomolgus, African greens, owls, chimpanzees, and marmosets. Transmission is by ingestion of the viral particles from feces. Humans and monkeys are usually asymptomatic. Prevention involves attention to hand washing and personal hygiene. Personnel working with monkeys that are experimentally infected with HAV should be given an HAV vaccine, which is available commercially.

Hepatitis B virus (HBV), a human hepadnavirus, causes a disease that was formerly known as serum hepatitis. Naturally occurring infections have primarily been reported in wild chimpanzees and gorillas.

Transmission is by parenteral inoculation, droplet exposure of mucous membranes, or contact exposure of broken skin with contaminated blood, saliva, semen, cerebrospinal fluid, or urine. Humans and monkeys are usually asymptomatic. A significant number (~8%) of infected people become chronic carriers and may eventually develop hepatocellular carcinoma. Personnel working with chimpanzees should be given an HBV vaccine.

Hepatitis C virus (HCV), a unique virus that is related to both flaviviruses and pestiviruses, causes a hepatic disease that was previously referred to as non-A, non-B hepatitis (NANBH). Transmission is parenteral and is similar to that for HBV. It appears that there are no naturally occurring cases of this viral disease in nonhuman primates, and only experimentally infected chimpanzees pose a zoonosis hazard to personnel. There is no vaccine available to prevent this disease.

Hepatitis D virus (HDV) is a defective, incomplete DNA virus that requires the presence of a hepadnavirus (HBV) antigen for replication. Transmission is similar to that for HBV. Only humans or chimpanzees that are infected with a hepadnavirus can become infected.

Hepatitis E virus (HEV), an enterovirus, causes NANBH via fecal–oral transmission. There are no reports of naturally occurring outbreaks of this disease in monkeys, but experimental infections have been established in owl monkeys, cynomolgus monkeys, and tamarins.

☞ Filoviruses

A simian Ebola-like filovirus has been identified as the cause of an acute, fatal hemorrhagic disease of cynomolgus monkeys newly imported from the Philippines. The virus is related to, but antigenically distinct from, the Ebola virus that has caused several outbreaks of hemorrhagic fever in humans in Africa. The reservoir host is thought to be a rodent. Clinical signs in monkeys include fever, depression, coma, and death. At necropsy, hemorrhages are seen throughout the organs and bloody fluid is present in body cavities. Several humans involved with these monkeys did seroconvert, but none developed clinical signs of disease.

Simian hemorrhagic fever (SHF) is caused by another filovirus. Macaques are susceptible to the disease with 100% mortality. Patas monkeys *(Erythrocebus patas)*, baboons, and African green monkeys can be asymptomatic carriers. Humans do not appear to be susceptible to this virus. Clinical signs include epistaxis, ecchymosis, ataxia, anorexia, and lethargy. Clinical pathology findings such as abnormal coagulation factors and fibrin degradation products are primarily caused by disseminated intravascular coagulation. Elevations in liver enzymes, blood urea nitrogen, and creatinine are due to hepatic and renal involvement. The pathognomonic gross lesions are duodenal necrosis and splenic infarction. This viral disease underlies the importance of strict separation of species, especially Asian and African monkeys.

Encephalomyocarditis Virus

Encephalomyocarditis virus (EMCV) is a picornavirus that has been shown to cause myocarditis in nonhuman primates, elephants, pigs, and other species. The reservoir host is thought to be a rodent. Sudden death and frothy exudate from the nose and mouth are the primary clinical signs seen in nonhuman primates. Gross findings include pericardial effusion and pale streaks in the myocardium. Histologically, there is necrosis of the myofibers with inflammation and edema. Controlling rodent populations around outdoor-housed nonhuman primates may be important in preventing infections.

☞ ## Retroviruses

The Retroviridae family consists of three subfamilies—Oncovirinae, Lentivirinae, and Spumavirinae. To date, only oncoviruses and lentiviruses have been shown to cause clinical disease in nonhuman primates. There are endogenous and exogenous viruses within the Retroviridae family. Endogenous viruses have become incorporated into the host's genomic material and are transmitted vertically. Exogenous viruses exist outside of the host and are transmitted horizontally.

Simian T-cell leukemia virus (STLV) is an exogenous type C oncovirus and is 90%–95% homologous to the human T-cell leukemia virus (HTLV) that induces adult T-cell leukemia/lymphoma and other disorders. Naturally occurring infections have been reported in baboons, patas monkeys, African green monkeys, macaques, and chimpanzees. Transmission is by sexual contact or parenteral inoculation. Most animals remain asymptomatic; however, a leukemia/lymphoma syndrome has been reported in baboons, African green monkeys, and macaques. Diagnosis is by serology and identification of the virus in tumor cells by molecular biologic techniques. The STLV infection is an important model for studying HTLV infections in humans.

Simian retroviruses (SRVs) consist of both endogenous and exogenous type D oncoviruses. To date, all type D viruses appear to be of nonhuman primate origin. The endogenous viruses are nonpathogenic.

There are numerous SRV exogenous serogroups that infect many different species of macaques. The prototype type D oncovirus is the Mason-Pfizer monkey virus. Simian retroviruses are shed in the saliva; thus, transmission requires close contact such as biting, licking, and grooming. Simian retrovirus infections in macaques may be asymptomatic or can induce immunosuppression and chronic wasting, which is referred to as simian autoimmune deficiency syndrome (SAIDS). Opportunistic infections, diarrhea, necrotizing gingivitis referred to as NOMA, and retroperitoneal fibromatosis are other possible sequelae to SAIDS. Clinical pathology findings include neutropenia, anemia, and terminal lymphopenia. Although SAIDS in monkeys is similar to AIDS in humans, SRV is not related to HIV and is not infectious to humans. Infected animals may occasionally remain seronegative despite active shedding of the virus. Thus, diagnosis of SRV infections must include repeated serologic screening by enzyme-linked immunosorbent assays (ELISAs), plus viral isolation from peripheral blood mononuclear cells.

Simian immunodeficiency viruses (SIVs) are lentiviruses that are closely related to HIV-2 but also share similarities with HIV-1. HIV-1 is the primary etiologic agent of AIDS worldwide; HIV-2 is less virulent than HIV-1 and is the agent which causes AIDS in western Africa. Multiple SIV serotypes have been isolated from naturally occurring infections in several African primates including *Cercopithecus* spp., *Papio* spp., *Cercocebus* spp., and *Pan troglodytes*. African primates are persistently infected but remain asymptomatic. The naturally occurring route of transmission is unknown but probably requires direct contact. Macaque monkeys infected with SIV develop a syndrome similar to AIDS with chronic wasting and immunosuppression. The SIV isolates from sooty mangabeys (SIV_{SMM}) and rhesus monkeys (SIV_{MAC}) are especially virulent to macaques. Clinical signs include weight loss, diarrhea, anemia, thrombocytopenia, and those associated with opportunistic infections. The most common opportunistic infections of both SRV and SIV are cytomegalovirus, *Candida* spp., *Mycobacterium avium-intracellulare complex*, *Cryptosporidium* spp., *Pneumocystis carinii*, *Trichomonas* spp., adenovirus, Epstein-Barr virus, and simian virus 40. Diagnosis of SRV infections is by serologic screening with ELISA or viral isolation (see Chapter 10, Serologic Testing and Quality Control).

Rabies

Rabies occurs occasionally in nonhuman primates. Free-ranging or outdoor-housed monkeys are particularly at risk for contracting rabies. If they are vaccinated against rabies, a killed vaccine should be used.

Miscellaneous Viral Infections

Other viral infections that have been reported in nonhuman primates include yellow fever, chickenpox, Epstein-Barr virus, adenovirus, papillomavirus, papovavirus, lymphocytic choriomeningitis, and cytomegalovirus.

PARASITIC DISEASES

Protozoa

Entamoeba histolytica is pathogenic for all primates, although it is less pathogenic for monkeys and apes than for humans. Asymptomatic carriers are common. Clinical diarrhea is occasionally seen. Special techniques may be needed to recover and identify the organism, as it is not ordinarily detected by routine fecal flotation. The most common lesions are gut ulceration and hepatic abscesses. Ulcers in the gut typically have a flask shape. Recommended treatments include diiodohydroxyquin, iodoquinol, and metronidazole.

Balantidium coli is frequently found in fecal specimens of various nonhuman primate species, especially the anthropoid apes. The pathogenicity of the organism for nonhuman primates has not been clearly established, but ulcerative lesions in the large intestine have been reported with concurrent infection. Infections in humans may result in severe diarrhea and dysentery. Recommended treatments for elimination of *B. coli* include iodoquinol and diiodohydroxyquin.

Both OW monkeys and NW monkeys as well as apes can contract malaria through infection with various *Plasmodium* spp. Various species of anopheline mosquitoes transmit malaria. Infections are usually asymptomatic in nonhuman primates. The life cycle in monkeys occurs in the hepatocytes and red blood cells. Some *Plasmodium* spp. will cause cyclic bouts of fever and anemia due to lysis of red blood cells caused by multiplication of the protozoan organisms. Gross findings include gray lungs, liver, and spleen due to malarial pigment in the macrophages. Infected animals may serve as a source of infection for humans if the required species of mosquito vectors are present or via parenteral inoculation. If treatment is necessary, Centers for Disease Control and Prevention recommendations for pediatric treatment of malaria should be followed.

Hepatocystis spp. are protozoans that are related to *Plasmodium* spp. These organisms infect African and Asian OW monkeys, primarily baboons, African green monkeys, and macaques. Transmission is through the bite of a midge, the intermediate host. Infected monkeys remain asymptomatic because replication of the organism occurs only in the hepatocytes. Gross findings include 2- to 4-mm opaque cysts or scars in the liver. Treatment is not necessary.

Nematodes

☞ *Oesophagostomum* spp., or nodular worms, are the most common helminth parasites affecting OW primates. The infection is usually asymptomatic, but heavy worm burdens can cause diarrhea and adhesions. The parasite produces firm, smooth, black or white nodules in the wall of the colon. Both the eggs and the adult worms resemble canine hookworms. Thiabendazole and ivermectin can be effective treatments.

Strongyloides fulleborni and *Strongyloides cebus* are very common parasites of nonhuman primates. Infections are frequently asymptomatic, but heavy infections can cause severe diarrhea and coughing from migration of the larvae through the lungs. Apes are more prone to develop severe clinical disease. Thiabendazole and ivermectin are effective in treating strongyloidosis.

Adult *Dipetalonema* spp. are commonly seen in the peritoneal cavity of NW monkeys and will occasionally be found in OW monkeys. Microfilariae appear in the blood. Although often found in large numbers, the parasite appears to cause only mild proliferative lesions in the peritoneal cavity and treatment is not indicated.

Enterobius vermicularis, the common pinworm of humans, is commonly found in captive chimpanzees. Cross-infection between chimpanzees and humans occurs readily. Pinworm infections in simian primates are usually not serious but can cause perianal pruritus and restlessness. Heavy infections, however, are occasionally fatal. The ova are more readily detected by application of cellophane tape to the perianal area than by fecal flotation. The treatment of choice is pyrvinium pamoate.

Tapeworms

Larval cestodes are seen with some frequency in nonhuman primates including cysticercus larvae (*Taenia* spp.), coenurus larvae (*Multiceps* spp.), and hydatid larvae (*Echinococcus granulosa*). These are usually incidental findings at necropsy or surgery, as there are rarely clinical signs of infection. Transmission is by ingestion of infective eggs or intermediate hosts, such as arthropods. Larvae may be found in subcutaneous tissues, muscles, and abdominal, peritoneal, or cranial cavities.

☞ ## Acanthocephalans

Prosthenorchis elegans and *P. spirula* are the thorny-headed worms of NW primates. The adults burrow deeply into the mucosa of the terminal ileum, cecum, or colon, causing abscesses, granulomas, and occasionally peritonitis. A large population of worms can cause intestinal blockage. The cockroach serves as an intermediate host. The use of praziquantel will reduce the population of adults but will not eliminate all the parasites.

Arthropods

The lung mite, *Pneumonyssus simicola,* is the most important arthropod infestation of OW primates. Although previously a common finding in wild macaques, the use of anthelmintics in captive-breeding programs has almost eliminated this mite. Affected animals are usually asymptomatic. At necropsy, pale yellow foci containing the mites are found throughout the lungs, and in some cases, cavitation of the lungs is seen. The lesions of lung mites may grossly resemble those of tuberculosis. Histologically, the presence of brown-to-black pigment and a focal bronchiolitis are characteristic of lung mite infestation. Radiographically, diffuse interstitial densities or discrete opaque densities may be seen throughout the lung lobes. Secondary bacterial bronchopneumonia may develop. Ivermectin appears to be an effective treatment.

Ectoparasites of nonhuman primates include lice and mites. Several of the more common external parasites reported in nonhuman primates are *Sarcoptes scabiei, Demodex* spp., *Pedicinus* spp. and *Psorergates simplex.* Topical organophosphate insecticides and pyrethrins, as well as parenteral ivermectin, are effective in treating external parasites.

Pentastomids

The nymphs of *Armillifer* spp. and others are often found encysted in the peritoneal cavity of nonhuman primates. Adult pentastomids live in the lungs of large snakes. Monkeys are the intermediate host and are infected by swallowing food contaminated by snake feces. There are usually no clinical signs, but peritonitis following penetration of the intestinal wall by immature stages of a pentastomid has been reported.

MYCOTIC DISEASES

Dermatophytosis

Ringworm in nonhuman primates is caused by several *Microsporum* spp. and *Trichophyton* spp. Systemic treatment with griseofulvin is suggested.

Systemic Mycoses

Candidiasis occurs in monkeys that are immunosuppressed, debilitated, or on long-term antibiotic therapy. Thrush is the most common form of *Candida albicans* and is seen as a white velvety overlay in the mouth and throat.

Pneumocystis carinii is another fungal organism that is primarily seen as an opportunistic infection in immunosuppressed monkeys with SRV or SIV infections. Clinical signs include fever, dyspnea, and coughing. Fungal cysts can be identified with special stains such as Gomori's methenamine silver.

Histoplasma capsulatum var *duboisii* is the etiologic agent of African histoplasmosis. Histoplasmosis has been reported in baboons. Transmission is from inhalation of spores from soil contaminated with bird or bat excreta. Organs affected include the skin, lymph nodes, and bones.

Nocardiosis in nonhuman primates is most commonly seen as a granulomatous disease of the lungs resembling tuberculosis. Nocardiosis can be differentiated from tuberculosis by the absence of involvement of hilar lymph nodes.

Moniliasis and aspergillosis rarely occur in animals not previously debilitated from other causes. Naturally occurring infection with *Coccidioides immitis* (coccidioidomycosis) is limited to arid portions of the southwestern United States. *Blastomyces dermatitidis* is occasionally seen in monkeys housed outdoors. Rare reports of systemic *Cryptococcus neoformans* infections in nonhuman primates exist in the literature.

MISCELLANEOUS CONDITIONS

☞ Acute Gastric Dilation

Acute gastric dilation occurs with some frequency in macaques and baboons. The exact etiology is unknown, but there is evidence that clostridial organisms are involved. *Clostridium perfringens* is usually isolated from the colon contents of animals dying of bloat; however, the condition has not been reproduced by administration of the organism.

236

Excessive food intake and excessive water intake are considered predisposing causes. Large amounts of raw vegetables or fruits may be particularly problematic. The condition is most often seen in greedy animals or animals in which full feeding was resumed after a period of restricted feeding. Most deaths occur at night following the evening feeding.

Gaseous distention of the stomach develops rapidly. The abdominal distention is extreme and may be accompanied by an accumulation of subcutaneous gas. Ingesta may be seen in the oral cavity, but neither frank vomiting or bloody diarrhea are usual features of acute gastric dilatation.

Mortality is high unless the problem is detected early and vigorous treatment is instituted. Recommended treatment consists of passing a gastric tube to relieve the gas and excess fluid contents until peristalsis is resumed. Supportive therapy in the form of intravenous fluids and analgesics should be administered. The use of antibiotics and steroids is also thought to increase the chances of survival. Bloat in primates is prevented by multiple feedings of small quantities of food plus full access to water.

☞ Trauma

Bite wounds are the most frequent problems seen in group-housed primates. Wounds are often very extensive. Fresh lacerations should be thoroughly cleaned and sutured using a subcuticular pattern to bury the suture. Bandages are difficult, if not impossible, to keep in place and self-mutilation following injury often poses a problem. Crushing injuries of the muscles may release large amounts of methemoglobin, which can lead to acute renal failure if left untreated. Intravenous fluid therapy should be aggressive to help diurese the kidneys; otherwise, treatment is essentially the same as for other species. Primates should receive tetanus antitoxin after penetrating injuries if they have not been previously immunized.

☞ Metabolic Bone Disease

Metabolic bone disease, referred to as simian bone disease, cage paralysis, or osteodystrophia fibrosa, results from a deficiency of vitamin D and an imbalance in the calcium:phosphorus ratio. This disease syndrome is due to a nutritional secondary hyperparathyroidism, which results in bone resorption and fibrous replacement. A deficiency of vitamin D alone results in rickets in young animals and osteomalacia in adult animals. In rickets, calcification of the cartilage never occurs. In osteomalacia, calcium resorption causes decalcified bones.

237

Vitamin D deficiencies are most frequently seen in NW monkeys that cannot utilize vitamin D_2 and thus require a diet containing vitamin D_3. Clinical signs include decreased activity, pain, paresis, soft bones, kyphosis, deformities of long bones, multiple fractures, and high levels of serum alkaline phosphatase. Radiographs show thinning of cortical bone. Treatment should be aimed at correcting the diet by providing vitamin D_3, calcium, and a proper calcium:phosphorus ratio. A full-spectrum light source will also aid in the production of adequate vitamin D_3 levels. Appropriate treatment with 5000 IU of vitamin D_3/kg/wk plus a high calcium and protein diet will prevent further progression of simian bone disease.

☞ Scurvy

Without an adequate dietary supply of vitamin C, scurvy develops in nonhuman primates. The usual clinical signs are swelling of the epiphyses of long bones and hemorrhage of the gums, eyes, and periosteum. Cephalohematomas are a unique clinical manifestation seen in squirrel monkeys. Treatment consists of administration of 25 mg/kg/d of vitamin C until clinical signs disappear. Response to therapy is usually rapid, with clinical signs resolving in several weeks. Prevention of scurvy is dependent upon feeding fresh foods that have been properly stored.

Endometriosis

Endometriosis is a condition in which endometrial glands and stroma are found in abnormal locations, most commonly on the serosal surface of pelvic organs. Endometriosis is commonly seen in rhesus monkeys, particularly following hysterotomy. Clinical signs may be nonexistent or may consist of irregular menstrual cycles or infertility. Abdominal masses may occasionally be palpable, especially when adhesions have developed. The pathogenesis of this disease in humans and nonhuman primates is unresolved. Treatment usually consists of surgical removal of the abnormally placed endometrial tissue, ovariectomy, and possibly hormonal therapies such as medroxyprogesterone. Extremely advanced cases may warrant euthanasia.

Fatal Fasting Syndrome of Obese Macaques

This syndrome is seen in obese macaques. Clinical signs include anorexia, lethargy, and sudden death. Histologically, there is fatty change in both the liver and kidney. The mechanism of action is unknown but may be similar to hepatic lipidosis of cats.

Arthritis

Arthritis is a common, old-age disease of rhesus monkeys. Clinical signs include enlarged joints, muscle contracture, and wasting. Interphalangeal and knee joints are most commonly affected. Deposition of calcium pyrophosphate crystals within the joint is observed histologically. Treatment with polysulfated glycosaminoglycans may be beneficial in alleviating clinical signs.

Colonic Carcinoma of Tamarins

Tamarins, especially the cotton-top tamarin, have a high incidence of chronic ulcerative colitis and associated colonic carcinomas. Exact etiology is unknown. Clinical signs include diarrhea, weight loss, intestinal obstruction, and a palpable abdominal mass.

☞ Dental Diseases

Periodic removal of dental deposits with a scaler is recommended to prevent periodontal disease. Dental caries are more likely to be seen in pet monkeys fed sweets than in research monkeys. Abscesses of the upper canine teeth are not uncommon in squirrel monkeys. Treatment consists of extraction of the involved tooth and irrigation with an antibacterial solution or performance of a root canal.

Extreme caution should be taken when performing dental work on nonhuman primates, especially macaques, as the possibility of aerosols or splatter of blood is significant. Personnel involved in the dental work should wear protective clothing including gloves, masks, and goggles or a face shield.

■ GENERAL REFERENCES

Sources consulted to compile the material in this chapter include *Nonhuman Primates in Biomedical Research,* edited by B. T. Bennett, C.R. Abee, and R. Henrickson (1995, Academic Press, Inc., San Diego, CA 92101); *Veterinary Clinics of North America: Small Animal Practice, Exotic Pet Medicine II,* Vol. 24 (1), edited by K.E. Quesenberry and E.V. Hillyer (1994, WB Saunders Co., The Curtis Center, Independence Square West, Philadelphia, PA 19106-3399); *Laboratory Animal Medicine,* edited by J.G. Fox, B.J. Cohen, and F.M. Loew (1984, Academic Press, Inc., Orlando, FL 32887); *The UFAW Handbook on the Care and Management of Laboratory Animals,* 6th edition, edited by T.B. Poole (1987, Churchill Livingstone Inc., 1560 Broadway, New York, NY 10036); and *Pathology of Nonhuman Primates,* notes from the Armed Forces Institute of Pathology (AFIP) course Pathology of Laboratory Animals (POLA) by Gary Baskin (1995).

■ TECHNICAL REFERENCES

Banish, L.D., R. Sims, M. Bush, D. Sack, and R.J. Montali. 1993. Clearance of *Shigella flexneri* carriers in a zoologic collection of primates. *J Am Vet Med Assoc* 203(1): 133–136.

Canadian Council on Animal Care (CCAC). 1984. *Guide to the Care and Use of Experimental Animals*, vols. I and II. Ottawa, Ontario: Canadian Council on Animal Care.

Centers for Disease Control (CDC). 1990. Recommendations for the prevention of malaria among travelers. *Morb Mortal Wkly Rep* 39.10.

Clifford, D.H. 1984. Preanesthesia, Anesthesia, Analgesia, and Euthanasia. In *Laboratory Animal Medicine,* ed. J.G. fox, B.J. Cohen, and F.M. Loew, pp. 541–543. Orlando, FL: Academic.

de Stefani Munao Diniz, L., M. Iwasaki, and B.W. de Martin. 1983. Clinical aspects of tuberculosis in a chimpanzee. *Vet Med Small Anim Clin* 78: 1289–1291.

Dysko, R.C. and D.E. Hoskins. 1995. Collection of biological samples and therapy administration. In *Nonhuman Primates in Biomedical Research,* ed. B.T. Bennett, C.R. Abee, and R. Henrickson, pp. 270–271. San Diego: Academic.

Feeser, P. and F. White. 1992. Medical management of *Lemur catta Varecia varegata,* and *Propithecus verreauxi* in natural habitat enclosures. In *Proceedings of the Annual Meeting of the American Association of Zoo Veterinarians,* pp. 320–323.

Fineg, J., W.C. Hanly, J.R. Prine, D.C. Van Riper, and P.W. Day. 1977. Isoniazid therapy in the chimpanzee. *Lab Anim Care* 16(5): 436–446.

Flecknell, P.A. 1985. The management of post-operative pain and distress in experimental animals. *Anim Tech* 36(2): 97–103.

Flecknell, P.A. 1987. *Laboratory Animal Anesthesia.* London: Academic.

Fraser, C.M. 1991. Management, husbandry, diseases of laboratory animals: diseases of nonhuman primates. In *The Merck Veterinary Manual,* 7th ed, pp. 1032–1036. Rahway, NJ: Merck.

Hainsey, B.M., G.B. Hubbard, M.M. Leland, and K.M. Brasky. 1993. Clinical parameters of the normal baboons (*Papio* species) and chimpanzees (*Pan troglodytes*). *Lab Anim Sci* 43(3): 236–243.

Hawk, C.T. and S.L. Leary. 1995. *Formulary for Laboratory Animals.* Ames: Iowa State University Press.

Hawkins, J.V., C.E. Jaquish, R.L. Carlson, et al. 1992. *Trichospirura leptostoma* infection in *Callithrix jacchus* (common marmoset): disease and treatment [abstr]. *Contemp Topics* 31(4): 26.

Heard, D.J. 1993. Principles and techniques of anesthesia and analgesia for exotic practice. *Vet Clin North Am Small Anim Pract* 23(6): 1301–1327.

Hollihn U. 1988. Krankheiten der Primaten [Diseases of Primates]. In *Kompendium Der Heimtierkrankheiten,* ed., E. Weisner. Stuttgart: Gustav Fischer.

Holmes, D.D. 1984. *Clinical Laboratory Animal Medicine.* Ames: Iowa State University Press.

Holmes, G.P., L.E. Chapman, J.A. Stewart, et al. 1995. Guidelines for the prevention and treatment of B-virus infections in exposed persons. *Clin Infect Dis* 20: 421–439.

Hotchkiss, E.C. 1995. Use of cisapride for the treatment of intestinal pseudoobstruction in a stumptail macaque (*Macaca arctoides*). *J Zoo Wildl Med* 26(1): 98–101.

Hughes, H.C. 1981. Anesthesia of laboratory animals. *Lab Animal* 10(5): 40–56.

Ialeggio, D.M. 1989. Practical medicine of primate pets. *Compend Contin Educ Pract Vet* 11: 1252–1259.

Isaza, R., B. Baker, and F. Dunker. 1992. Medical management of inflammatory bowel disease in a spider monkey. *J Am Vet Med Assoc* 200(10): 1543–1545.

Izard, M.K., S.J., Heath, Y. Hayes, and E.L. Simons. 1991. Hematology, serum chemistry values, and rectal temperatures of adult greater galagos (*Galago garnetti* and *G. crassicaudatus*). *J Med Primatol* 20(3): 117–121.

Jenkins, W.L. 1987. Pharmacologic aspects of analgesic drugs in animals: an overview. *J Am Vet Med Assoc* 191(10): 1231–1240.

Johnson, D.K., R.J. Russell, and J.A. Stunkard. 1981. *A Guide to the Diagnosis, Treatment, and Husbandry of Nonhuman Primates.* Edwardsville, KS: Veterinary Medicine.

Johnson-Delaney, C.A. 1994. Primates. *Vet Clin North Am Small Anim Pract* 24(1): 121–156.

Junge, R.E., K.G. Mehren, T.P. Meehan, et al. 1992. Hypertrophic osteoarthropathy and renal disease in three black lemurs (*Lemur macaco*). In *Proceedings of the Annual Meeting of the American Association of Zoo Veterinarians,* pp.324–330.

Kelly, D.J., J.D. Chulay, P. Mikesell , and A.M. Friedlander. 1992. Serum concentrations of penicillin, doxycycline, and ciprofloxacin during prolonged therapy in rhesus monkeys. *J Infect Dis* 166(5): 1184–1187.

Koehn, C.J. 1966. The feeding of baboons, *Papio cynocephalus* and *P. doguera*. *Lab Anim Care* 16(2): 178–184.

Krasnow, S.W. 1987. Primate nutrition [ACLAM notes]. Privately published, Jan. 12, 1987.

Line, A.S. 1993. Comments on Baytril antimicrobial therapy and considerations for intramuscular antibiotic therapy in captive primates. *Lab Primate Newsl* 32: 3.

Marks, S.K. 1994. Disease review: balantidiasis. A report of the American Association of Zoo Veterinarians Infectious Disease Committee. Philadelphia: American Association of Zoo Veterinarians.

Martin, D.P. 1986. Primates: feeding and nutrition. In *Zoo and Wild Animal Medicine,* ed. M.E. Fowler, pp. 661–663. Philadelphia: WB Saunders.

Melby, E.C. and N.H. Altman. 1976. *CRC Handbook of Laboratory Animal Science,* vol. 3. Cleveland: CRC Press.

NRC (National Research Council). 1996. *Guide for the Care and Use of Laboratory Animals.* Washington, DC: National Academy Press.

Paul-Murphy, J. 1992. Preventative medicine program for nonhuman primates. In *Proceedings of the North American Veterinary Conference,* pp.736–738.

Pernikoff, D.S. and J. Orkin. 1991. Bacterial meningitis syndrome: an overall review of the disease complex and considerations of cross infectivity between great apes and man. In *Proceedings of the American Association of Zoo Veterinarians,* pp.235–241.

Regional Primate Research Center at the University of Washington, Colony Division. Antibiotics routinely used for treatment. [Privately published]. Seattle, 1987.

Rosenberg, D.P. 1991. Nonhuman primate analgesia. *Lab Animal* 20(9): 22–33.

Sainsbury, A. Primates. 1991. In *Manual of Exotic Pets,* ed. P. Benyon and J. Cooper, pp. 111–121. Ames: Iowa State University Press.

Sanders, E.A., R.D. Gleed, and P.W. Nathanielsz. 1991. Anesthetic management for instrumentation of the pregnant rhesus monkey. *J Med Primatol* 20(5): 223–228.

Schultz, C.S. 1989. Formulary—Veterinary Hospital Pharmacy, Washington State University. Pullman, WA: Washington State University Press, p. 156.

Swenson, R.B. 1993. Protozoal parasites of great apes. In *Zoo and Wildl Animal Medicine—Current Therapy 3,* pp. 352–355. Philadelphia: WB Saunders.

Weller, R.E., J.F. Baer, et al. 1992. Renal clearance and excretion of endogenous substances in the owl monkey. *Am J Primatol* 28(2): 115–123.

White, G.L. and J.F. Cummings. 1979. A comparison of ketamine and ketamine-xylazine in the baboon. *Vet Med Small Anim Clin* 74(3): 392–394, 396.

Whitney, R.A., Jr. 1979. Primate medicine and husbandry. *Vet Clin of North Am Small Anim Pract* 9(3): 429–445.

Whitney, R.A., Jr., J.B. Mulder, and D.K. Johnson. 1977. Nonhuman primates: bacterial diseases. In *Nonhuman Primates,* ed. G.L. Van Hoosier., Jr., pp. 77–94. Seattle: ACLAM.

Wissman, M, and B. Parsons. 1992. Surgical removal of a lipoma-like mass in a lemur (*Lemur fulvus vulvu*). *J Small Exotic Anim Med* 2: 8–12.

Wolf, R.H., S.V. Gibson, E.A. Watson, and G.B. Baskin. 1988. Multidrug chemotherapy of tuberculosis in rhesus monkeys. *Lab Anim Sci* 38(1): 25–33.

Wolff, P.L.1990. The parasites of New World primates: a review. In *Proceedings of the American Association of Zoo Veterinarians,* pp.87–94.

Woolfson, M.W., J.A. Foran, H.M. Freedman, P.A. Moore, L.B. Shulman, and P.A. Schnitman. 1980. Immobilization of baboons (*Papio anubis*) using ketamine and diazepam. *Lab Anim Sci* 30(5): 902–904.

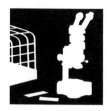

SEROLOGIC TESTING AND QUALITY CONTROL

As DEPICTED IN Figure 10.1, there are numerous environmental factors that can act as nonexperimental variables and affect the biologic responses of laboratory animals. These environmental factors are generally divided into three categories: physical, chemical, and microbial. Genetic factors also play an important role in determining the biologic responses of individual animals.

10

Environmental Factors

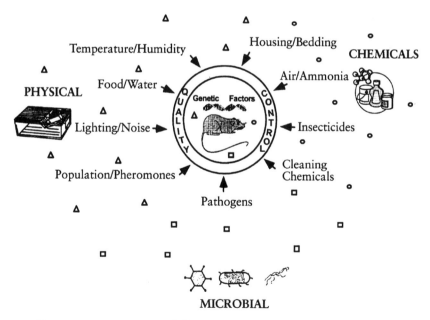

Figure 10.1. Environmental factors that can act as nonexperimental variables and affect the biologic responses of laboratory animals.

Physical factors include macroenvironmental or microenvironmental conditions, as well as stress. Cage design, temperature, relative humidity, ventilation, lighting, and noise are several of the more important environmental variables. Physical factors can affect animals directly and indirectly. According to the *Guide for the Care and Use of Laboratory Animals,* regulation of body temperature within normal variation is necessary for the well-being of homeotherms. Exposure of unadapted animals to temperature extremes may produce physiologic effects which could be life threatening. Low environmental humidity causes ringtail in rat pups and epistaxis in some species of nonhuman primates. Excess noise levels can cause audiogenic seizures in DBA mice, and too high a light intensity can cause retinal degeneration in albino rodents. Stressors such as housing method, cage population, and transportation can indirectly affect animals. Cage designs should take into account an animal's space and social needs in order to create a less stressful environment.

Chemical variables include exposures to insecticides, cleaning agents, and contaminants in food, water, or bedding. Chemicals may cause direct damage to animal tissues and organs or may have indirect effects such as the upregulation of hepatic microsomal enzymes.

Microbes are one of the most obvious factors. Pathogenic organisms frequently cause clinical disease that directly impacts the biologic responses of affected animals. Many organisms cause latent or subclinical infections in animals. Although there are no overt clinical signs of illness, latent microbial infections often cause subtle changes in the physiologic responses of infected animals. Table 10.1 summarizes major rodent infectious agents and their adverse effects.

Genetic composition often determines the biologic responses of individual animals within a species. Different strains of mice will have different responses to anesthetics and different abilities to mount an immune response to pathogenic organisms. For examples, DBA/1J mice are very susceptible to Sendai virus, whereas, SJL/J mice are highly resistant to developing clinical disease from Sendai virus infection. Likewise, LEW rats are more susceptible to infection with sialodacryoadenitis virus than are F344 rats. An animal may inherit a disease condition such as von Willebrand's, diabetes mellitus, or cataracts.

In a research setting, it is important to keep nonexperimental variables to a minimum. Animals to be used in research should be of the healthiest status possible and obtained from companies that monitor and can ensure their genetic and microbial status. Close attention must be given to maintaining an animal's environmental parameters within the generally recommended ranges. These ranges are outlined in the

Table 10.1. Major rodent infectious agents

Organism	Host	Adverse effects
Mouse hepatitis virus (MHV)	Mouse	Immunosuppression; alters hepatic enzymes; alters phagocytic and tumoricidal activities; increased susceptibility to other indigenous pathogens; activation of natural killer cells and production of interferon
Sendai virus	Mouse, rat, hamster, guinea pig	Immunosuppression; alters host response to transplantable tumors; wound healing delayed; neonatal and adult deaths; interruption in breeding
Sialodacryoadenitis virus/ Rat coronavirus (SDAV/RCV)	Rat	Interferes with studies involving eyes, salivary glands, respiratory tract; reduced reproductive rate; slow growth rate of young
Parvovirus (MPV, RPV)	Mouse, rat	Immunosuppression; lymphocytotrophic
Theiler's murine encephalomyelitis virus (TMEV, GDVII)	Mouse, rat	Neuropathic; can interfere with studies of unrelated viruses in mice
Pneumonia virus of mice (PVM)	Mouse, rat, hamster, guinea pig	Chronic illness in immunocompromised animals
Minute virus of mice (MVM)	Mouse	Immunosuppression; low ascites production
Adenoviruses (MAd-1 and MAd-2)	Mouse, rat	Lesions in kidneys of mice; more susceptible to kidney problems
Lactic dehydrogenase-elevating virus (LDV)	Mouse	Immunosuppression; tumor growth enhanced early in infection; prevents development of experimental allergic encephalomyelitis in NZB mice; alters incidence and behavior of spontaneous neoplasms; tumor contaminant
Lymphocytic choriomeningitis virus (LCMV)	Mouse, rat, hamster, guinea pig	Immunosuppression; delayed rejection of tumor allografts; mortality; infectious to humans and can cause serious disease; biologic material contaminant
Rotaviruses (EDIM and IDIR)	Mouse, rat	Severe diarrhea, reduced weight gains, increased neonatal mortality
Reovirus-3	Mouse, rat, hamster, guinea pig	May interfere with research involving transplantable tumors and cell lines; tumor contaminant
Mouse cytomegalovirus (MCMV)	Mouse	Can cause severe immunomodulation; increases suceptibility to other pathogens
Toolan's and Kilham's rat virus (H-1, KRV)	Rat	Immunosuppression; hepatocellular necrosis; induces interferon production; skeletal defects in newborns
Polyomavirus	Mouse	Wasting disease and paralysis in nude (nu/nu) mice; tumor contaminant
K virus	Mouse	Tumor contaminant; reported to transform cells in vitro; increases severity of other concurrent infections

Table 10.1. *(Continued)*

Organism	Host	Adverse effects
Ectromelia virus	Mouse	High mortality of animals; can alter phago-cytic response; tumor contaminant
Hantaviruses	Small mammals, rodents	Infectious to humans and can cause fatal hemorrhagic disease
Mycoplasma pulmonis and *M. arthriditis*	Mouse, rat	Respiratory disease resulting in morbidity and mortality; alters ciliary function, cell kinetics; changes response to carcinogens; can induce spontaneous polyarthritis
Cilia-associated respiratory bacillus (CAR bacillus)	Mouse, rat, rabbit	Respiratory disease resulting in morbidity and mortality; interferes with research involving the respiratory tract; causes a loss of respiratory cilia; enhances severity of other concurrent infections
Encephalitozoon cuniculi (ECUN)	Mouse, rat, hamster, guinea pig, rabbit	Histologic changes in brain and kidney complicate interpretation of studies; mice are immunosuppressed; tumor contaminant
Pinworms (*Aspicularis tetraptera, Syphacia obvelata,* and *S. muris*)	Mouse, rat, hamster, gerbil	Reduces the occurrence of adjuvant-induced arthritis; change in physiologic parameters

Source: Adapted from Rodent Health Surveillance Program, University of Miami. Information compiled from *Infectious Diseases of Mice and Rats* by the National Research Council (1991, National Academy Press, Washington, DC), *Viral and Mycoplasmal Infections of Laboratory Rodents: Effects on Biomedical Research* by P.N. Bhatt, R.O. Jacoby, H.C. Morse III, and A.E. New (1988, Academic Press, Orlando, FL), and *"Orphan" Parvovirus Update* by Charles River Laboratories (1995, Wilmington, MA).

Guide for the Care and Use of Laboratory Animals. Chemical contaminants must be monitored and eliminated when possible.

Animals should be screened for pathogenic microorganisms. Viral and mycoplasmal infections are common in conventionally housed rodents and are recognized to be important complicating factors for biomedical research. Biologic materials, such as tissue cultures and tumor lines, can become contaminated and serve as a nidus of infection. Genetic monitoring is imperative for large production colonies to avoid the possibility of contamination or genetic drift within a strain. A standardized method should be in place to monitor quality control.

A quality-control program safeguards the health of animals and of personnel. A well-trained staff capable of recognizing signs of illness is an important component of a quality-control program. Serologic testing can be used as a diagnostic tool and as a health surveillance instrument. Health surveillance and environmental monitoring identify what is present. Clinically ill animals and/or sentinel animals can be used to monitor the health status of a colony. Sentinel animals can be extra animals of the same strain or stock of animal that is being monitored, or they may be a strain that is known to be more sensitive to the agent for which you are monitoring. An established protocol should be followed when collecting and processing samples for testing if the results are to be meaningful. Disease prevention comes through proper management of data and of personnel including animal care staff and researchers. Test results should be interpreted using scientific and professional judgment. Any action taken should be based on sound quality-control principles.

A number of companies and universities have diagnostic laboratories that can run a variety of tests. Serology screening panels that test for a number of viral agents are routinely used to monitor the health status of rodent colonies. Mouse antibody production (MAP) and rat antibody production (RAP) tests are used to check tumors for viral contamination. The primary test method used for serology testing is the enzyme-linked immunosorbent assay (ELISA). Indirect fluorescent antibody (IFA), hemagglutination inhibition (HAI), Western blot analysis, and polymerase chain reaction (PCR) are alternative testing methods. Food, water, and bedding samples can also be tested for chemical and microbial contamination. Replicate organism detection and counting (RODAC) plates can be used to test the effectiveness of cleaning agents on inanimate objects or surfaces. Table 10.2 is a partial listing of commercial and university comprehensive animal diagnostic laboratories. Table 10.3 is a partial listing of laboratories that perform nonhuman primate diagnostic testing. The information provided is strictly a point of reference and in no way indicates author preferences. Other diagnostic laboratories may be available in your area.

Table 10.2. Comprehensive diagnostic laboratories

Company/University	Contact information	Comments
Anmed/Biosafe, Inc.	7642 Standish Place Rockville, MD 20855 Phone: 301-762-0366 Fax: 301-762-7438	Animal health screening, disease diagnosis, histopathology, environmental monitoring, biotechnical services

Charles River Laboratories	251 Ballardvale St.
	Wilmington, MA 01887
	Phone: 508-658-6000
	    800-522-7287
	Fax: 508-658-7132
	    800-992-7329
	URL: http://www.criver.com
		Comprehensive health monitoring, serology testing services, serology reagents and test kits

Massachusetts Institute of Technology	Division of Comparative Medicine 77 Massachusetts Avenue Cambridge, MA 02139 Phone: 617-253-1757 Fax: 617-258-5708	Rodent and rabbit serology, Aleutian disease screen, necropsy and microbiology
MA BioServices, Inc.	Laboratory Animal Health Services Division 9900 Blackwell Road Rockville, MD 20850-3349 Phone: 301-738-1000 800-804-3586 Fax: 301-838-0371	Rodent serology, simian virus laboratory tests, genetic testing, toxicology services
University of Miami	Division of Comprehensive Pathology Rodent Health Surveillance 1550 Northwest 10th Avenue PAP 105 Miami, FL 33136 Phone: 305-243-6700 800-596-7390 Fax: 305-243-5662	Rodents, exotics, nonhuman primates, and avian serology, histology, and microbiology
University of Missouri	Research Animal Diagnostic and Investigative Laboratory 1600 E. Rollins Columbia, MO 65211 Phone: 573-882-5983 800-669-0825 Fax: 573-884-7521	Screen for CAR bacillus, Tyzzer's, *Helicobacter, Treponema, Encephalitozoon;* rodent serology and necropsy

Table 10.3. Nonhuman primate diagnostic testing laboratories		
Company	Contact information	Comments
Southwest Foundation for Biomedical Research	Department of Virology and Immunology 7620 N.W. Loop 410 San Antonio, TX 78227 Phone: 210-674-1410 ext. 240 Fax: 210-673-3529 http://www.sfbn.org/bvirus	B-virus screens for nonhumans and humans
Virus Reference Laboratory	7540 Louis Pasteur San Antonio, TX 78229 Phone: 210-614-7350 Fax: 210-614-7355	Simian diagnostic laboratory, antibody assays, virus isolation, microbiology, polymerase chain reaction

■ GENERAL REFERENCES

Sources consulted to compile the information in this chapter include *Laboratory Animal Medicine* edited by J.G. Fox, B.J. Cohen, and F.M. Loew (1984, Academic Press, Inc., Orlando, FL 32887); *Guide for the Care and Use of Laboratory Animals* by the Institute of Laboratory Animal Resources Commission of Life Sciences National Research Council (1996, National Academy Press, Washington, DC 20418); *Viral and Mycoplasmal Infections of Laboratory Rodents, Effects on Biomedical Research* edited by P.N. Bhatt, R.O. Jacoby, H.C. Morse III, and A.E. New (1996, Academic Press, Inc., Orlando, FL 32887); *Infectious Diseases of Mice and Rats* by National Research Council (1991, National Academy Press, Washington, DC 20418); *Companion Guide to Infectious Diseases of Mice and Rats* by National Researach Council (1991, National Academy Press, Washington, DC 20418); and *Manual of Microbiologic Monitoring of Laboratory Animals,* 2nd edition, edited by K. Waggie, A.M. Allen, and T. Nomura (1994, National Institutes of Health).

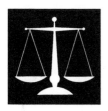

REGULATIONS AND POLICIES GOVERNING THE CARE AND USE OF LABORATORY ANIMALS

11

Numerous regulations, policies, and guidelines impact the care and use of animals in research, teaching, and testing. Federal regulations such as the Animal Welfare Act, the Public Health Service Policy, and the Good Laboratory Practice Act are mandatory and must be adhered to. Several organizations exist that provide for voluntary membership and/or accreditation. This chapter outlines the basic federal regulatory requirements as well as other important guidelines. Depicted in Figure 11.1 are several of the more prevalent documents used in the regulation of laboratory animals.

Animal Welfare Act

The Animal Welfare Act (AWA), passed in 1966, was the first law that protected nonfarm animals in the United States. It was originally known as the Laboratory Animal Welfare Act, or PL-89-544, and was amended in 1970, 1976, 1985, and 1990. The requirements of the AWA are set forth under Regulations and Standards in the Code of Federal Regulations (CRF) and can be found in Title 9, C.F.R., Chapter 1, Subchapter A—Animal Welfare, Parts 1, 2, and 3. The responsibility for administering the AWA was delegated within the United States Department of Agriculture (USDA) to the Animal and Plant Health Inspection Service (APHIS)—Regulatory Enforcement and Animal Care (REAC). Unannounced site visits are done at least once yearly. The regulations apply to animal research facilities, animal dealers and exhibitors, operators of animal auction sales, and carriers and intermediate handlers of animals in shipment. The regulations include humane handling, care,

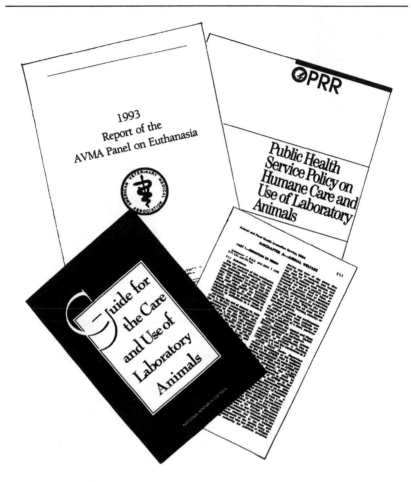

Figure 11.1. Documents used in the regulation of laboratory animals.

identification, record keeping, treatment, and transportation of animals.

The purpose of the original Act was to protect owners of dogs and cats from theft of their pets, prevent the sale or use of dogs and cats that had been stolen, and ensure that certain animals intended for use in research facilities were provided humane care and treatment. The law required licensure of individuals or corporations that bought or sold dogs or cats for laboratory activities. Organizations that used dogs or cats in biomedical activities were required to register. The original Act covered nonhuman primates, guinea pigs, hamsters, rabbits, dogs, and cats. It applied only to animals being held before or after actual research and testing and not during the time the animals were being used.

The Act was amended in 1970, PL-91-579, and given the official title of The Animal Welfare Act. The amendments broadened the coverage of the law to include any warm-blooded animal designated by the Secretary of Agriculture. The standards for animal care were extended to apply to animals throughout their stay in the research facility. The Act did not allow the Secretary of Agriculture to promulgate rules, regulations, or orders with regard to the actual research. It did require, however, that every research facility show at least annually that professionally acceptable standards governing care, treatment, and use of animals were being followed. Research facilities were also required to file an annual report listing the number of animals used or held for research and whether the animals required or received anesthetics, analgesics, or tranquilizers. The annual report due date is December 1 and covers the period October 1 through September 30 of the preceding year.

In 1976, the AWA was further amended, PL-94-279, to redefine the regulation of animals during transportation and to combat the use of animals for fighting. All carriers and intermediate handlers who were not required to be licensed under the AWA were required to register with the USDA. The Secretary of Agriculture also promulgated regulations that specifically excluded rats and mice bred for use in research, birds, horses, and farm animals intended for use as food or fiber or used in studies to improve production of food and fiber.

In 1985, the AWA was changed with the passage of the Food Security Act, PL-99-198. The Food Security Act contained an amendment entitled the Improved Standards for Laboratory Animals Act. This amendment requires the chief executive officer of each research facility to appoint an Institutional Animal Care and Use Committee (IACUC). The IACUC must consist of at least three members including a doctor of veterinary medicine with experience or training in laboratory animal medicine and one member who is not affiliated with the institution. The IACUC is charged to act as an agent of the research facility to assure compliance with the AWA. Once every 6 months, the IACUC is required to inspect all animal facilities and study areas and to review the research facility's program to assure that the care and use of the animals conform with the regulations and standards. The IACUC must file a report of its inspection with the institutional official of the research facility. If significant deficiencies or deviations are found during the inspection and review and are not corrected according to the IACUC's specific plan, the USDA and any federal funding agencies must be notified in writing. The IACUC must review and approve all proposed activities or protocols involving the care and use of animals in research, testing, or teaching procedures. The IACUC must assure that the principal investigator considered alternatives to painful procedures and that the work being proposed does not unnecessarily duplicate previous experiments. The 1985 amendment also specifies that consultation with a doctor of veterinary medicine is necessary in planning any procedure that could cause pain to animals and that no animal may be used in more than one major operative procedure from which it recovers. Training of all personnel using animals in research facilities is mandated. The amendment sets standards for exercise of dogs and an environment adequate to promote the psychological well-being of nonhuman primates. In addition, the amendment established the National Agriculture Library's Animal Welfare Information Center (AWIC) to prevent unintended duplication of research.

The most recent amendment, called Protection of Pets, occurred in 1990. It was attached to the farm bill Food, Agriculture, Conservation and Trade Act, PL-101-624. This amendment mandates pounds and shelters to hold any live dog or cat for a minimum period of 5 days before releasing the animal to a Class B dealer.

Failure to comply with the AWA regulations can lead to a warning with opportunity to make corrections. If the infraction is serious, civil or criminal prosecution and/or suspension of federal support for animal research may occur. For further information, contact USDA-APHIS at http://www.aphis.usda.gov/ac.

National Institutes of Health and Public Health Service Policy

The Health Research Extension Act, PL-99-158, revised the Public Health Service (PHS) policy originally initiated in 1971. The PHS policy relates to the use of animals in research and other biomedical activities that are supported by grants, contracts, and awards from the U.S. Public Health Service. The PHS includes the National Institutes of Health (NIH) and the Food and Drug Administration (FDA). The PHS policy extends to all vertebrates rather than just warm-blooded animals. Institutions must submit a written assurance to the Office for Protection from Research Risks (OPRR) that they are committed to follow the U.S. Government Principles for the Utilization and Care of Vertebrate Animals Used in Testing, Research, and Training (see Table 11.1) and the *Guide for the Care and Use of Laboratory Animals*. The institution must have a committee (IACUC), which consists of at least five members, to maintain oversight of its animal facilities and procedures. Institutions are required to establish a mechanism to review their animal facilities and procedures for conformance with the *Guide*. Voluntary accreditation by the Association for Assessment and Accreditation of Laboratory Animal Care (AAALAC International) is deemed to be the best method of demonstrating conformance to the *Guide*. Alternatively, the institutional IACUC could review the facilities and procedures annually. If improvements are needed, they are reported in the assurance statement. An annual report of progress must be submitted to OPRR.

Table 11.1.   U.S. government principles for the utilization and care of vertebrate animals used in testing, research, and training

   I. The transportation, care, and use of animals should be in accordance with the Animal Welfare Act (7 U.S.C. 2131 et seq.) and other applicable Federal laws, guidelines, and policies.

  II. Procedures involving animals should be designed and performed with due consideration of their relevance to human or animal health, the advancement of knowledge, or the good of society.

 III. The animals selected for a procedure should be of an appropriate species and quality and the minimum number required to obtain valid results. Methods such as mathematical models, computer simulation, and in vitro biological systems should be considered.

  IV. Proper use of animals, including the avoidance or minimization of discomfort, distress, and pain when consistent with sound scientific practices, is imperative. Unless the contrary is established, investigators should consider that procedures that cause pain or distress in human beings may cause pain or distress in other animals.

   V. Procedures with animals that may cause more than momentary or slight pain or distress should be performed with appropriate sedation, analgesia, or anesthesia. Surgical or other painful procedures should not be performed on unanesthetized animals paralyzed by chemical agents.

  VI. Animals that would otherwise suffer severe or chronic pain or distress that cannot be relieved should be painlessly killed at the end of the procedure or, if appropriate, during the procedure.

 VII. The living conditions of animals should be appropriate for their species and contribute to their health and comfort. Normally, the housing, feeding, and care of all animals used for biomedical purposes must be directed by a veterinarian or other scientist trained and experienced in the proper care, handling, and use of the species being maintained or studied. In any case, veterinary care shall be provided as indicated.

VIII. Investigators and other personnel shall be appropriately qualified and experienced for conducting procedures on living animals. Adequate arrangements shall be made for their in-service training, including the proper and humane care and use of laboratory animals.

  IX. Where exceptions are required in relation to the provisions of these Principles, the decisions should not rest with the investigators directly concerned but should be made, with due regard to Principle II, by an appropriate review group such as an institutional animal care and use committee. Such exceptions should not be made solely for the purposes of teaching or demonstration.

Good Laboratory Practice Regulations

Good Laboratory Practice (GLP) regulations were adopted in 1978. They apply to animal research and safety studies funded by the FDA. These regulations tighten the standards for research facilities that are engaged in product testing for the FDA. Quality assurance and standard operating procedures are very important components of the regulations. Laboratories must maintain extensive records of all steps of research and make them available to the FDA. The general concept is that inadequate animal facilities, treatment, or records are sufficient reasons to question the value or the validity of the data gathered.

State Regulations

In the United States, all 50 states and the District of Columbia have laws that protect animals. Most of these laws protect animals from cruel treatment and require that animals have access to food and water and be provided with shelter from extreme weather. Some states have public health and agriculture regulations that specifically cover animals used in research. A number of states regulate the release of impounded animals for research.

Association for Assessment and Accreditation of Laboratory Animal Care

The Association for Assessment and Accreditation of Laboratory Animal Care (AAALAC International) was organized by leading veterinarians and researchers in 1965. The AAALAC's mission is to promote high standards of animal care, use, and well-being and to enhance life sciences research and education through the accreditation process. It conducts voluntary peer review evaluation of laboratory animal care facilities and programs. The AAALAC's accreditation is the "gold standard" of the industry because it demonstrates that an organization has achieved standards beyond the minima required by law. The AAALAC relies on the *Guide for the Care and Use of Laboratory Animals* as its primary reference for evaluating laboratory animal care and use programs. For further information, contact AAALAC International, 11300 Rockville Pike, Suite 1211, Rockville, MD 20852-3035. Phone: 301-231-5353 Fax: 301-231-8282. E-Mail: accredit@aaalac.org.

Guide for the Care and Use of Laboratory Animals

The *Guide for the Care and Use of Laboratory Animals,* prepared by the Institute of Laboratory Animal Resources (ILAR) for the NIH, was first published in 1963 and most recently revised in 1996. "The purpose of the *Guide* is to assist institutions caring for and using animals in ways judged to be scientifically, technically, and humanely appropriate. The *Guide* is also intended to assist investigators in fulfilling their obligation to plan and conduct animal experiments in accord with the highest scientific, humane, and ethical principles." The *Guide* outlines and references the major components of an animal care and use program—institutional policies and responsibilities; animal environment, housing, and management; veterinary medical care; and physical plant. Personnel qualifications and training, occupational health and safety of personnel, preventive medicine, surgery including postsurgical care, and euthanasia are addressed in detail. The *Guide* states that unless a deviation is justified for scientific or medical reasons, the method of euthanasia should be consistence with the *1993 Report of the AVMA Panel on Euthanasia* (or later editions). The latest revision of the *Guide* puts emphasis on performance goals as opposed to engineering standards. Performance goals place more responsibility on the user, but tend to result in greater enhancement of animal well-being.

Occupational Health and Safety

Employees, students, and visitors in the course of their work with research animals may be exposed to hazards that could adversely affect their health. Physical and chemical hazards, allergens, zoonoses, and hazards from experiments are all potential problems. The *Guide for the Care and Use of Laboratory Animals* states that "an occupational health and safety program must be part of the overall animal care and use program. The program must be consistent with federal, state, and local regulations and should focus on maintaining a safe and healthy workplace." The type of program needed depends on the facility, what type of research activities are ongoing, hazards, and animal species involved. The Committee on Occupational Safety and Health in Research Animal Facilities, in the Institute of Laboratory Animal Resources of the National Research Council's Commission of Life Sciences, has written an implementation handbook called *Occupational Health and Safety in the Care and Use of Research Animals*. This book identifies principles for building an effective safety program and discusses the accountability of institutional leaders, managers, and employees for a program's success.

Animal Welfare Information Center

The Animal Welfare Information Center (AWIC) is part of the National Agricultural Library located in Beltsville, Maryland. It was estab-

257

lished in 1986 as mandated by amendments to the Animal Welfare Act. The AWIC is the focal point for those interested in obtaining information or publications covering many aspects of animal welfare. It combines personnel with subject expertise, state-of-the-art technology, and networking to assist those interested in learning more about methods for the humane care, use, and handling of animals in research, testing, and education. For further information, contact Animal Welfare Information Center, National Agriculture Library, Beltsville, MD 20705-2351; phone 301-504-6212; http://www.nal.usda.gov/awic.

■ GENERAL REFERENCES

Sources consulted to compile the information in this chapter include *Laboratory Animal Medicine* edited by J.G. Fox, B.J. Cohen, and F.M. Loew (1984, Academic Press, Inc., Orlando, FL 32887); *Essentials for Animal Research: A Primer for Research Personnel* by B.T. Bennett, M.J. Brown, and J.C. Schofield (1990, National Agricultural Library, Beltsville, MD 20705); *Guide for the Care and Use of Laboratory Animals* by the Institute of Laboratory Animal Resources Commission of Life Sciences National Research Council (1996, National Academy Press, Washington, DC); *Occupational Health and Safety in the Care and Use of Research Animals* by the Institute of Laboratory Animal Resources Commission of Life Sciences National Research Council (1997, National Academy Press, Washington, DC 20418); and the Animal Welfare Act, Title 9 C.F.R., Chapter 1, Subchapter A—Animal Welfare, Parts 1, 2, and 3.

NORMAL VALUES

THE FOLLOWING tables provide "normal" hematologic and biochemical data for each species covered in the text. The values should be used as guidelines, for there are many inherent variables in reporting such data. Sample collection method, the breed, strain, or stock, health status, age, sex, environment, and analytic techniques are but a few of the many variables that can affect specific clinical laboratory values.

Table A.1. Hematologic data

Species	RBC (10^6/mL)	PCV (%)	Hb (g/dL)	Platelets (10^3/mL)
Mouse[a]	7.0–12.5	39–49	10.2–16.6	800–1100
Rat[a]	7–10	36–48	11–18	500–1300
Gerbil[a]	8–9	43–49	12.6–16.2	400–600
Hamster[a]	6–10	36–55	10–16	200–500
Guinea Pig[a]	4.5–7	37–48	11–15	250–850
Chinchilla[b]	6.6–10.7	40	11.7–13.5	254–298
Rabbit[a]	4–7.2	36–48	10–15.5	200–1000
Ferret[c]	6.8–12.2	42–61	15–18	297–910
Rhesus monkey[d]	4.5–6	39–43	12.7	130–144
Squirrel monkey[d]	7.1–10.9	43–56	12.9–17	112

[a]From Harkness and Wagner (1995). [b]Adapted from Newberne, Casella, Kraft, and Strike in Merry (1990). [c]From Bernard et al. (1984). [d]From Johnson-Delaney (1994). RBC = red blood cells; PCV = packed cell volume; Hb = hemoglobin.

Table A.2. Hematologic data

Species	WBC (10^3/μL)	Neutrophils (%)	Lymphocytes (%)	Monocytes (%)	Eosinophils (%)	Basophils (%)
Mouse[a]	6–15	10–40	55–95	0.1–3.5	0–4	0–0.3
Rat[a]	6–17	9–34	65–85	0–5	0–6	0–1.5
Gerbil[a]	7–15	5–34	60–95	0–3	0–4	0–1
Hamster[a]	3–11	10–42	50–95	0–3	0–4.5	0–1
Guinea pig[a]	7–18	28–44	39–72	3–12	1–5	0–3
Chinchilla[b]	7.6–11.5	23–45	51–73	1–2	0.5–2.6	0–1
Rabbit[a]	7.5–13.5	20–35	55–80	1–4	0–4	2–10
Ferret[c]	4–19	11–84	12–54	0–9	0–7	0–2
Rhesus monkey[d]	11.5–12.4	20–56	40–76	0–2	1–3	0–1
Squirrel monkey[d]	5.1–10.9	36–66	27–55	0–6	0–11	<1

[a]From Harkness and Wagner (1995). [b]Adapted from Newberne, Casella, Kraft, and Strike in Merry (1990). [c]From Bernard et al. (1984). [d]From Johnson-Delaney (1994). WBC = white blood cells.

■ REFERENCES FOR NORMAL VALUES

Anderson, N.J. 1994. Basic husbandry and medicine of pocket pets. In *Saunders Manual of Small Animal Practice*, ed. S.J. Birchard and R.G. Sherding, pp. 1368–1369. Philadelphia: WB Saunders.

Bernard, S.L., J.R. Gorham, and L.M. Ryland. 1984. Biology and Diseases of Ferrets. In *Laboratory Animal Medicine*, ed. J.G. Fox, B.J. Cohen, and F.M. Loew, pp. 387. New York: Academic.

Canadian Council on Animal Care (CCAC). 1980. *Guide to the care and use of experimental animals—Volume 1*, pp.87. Ottawa, Ontario: Canadian Council on Animal Care.

Carpenter, J. W., T.Y. Mashima, and D.J. Rupiper. 1996. *Exotic Animal Formulary*, pp. 204, 225, 243, 278. Manhattan, KS: Greystone.

Fox, J.G., L. Hotaling, B.O. Ackerman, and K. Hewes. 1986. Serum chemistry and hematology reference values in the ferret (*Mustela putorius furo*). *Lab Anim Sci* 36:583.

Harkness, J.E. and J.E. Wagner. 1995. *The Biology and Medicine of Rabbits and Rodents*, 4th ed. Philadelphia: Williams & Wilkins.

Johnson-Delaney, C. A. 1994. Primates. *Vet Clin North Am Small Anim Pract* 24:121–156.

Lee, E.J., W.E. Moore, H.C. Fryer, et al. 1982. Haematological and serum chemistry profiles of ferrets (*Mustela putorius furo*). *Lab Anim* 16:133.

Loeb, W. And F. Quimby. 1987. *The Clinical Chemistry of Laboratory Animals*, pp. 429–431. Elmstord, NY: Pergamon.

Manning, P.J., N.D.M. Lehner, M.A. Feldner, and B.C. Bullock. 1969. Selected hematologic, serum chemical, and arterial blood gas characteristics of squirrel monkeys (*Saimiri sciureus*). *Lab Anim Sci* 19: 831–837.

McClure, H.M. 1975. Hematologic, blood chemistry and cerebrospinal fluid data for the rhesus monkey. In *The Rhesus Monkey, Volume 2*, ed. G.H. Bourne, pp. 409–429. New York: Academic.

Merry, C.J. 1990. An Introduction to chinchillas. *Vet Tech* 11(5): 315–321.

Mitruka, B.M. and H.M. Rawnsley. 1977. *Clinical Biochemical and Hematological Reference Values in Normal Experimental Animals*. Mason, New York.

Quesenberry, K.E. 1994. Rabbits. In *Saunders Manual of Small Animal Practice*, ed. S.J. Birchard and R.G. Sherding, pp. 1346. Philadelphia: WB Saunders.

Ringler, D.H. and L. Dabich. 1979. Hematology and Clinical Biochemistry. In *The Laboratory Rat, Volume I, Biology and Diseases*, ed. H.J. Baker, J.R. Lindsey, and S.H. Weisbroth, pp. 105–121. New York: Academic.

Whitney, R.A. Jr., D.J. Johnson, and W.C. Cole. 1973. *Laboratory Primate Handbook*. New York: Academic.

Table A.3. Serum biochemical data

Species	BUN (mg/dL)	Creatinine (mg/dL)	Glucose (mg/dL)	ALT (IU/L)	AST (IU/L)	AP (IU/L)	Total bilirubin (mg/dL)	Cholesterol (mg/dL)
Mouse[a,b]	12–28	0.3–1	62–175	26–77	54–269	45–222	0.1–0.9	26–82
Rat[a,b,c]	15–21	0.2–0.8	50–135	16–89	192–262	16–125	0.2–0.55	40–130
Gerbil[a,d]	17–27	0.6–1.4	50–135	—	—	12–37	0.2–0.6	90–150
Hamster[a,b]	12–25	0.91–0.99	60–150	22–128	28–122	45–187	0.25–0.6	25–135
Guinea pig[a,b,c]	9–31.5	0.6–2.2	60–125	10–25	45.5–48.2	18–28	0.3–0.9	20–43
Chinchilla[b,e]	10–25	0.4–1.3	60–120	10–35	96	3–47	0.6–1.28	40–100
Rabbit[a,e]	15–23.5	0.8–1.8	75–150	14–80	14–113	4–16	0.25–0.74	35–60
Ferret[f]	12–43	0.2–0.6	62.5–134	78–149	57–165	30–120	0–0.1	119–209
Rhesus monkey[e,g]	14.2–19.6	0.1–2.8	53–87	145–171	20–34	—	0.1–0.66	94–162
Squirrel monkey[e]	23–39	—	52–108	59–99	56–118	—	0.1–0.53	127–207

[a] From Harkness and Wagner (1995).
[b] From Anderson (1994).
[c] Adapted from Loeb and Quimby (1989).
[d] From Canadian Council on Animal Care (1980).
[e] From Carpenter et al. (1996).
[f] Adapted from Fox et al. (1986) and Lee et al. (1982).
[g] From McClure (1975).
BUN = blood urea nitrogen; ALT = alanine transferase; AST = aspartate transferase; AP = alkaline phosphate.

Table A.4. Serum biochemical data								
Species	Protein (g/dL)	Albumin (g/dL)	Globulin (g/dL)	Calcium (mg/dL)	Phosphorus (mg/dL)	Sodium (mEq/L)	Potassium (mEq/L)	Chloride (mEq/L)
Mouse[a,b]	3.5–7.2	2.5–4.8	0.6	3.2–8.5	2.3–9.2	112–193	5.1–10.4	82–114
Rat[a-c]	5.6–7.6	3.8–4.8	1.8–3	5.3–13	5.3–8.3	135–155	4–8	94–116.3
Gerbil[a,b,k]	4.3–12.5	1.8–5.5	1.2–6	3.7–6.2	3.7–7	144–158	3.8–5.2	93–118
Hamster[a,b,d]	4.5–7.5	2.6–4.1	2.7–4.2	5–12	3.4–8.2	128–144	3.9–5.5	93–98
Guinea pig[a,b]	4.6–6.2	2.1–3.9	1.7–2.6	5.3–12	3–12	132–156	4.5–8.9	98–115
Chinchilla[e,f]	3.8–5.6	2.3–4.1	0.9–2.2	5.6–12.1	4–8	130–155	5–6.5	105–115
Rabbit[a,g]	2.8–10	2.7–4.6	1.5–2.8	5.6–12.5	2.7–7.3	131–155	3.6–6.9	92–112
Ferret[h]	5.3–7.2	3.3–4.1	1.8–3.1	8.6–10.5	5.6–8.7	146–160	4.3–5.3	102–121
Rhesus monkey[i]	4.9–9.3	2.8–5.2	1.2–5.8	6.9–13	3.1–7.1	102–166	2.3–6.7	84–126
Squirrel monkey[j]	6.6–7.8	3.5–4.5	2.6–3.6	9.5–10.5	3.2–6.6	143.1–152.9	3.6–5.4	107.6–118.4

[a] From Harkness and Wagner (1995).
[b] From Anderson (1994).
[c] Ringler and Dabich (1979).
[d] Mitruka and Rawnsley (1977).
[e] Adapted from Merry (1990).
[f] From Carpenter et al. (1996).
[g] From Quesenberry (1994).
[h] Adapted from Fox et al. (1986) and Lee et al. (1982).
[i] McClure (1975).
[j] Adapted from Manning et al. (1969).
[k] From Canadian Council on Animal Care (1980).

ORGANIZATIONS IN LABORATORY ANIMAL MEDICINE

American Society of Laboratory Animal Practitioners

THE AMERICAN SOCIETY OF LABORATORY ANIMAL PRACTITIONERS (ASLAP) was founded in 1966 as a professional organization to exchange ideas, experiences, and knowledge among veterinarians engaged or interested in the practice of laboratory animal medicine. The objectives of ASLAP are to 1) provide a mechanism for the exchange of scientific and technical information among veterinarians engaged in laboratory animal practice, 2) encourage the development and dissemination of knowledge in areas related to laboratory animal practice, 3) act as a spokesperson for laboratory animal practitioners within the AVMA House of Delegates and to work with other organizations involved in the care and use of laboratory animals in representing our interests and concerns to the scientific community and the public at large, and 4) actively encourage its members to provide training for veterinarians in the field of laboratory animal practice at both the predoctoral and postdoctoral levels and lend their expertise to institutions conducting laboratory animal medicine training programs. For further information contact: Dr. Bradford S. Goodwin, Jr., ASLAP Secretary-Treasurer, University of Texas Medical School, CLAMC Room 1.132, 6431 Fannin St., Houston, TX 77030-1503. Phone: 713-792-5127; Fax: 713-792-5796. E-mail: bgoodwin@admin4.hsc.uth.tmc.edu.

American College of Laboratory Animal Medicine

The American College of Laboratory Animal Medicine (ACLAM) was founded in 1957 to encourage education, training, and research in laboratory animal medicine; to establish standards of training and experience for veterinarians professionally concerned with the care and health of laboratory animals; and to recognize qualified persons in laboratory animal medicine by certification examination and other means. The ACLAM is a specialty board recognized by the American Veterinary Medical Association. For further information contact: Dr. Charles W. McPherson, Executive Director, American College of Laboratory Animal Medicine, 200 Summerwinds Drive, Cary, NC 27511. Phone: 919-859-5985; Fax: 919-851-3126. E-mail: cwmaclam@aol.com ACLAM's homepage: http://chopin.osp.uh.edu/~rocky/aclam/hdg1055.htm.

INDEX